An aid to the MRCP viva

M Afzal Mir
Senior Lecturer in Medicine,
University of Wales, and
Honorary Consultant Physician,
University Hospital of Wales, Cardiff

E Anne Freeman
Consultant Physician in Geriatric Medicine,
St Woolos Hospital, Newport, Gwent

Robert E J Ryder
Consultant Physician
Dudley Road Hospital, Birmingham

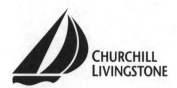

CHURCHILL
LIVINGSTONE

EDINBURGH LONDON MADRID MELBOURNE NEW YORK AND TOKYO 1992

CHURCHILL LIVINGSTONE
Medical Division of Pearson Professional Ltd

Distributed in the United States of America by
Churchill Livingstone Inc., 650 Avenue of the Americas,
New York, N.Y. 10011, and by associated companies,
branches and representatives throughout the world.

First published 1992
    Reprinted 1993
    Reprinted 1996

ISBN 0-443-04659-X

British Library Cataloguing in Publication Data
A catalogue record for this book is available from the British Library.

Library of Congress Cataloging in Publication Data

Mir, M A (Mohammad Afzal)
    An aid to the MRCP viva/M A Mir, E A Freeman, R E J Ryder.
        p. cm.
    Includes index.
    ISBN 0-443-04659-X
    1. Internal medicine-Examinations, questions, etc. I Freeman, E A (Eleanor Anne) II.
Ryder, R E J (Robert Elford John)
III. Title.
    [DNLM: 1. Clinical Competence – standards. 2. Clinical Medicine – examination
questions. 3. Physical Examination – examination questions. WB 18 M671a]
RC58.M57 1992
616.0076 – dc20
DNLM/DLC
for Library of Congress

Produced by Longman Singapore Publishers Pte Ltd
Printed in Singapore

Preface

There was absolutely no feedback when I answered a question, just more questions.[1]

The viva part of the examination for the membership of the Royal College of Physicians (MRCP) is by far the most evolved test of clinical knowledge and competence. Until about 30 years ago, the viva was regarded as a final handshake for those candidates who had been successful in the written and clinical sections of the examination, and very few questions were asked to test their clinical knowledge. Indeed, the very advisability of the retention of such an encounter was in doubt.

During the last three decades the viva has assumed an increasing importance as an integral part of the MRCP examination. A candidate can fail the entire examination if he or she fails the viva and does not compensate for this by scoring additional marks in the clinical and written sections. Conversely, a marginal failure in the clinical section can be compensated for by a good performance in the viva and/or written parts of the examination. The viva examination provides the examiners with considerable scope for testing the candidates' ability to deal with medical emergencies and referrals from within or outside the hospital, for judging their skills of communication and interaction, and for assessing the depth of their knowledge in key clinical problems. In a subject as vast and diverse as general medicine the range of likely questions that can be asked in the viva is equally vast.

However, the examiners, who are practising experts themselves, tend to ask questions from their own clinical repertoire that reflect their day-to-day concerns. For this reason, we have used a journalistic approach to the field and have built this book around an extensive survey conducted over several years. The survey has enabled us not only to identify the chief medical problems that should occupy the attention of postgraduate medical

---

[1] p. 190

practitioners, but it has also allowed us to focus on the principal difficulties of the candidates and to address these. Thus, in Section 1 we have concentrated on how to prepare for the viva examination, what books and journals should be consulted, what psychological approach should be adopted, how to conduct oneself in the viva, how to interact with the examiners, and how to maintain unobtrusive verbal and nonverbal language. Section 2 represents our dissection of the viva questions (99% of these are derived from our surveys), identifies various recognisable groups of questions, and presents our approach to handling different categories of questions. Our 'model answers', given in an indented form and presented by a hypothetical candidate in the first person, are not exhaustive in relation to the topics selected by the examiners; rather, we have attempted to get under the skin of the questioner and have endeavoured to identify and address his chief concern. In Section 3 we have reproduced 80 actual viva experiences (with some minor corrections) as reported to us by the candidates, together with our comments wherever appropriate. Once again, in most cases these comments have been kept brief and pertinent to the answer required by the examiner; they are not designed to give a deep knowledge of the subject. In the final section we pass on a *pot pourri* of experiences, tips and advice from some of the candidates in our survey, which we felt would add some spice to the experience of our readers.

We have used a novel, unorthodox and somewhat animated method of classifying the questions in Section 2. This is an attempt to help candidates to learn the 'game plan' of the examiners, to focus on the line of play, and to deliver coherent, unambiguous and polished answers. Further, this light-hearted method has enabled us to unload the clinical information without overburdening the busy and anxious candidate. Additional information is provided in the footnotes, which can be used if the question is started differently by the examiners. As many candidates experience difficulties with the questions on statistics, we have provided definitions and brief explanations of some commonly used tests in Appendix I. Appendix II has been devoted to eponyms which are a favourite with some examiners and so the candidate has his or her chance to impress them. In Appendix III we have summarised, under different specialities, the majority of the questions derived from a series of six surveys, giving the candidate a 'syllabus' to work on.

Acknowledgements

We are indebted to all the candidates who spared their time and effort to complete and return our ten-page questionnaires. Without their contributions this book would never have been started! We referred most of the controversial questions discussed in this book to many clinicians in this and other countries, and we would like to record our grateful thanks to all of them. Our thanks are due to Professor Reginald Hall who, despite his numerous pressing engagements, read the entire manuscript at an early stage and gave us valuable advice. We are indebted to Professor Phillip Routledge and Dr Margaret Elmes for their advice in their fields of interest. We are grateful to Susan Morgan for typing several drafts of the manuscript.

Most of all we thank our long-suffering families, without whose forbearance, encouragement and help the book would never have been finished.

Contents

Section 1
Preparation

One should do busy medical jobs.
In the end experience counts for
more than knowledge.[1]

When a man (or a woman) knows
he is to be hanged in a fortnight,
it concentrates his mind
wonderfully.[2]

---

[1] p. 134
[2] Samuel Johnson (1709 – 1784)

The heights by great men reached and kept
Were not attained by sudden flight,
But they, while their companions slept
Were toiling upward in the night[1]

The best preparation for the viva, as indeed for the other sections of the MRCP examination, is to work under the supervision of a good clinician who is also a good teacher. A good clinical teacher will discuss with you the diagnostic and therapeutic problems you encounter in emergency situations, supervise and contribute constructively to the problems referred to you by your surgical or obstetric colleagues, and teach you when and how to look for help from the literature. Unfortunately, such guidance is not usually available and you have to consider alternative avenues and sources of help. Although by the time you come to taking the coveted membership examination you will have tapped some of these sources and built a fund of knowledge, it is still worth considering some of the basic principles of preparation.

---

[1] H W Longfellow (1807–1882)

Learn as you work

My viva was merely a commonsense discussion of regularly encountered clinical scenarios[2]

This simple and straightforward advice, well-known to almost all candidates, is not followed in practice by most doctors one meets in various postgraduate courses. The commonest mistake made by many candidates is that they do not read about the clinical problems they encounter in everyday practice, and leave the bulk of their reading to the last few months before the examination. The result is that there is far too much to read in too little time, and confusion, compounded by anxiety, sets in. A more organised approach to acquiring specific and clear knowledge is to read a standard textbook about each condition after you have seen a patient. This practice enables you to remember both the clinical features that are present as well as those that are not present in your patient, using his or her clinical picture as a reference or a 'memory pillar', which helps you to remember what you read in the book. Having organised the material in your mind, you should practise presenting the clinical scenario of the patient and your plan of management to a hypothetical examiner. It is a sound practice, not only for the examination but also for developing good habits, to imagine that you are in the dock defending your clinical decisions. For every therapeutic intervention consider its worst side effect and how you would justify your decision. This thoughtful and incisive approach to your clinical practice will not only save you from unnecessary litigation, but also enables you to build a huge repertoire of clinical information from which you are able to answer awkward questions.

Asking yourself 'why' at every stage of your clinical practice will enable you to obtain useful information from appropriate books and senior colleagues, discipline you in formulating your thoughts, and help you to become articulate in voicing your response. For as many patients as possible that you see in the ward or clinic, prepare a summary of the clinical picture and the planned investigations and management that you would present to the examiner. While you are walking or having a restful bath, go over your prepared summaries and practise answering questions that might arise from them. This practice will help to keep you in a high state of alertness, ready to answer apparently unexpected questions.

Reading list

Know the basics well[3]

In answer to our question, 'What is your reading list?', the overwhelming majority of successful candidates indicated that they used one of the smaller textbooks regularly, and one of the bigger ones as a reference book. This is a good practice, as reading a smaller textbook is time-effective, provides enough information on most common conditions, and is less

---

[2] p. 229
[3] p. 136

likely to generate confusion. A recommended title is Davidson's *Principles and Practice of Medicine*. You should also use one of the bigger books since some topics, likely to feature in the written and viva examinations, are either not covered or are sparsely dealt with in the smaller books. The selection of any one of the major textbooks available is one of personal preference as all of them are reasonably comprehensive. Cecil's *Textbook of Medicine* is well-written and a new edition is printed every two years. An English multiauthor book, the *Oxford Textbook of Medicine*, is now available and, despite a few indifferently written sections, is well worth reading and quite suitable for the membership examination.

It is advisable to read the monthly *Medicine International* and the *Hospital Update*, and to cultivate the habit of reading the editorials in the three general journals, *The New England Journal of Medicine*, the *Lancet* and the *British Medical Journal*. The Royal College of Physicians publishes its own journal from London which is distributed to members and fellows (the examiners!). It is always worth reading, and often has informative articles on topical issues. As we have illustrated in Section 2, it is also profitable to watch both the medical and the lay press for newsworthy medical topics, particularly as the examination approaches. The *Prescribers' Journal* and the *Drug and Therapeutics Bulletin* are most time-effective, as you can get a lot of updated information in a short time. Useful information about current topics can also be obtained by leafing through some of the specialist journals, such as *Cardiology*, *Rheumatology*, etc., which are distributed free to doctors. Finally, although various medical emergencies are covered in all textbooks, it is a mistake to go to the viva examination without reading one of the smaller books specifically devoted to emergency medicine.[4]

'Mock' viva practice

An impression of being at the sharp end managing real problems seems to be important[5]

Simulated sessions are important for improving one's ability to cope with the viva. Not only can such sessions improve your spontaneity and sharpen your attention in responding to questions, but they also reveal your areas of unpreparedness and whether you have any mannerisms which may distract, or even annoy, the examiner. If you join a membership course you may get some experience with 'mock' sessions, but you should also arrange more sessions yourself by asking a senior colleague to put you on the spot! Even if your mock examiner is not an expert interviewer (neither are many examiners!), the encounter will at least give you an opportunity to assess your own ability in responding to questions.

In Cardiff we have found that the most useful and informative mock sessions are those which are conducted in front of a video camera and then

---

[4] Brown A F T 1990 Accident and emergency diagnosis. Redwood Burn Ltd., Wiltshire
Jenkins J L, Loscalzo J (eds) 1986 Manual of emergency medicine. Little, Brown & Co., Boston
Robson R, Stott R 1989 Medical emergencies: diagnosis and management, 5th edn. Heinemann Medical Books, London
[5] p. 126

played back to the candidates in the presence of a 'hawkish' assessor. Candidates need a sturdy personality and a thick skin to benefit from these, and those who have an inferiority complex about their physical appearance or presentation should avoid them altogether, as they are likely to regard the ensuing discussion as public humiliation! Those candidates who can endure a 'mock' video viva show remarkable improvement in their demeanour and presentation.

Single 'mock' exercises, even when conducted by an expert 'hawk', have a limited usefulness in improving one's reflexes, reaction time and presentation, unless these are supplemented by a thoughtful and introspective analysis by the examinee, together with further examination practices. You should arrange as many sessions as you can with the help of a consultant, senior registrar or fellow examinee, invite criticism after each session, and try to improve your imperfections. In Section 2 we have presented some model answers, and candidates may find it useful to adapt these to use in their mock examinations, to improve their spontaneity in responding and fluidity in presenting their responses. In studying Section 3, in which we have presented some real experiences as reported to us by candidates, try to imagine yourself at the receiving end and practise your answers to the examiners' questions. Finally, a vast list of viva questions is given in Appendix III, and you could practise answering these to a mirror and into a dictaphone.

The real viva examination

Vivas are hit-and-miss affairs and the onus is on the examiners to enable you to show your knowledge. If they fail to do this, then they are bad interviewers and you are unlucky![6]

If you have prepared along the lines suggested above, you should have little to be afraid of when going for your viva examination. Unfortunately, many candidates do not give the viva its due importance and mistakenly believe that a bad performance in the viva will not mean a failure in the entire examination. The Colleges' guidelines are unequivocal about this, and state that a clear failure in the Oral Section, uncompensated by a better performance in the other two sections, will mean that the candidate has to take the entire examination again. On the other hand, scoring extra marks in the viva can save you from failure even if you have marginally failed in one of the other sections. An indifferent attitude to the viva followed by an indifferent performance can often prove to be a self-fulfilling prophesy resulting in failure. Thus, the only way forward is to go fully prepared for all three stages of the viva examination.

---

[6] p. 246

1. Before the viva

I felt the questions were on very reasonable topics but they could have been delivered more clearly...[7]

Adopt the right mental approach and go with a positive attitude. Approach the examination with the knowledge that the *vast majority* of the questions are straightforward and the examiners are not going to trick you or ask you something you have never heard of. It is worth reminding yourself that even if the examiners ask something about a rare or exotic condition there is no shame in admitting your ignorance. A close scrutiny of the experiences in Section 3 will reassure you that candidates have passed the viva even when they could not answer one or two questions. After all, the viva is not a simple test of recall of information; rather, the examiners' task is to assess your ability to cope with familiar as well as unfamiliar clinical situations.

Your psychological tuning should be complemented by an appropriate physical appearance; whatever your gender you should dress conservatively but smartly in the knowledge that it is an occasion when *you are being tested*. As the viva may follow long and gruelling clinical sections, you should make an effort to look fresh and interested in the proceedings. If you are obliged to wait, then do so with good grace and do not fight with the poor invigilators who are themselves often harassed and helpless. It is very important to keep calm and suppress any signs of anxiety.

2. During the viva examination

This examiner did not smile. He seemed cold and inflicted fear on me![8]

When your turn comes, enter softly, approach the desk where the examiners are seated, greet them and sit when asked to do so. Do not grovel; treat the examiners as you would your senior colleagues. The viva is a formal examination in which your professional competence is being tested, therefore suppress all body language of familiarity. Do not offer your hand for a handshake unless one of the examiners clearly offers a hand (some do!), sit upright in the chair occupying the entire seat and avoid sitting either on the front edge (suggests anxiety), or reclining with legs spread in front entangling with the examiners' feet (the vivas are often held in small side rooms, with not enough space under the desk for three pairs of legs!). Some examiners are expert interviewers and may try to put you at ease by engaging in a preliminary chat about your journey or your experience in the clinical section of the examination. The examiners should be allowed to dictate the length of this chat; this is no time to go into a fugal discussion about your interesting short cases, nor should you bring in a fresh topic (e.g. weather, accommodation, food, etc.) to delay the serious questioning about some medical problems. There is a blurred line between

---

[7]   p. 220
[8]   p. 188

appearing relaxed on the one hand, and casual or careless on the other. The optimum effect can be achieved by sitting comfortably without reclining or leaning forwards on the desk sharing a look with the examiners at their papers!

Avoid tension

He asked me to demonstrate the precordial thump. I don't know if I just had a lot of adrenaline flowing, or whether there was more echo in the room, but my blow to the desk top sounded very loud indeed![9]

Our advice about answering questions is outlined in Section 2 but some general comments are presented here which you may find useful. Look at the examiner who is asking the question and show that you are *listening* as you would during a serious discussion. Keep body movements to a minimum and suppress mannerisms. While answering the question you may need to use your hands to make or emphasise a point, but do not make a fist (looks intimidating) or bang on the desk (creates tension). It is standard advice that as you deliver your response you should maintain eye contact with the questioner, but you may find it profitable to cast a few glances at the coexaminer, who may otherwise sink in a reverie, and your inviting look may evoke an encouraging nod from him. Maintain a moderate tempo and keep your answers *conversational* even when you are delivering a prepared spiel, which could otherwise easily sound like a sterile harangue. At such times, the answer can be softened with the use of some well-known qualifiers, such as 'as you said', 'as mentioned by you', 'as was the case in the clinical scenario described by you', etc.

Keep talking

I failed the viva, and I am sure this was because I was not sure enough of myself and my answers were often faltering and indecisive[10]

I tried not to let the examiners do any talking since that wouldn't have got me any marks[11]

By the time you come to the viva you have spent some years in medicine and gained a lot of knowledge. The secret of the viva is to reveal this to the examiners. Your aim should be to home in on a subject you know about and then *keep talking*. Many candidates answer a question with one or two sentences and then wait for another question. This both fails to reveal their knowledge – the object of the viva – and makes the examiner work harder! Thus, when asked what you would do if called to casualty to see a breathless patient, you should imagine yourself dealing with this patient, and go through at length what you would do. You should take charge and

---

[9] p. 177
[10] p. 151
[11] p. 203

outline your approach in full, bearing in mind that the examiner will not have been in casualty himself for many years!

When you have completed an answer finish on a soft cadence and look the examiner in the eye. This may need some effort since anxiety tends to generate a higher pitch, which can create a confusing signal at the end of an answer. The examiners may think that you have not finished and wait for more, and you may therefore think that you have left out something important and they are waiting to hear it. Avoid giving monosyllabic answers like 'Yes' and 'No' (these sound aggressive); even when agreeing with the examiner, such responses should be qualified with a brief explanation. Avoid 'ums' and 'ers', superfluous expressions such as 'what d'you call', 'what's the name', 'this thing', 'the thing is', and casual clichés such as 'till the cows come home', 'as long as my arm', 'rare as hen's teeth', etc. Use abbreviations sparingly, particularly when they are not universally recognised and the full expressions are easy to pronounce, e.g. left ventricular failure for LVF, acute myocardial infarction for AMI, etc.

Many candidates try to waffle out of a tricky situation instead of saying 'I am sorry, I do not know the answer to this question'. This is always unproductive and can often create unnecessary tension, since the examiners, being knowledgeable and experienced clinicians, see through such attempts. There is no profit in prolonging the discussion on a subject about which you know nothing. If you realise that you made a mistake, admit it, apologise but not too abjectly, put it out of your mind and start afresh with the next question. The more questions you answer satisfactorily the more likely you are to pass the examination.

Keep calm

Arguing on controversial subjects does not pay. It is fine to be honest but finer still to be right![12]

In general, it is not advisable to argue with the examiners, particularly when there is no 'right' or 'wrong' answer and you are only supporting a point of view (yours!). Even when you are certain that you are right, put your point across politely and with sensitivity. Do not interrupt the examiner either when he is asking the question (and you are eager to answer), or when he is contradicting you (and you do not like it!). Such exchanges raise the tempo of the viva and you will then seem excessively slow even when you take an appropriate pause before answering the next question. If the examiner butts in while you are talking, do not get agitated, thank him for reminding you or for making a 'helpful suggestion'! Be honest in confessing your ignorance, or in admitting it when you discover that you made a mistake, and push your point gently when you *know* you are right. The examiner may have a different point of view and he surely is entitled to that.

---

[12] A candidate

3. After the viva

I tripped over my chair on the way out, forcing the metal leg over the concrete floor with a noisy effect![13]

I left the room with silent dignity, but caught my foot in the mat.[14]

It is advisable that you should continue to talk and complete your answer (if you know it) even when the bell has been rung, and not look enquiringly in silence thereby precipitating the end of the viva. The examiners will, and should be allowed to, indicate the end of the viva by thanking you. You should respond warmly (but do not overdo it!), thank the examiners with a spontaneous smile (practise it in front of a mirror!) which does not look forced, contrived or synthetic, and rise gently from your chair. Leave the room at a normal pace and quietly close the door. Do not be in a hurry to leave the room and do not bang the door even if your experience in the viva has been less than pleasant. Think kindly of the examiners who shared the same experience!

---

[13] p. 109
[14] W W Grossmith (1854 – 1919)

Section 2
Viva question groups

The main problem was that the examiner always had one particular answer in mind, and it became an exercise in mind-reading![1]

---

[1] p. 108

1 Introduction

In asking a question on a particular subject, the examiners are either probing the depth of your knowledge, or your clinical judgement or your skills of management. The subject can be the same, but the way the question is phrased may indicate the specific objective that the examiners want to achieve. As far as possible, you should identify their objective quickly, because addressing the main concern of the examiner and giving an appropriate answer (i.e. getting on the same wavelength), can help to avoid the increasingly agitating enquiry 'What else?', and save time that could be used in answering other questions to demonstrate the breadth of your knowledge. Hearing the answer that he is looking for will put the examiner in a benevolent frame of mind. Some examples of possible presentations to the examiner are presented later on in this section. Here, we are concerned with illustrating how examiners can vary the same subject and expect different responses. For example, questions on the subject of weight loss can be asked in a variety of ways:

1. **'What are the principal causes of weight loss in the elderly?'**

One could answer this question by loosely classifying the possible causes in relation to appetite; loss of weight with increased appetite in one group, and loss of weight with decreased appetite in the other. Alternatively, the examiner may wish to probe your ability to plan investigations and therapeutic regimes, and ask you to imagine yourself in a clinic.

2. **'A 75-year-old man has been referred to your clinic with weight loss. What are your initial thoughts?'**

Put this way, the examiner is attempting to evaluate how you would cope with this referral situation. Obviously, you would want to get a more comprehensive and precise clinical history and then examine the patient. In accordance with everyday clinical practice, you would decide upon a provisional diagnosis, and the initial investigations you would undertake to confirm it. Thus, in putting you in a referral setting the examiner does not want a long list of the causes of weight loss but, rather, how you would set about tackling the clinical problem. Candidates often make the right decision subconsciously and respond in an appropriate manner, but analysing the question properly, and the motive of the questioner, may help improve your approach.

3. **'You see a 75-year-old frail and anxious male patient with weight loss. What do you think?'**[2]

A slight change in the wording with the addition of two adjectives makes it more like a diagnostic challenge and brings it down to a simple 'guess the diagnosis' situation. In outlining your answer you will be particularly concerned with those features in the history and examination which allow you to make a provisional diagnosis. The critical questions of appetite,

---

[2] See *Detective* Stories, p. 68

speed of the weight loss, polyuria and heat intolerance will enable you to decide which out of the four major diagnostic probabilities (thyrotoxicosis, neoplastic disease, diabetes mellitus, gastrointestinal tract disturbances) is the most likely one.

Unless you can guess what the examiner had in mind from a clue ('anxious' was probably suggestive) you can weigh your answer slightly towards the area you would most like to talk about. For example, you may feel that **thyrotoxicosis** is easier to deal with at the outset, and so you can adjust your response to aim at this. Any interchange along these lines will lead to a satisfactory and uninterrupted monologue from you and on to the next question. Firing questions back at the examiner (which may be necessary sometimes either to seek clarification or a *ghost-link*, see pp. 151 and 221) only tires the examiner, makes *him* talk and feel less amiable when deciding as to who should be given the marks for talking!

The three variations of the same question discussed above illustrate one of the main reasons underlying our attempt to classify the questions asked in the viva into different groups. You will be better prepared if you train your mind to think along these lines, and allow yourself a moment's reflection before deciding how to answer a particular question. Most of the questions will fall clearly into one of the several groups presented here, but sometimes there may be some ambiguity as to where a question belongs (e.g. *Ghost* or *Detective* Stories). Since the classification of questions is not the main purpose of the viva, and only a guide to streamlining one's answer, it is important not to waste too much time in resolving the uncertainty; as long as you have correctly judged the principal motive of the examiner, you should have little difficulty in satisfying his or her curiosity about your competence. However, judging which group the question belongs to from the phraseology will enable you to take control and deliver a good response, without having to engage in a verbal ping-pong with the examiner. In most cases the decision should be easy, and where a precise decision is not possible your thoughtful approach will usually get you there. It is with this knowledge that you should approach this section and devise a constructive way to decide the nature of each question.

Each group will be considered in turn, and examples are given that have actually occurred in the examination, as revealed in our survey. At the beginning of each group of questions we have given samples of how these might be answered ('model' answers); these are followed by questions, with our suggestions summarised briefly after each question. We have also provided other examples from the survey, which we have left for you to ponder your response. The factual details of some candidates' actual responses are given in Section 3.

1. REFERRALS

As the name implies, all the questions in this group are about problems *referred* to you, either in your capacity as a deputy to your consultant in the outpatient clinic, or as a medical registrar who is contacted by a registrar in another speciality about a difficult medical problem. This category of questions is not hard to recognise because the examiner always presents them somewhat like this:

'At a BUPA screening a patient was found to have raised serum lipids and he has been *referred* to your clinic. What do you do?'

or

'A patient was *referred* to you with rectal bleeding.'

or

'How do you investigate an obese patient?'

or

'What would you do with a patient who has been *referred* to you with a systolic murmur?'

In tackling referral questions, it is important to remember that the examiner's main concern is to see whether you have a logical approach in coping with day-to-day clinical problems. The examiners may not have a definite line of thought, or a single answer to their question in mind, and they are usually willing to follow your possible plan of action. Often, you have considerable freedom in fashioning your answer but your strategy has to be workable in practice! The best answers are often those based on personal experience, particularly if the outcome was successful. The examiners will challenge you whenever they suspect that you are guessing, or that you are uncertain about your answers. The referral questions broadly fall into two major subgroups: referrals from general practitioners, and referrals from nonmedical wards.

a. Referrals from general practitioners

1. **'A middle-aged man has been referred to you with a raised serum alkaline phosphatase discovered on routine screening. How do you proceed'?**

'Screening' has two possible implications: (1) the subject has no symptoms and (2) there is nothing abnormal in the liver function tests and serum urea and electrolyte levels as these are also measured in most screening protocols. However, making these assumptions without stating to the examiner that you have done so may prove hazardous, as he may conclude that you did not think of the relevant history and investigations. The answer should be adequately qualified:

■ 'I presume it is a lone finding unassociated with any symptoms and other abnormal laboratory findings, since screening implies that the subject was derived from a "normal" population, and that it would probably have included a check on serum urea and electrolytes, liver function tests and serum lipids. If so, gross **hepatobiliary disease** (biliary obstruction, sclerosing cholangitis, primary biliary cirrhosis, hepatic neoplasm, etc.) and gross **bone disease** (advanced multiple myeloma with extensive bone deposits, osteitis fibrosa cystica, neoplastic infiltration, etc.) are unlikely. Nonetheless, I would take a reasonably comprehensive history particularly about **alcohol intake**, bone pains and any **recent fractures**. My physical examination of the patient would include inspection for Paget's disease and palpation for **hepatomegaly**, and I would arrange X-rays of the skull and pelvis to look for any evidence of Paget's disease and bone secondaries, as in the early stages there may be no symptoms. I would obtain a full blood count for macrocytosis (alcoholism) and I may have to arrange additional tests such as isoenzymes of alkaline phosphatase, 5'-nucleotidase, leucine aminopeptidase and gamma glutamyl transpeptidase which should help to identify the source of the alkaline phosphatase, whether from a mild hepatic or bone disorder. In some cases of **bile duct stricture** (particularly when only a part of the lobe is involved), a raised level of alkaline phosphatase may be the only abnormality. Sometimes, there is a moderate increase in alkaline phosphatase in otherwise normal subjects.'

This answer is by no means comprehensive, as the questions about a single abnormal finding tend to be open-ended. This allows the examiners the scope to pick up any area of their choosing. However, your answer must reassure the examiner that you are aware of the many possible causes of the abnormality, and that you would employ a systematic approach and not embark on a vast array of investigations without further thought.

In the next example, the examiner was probing whether the candidate could distinguish between simple obesity and Cushing's syndrome.

2. **'How would you investigate an obese patient?'**

■ 'In most cases obesity is simply related to overeating over a long period; the history of weight gain begins in childhood and spurts of the gain are punctuated in females by the usual milestones of marriage (new recipes), pregnancies (eating for two) and bouts of depression (eating for comfort). However, there are a few rather rare conditions in which obesity is a presenting feature and in which a clinical diagnosis can be made, such as **Cushing's syndrome** (thin skin, truncal obesity, moon-shaped face, acne, buffalo hump, difficulty in standing up from a sitting position); **acromegaly** (coarse features, spade-like hands and feet, large tongue, thick skin, bitemporal hemianopia); **hypothyroidism** (puffy face, cold-intolerance, delayed relaxation of the tendon jerks, croaky voice, cold and pale skin); **islet cell tumour** (sweating, palpitations, weakness, anxiety, blurred vision, diplopia, confusion, psychiatric disorders, seizures); **polycystic ovary syndrome** (hirsutism, thick skin, irregular menses or amenorrhoea); **Laurence-Moon-Biedl syndrome** (hypogonadism, polydactyly); **pseudohypoparathyroidism** (rounded face, stocky build, short 4th or 5th metacarpals and metatarsals, mental retardation, delayed dentition, bowing of the radii and tibiae, hypocalcaemia) and **hypothalamic injury** (history of fractured skull or meningitis). In a small proportion of cases where there is doubt, even after a proper clinical assessment, the diagnosis can be confirmed for Cushing's syndrome (elevated 24-hour urinary free cortisol, 9 a.m. high ACTH if of pituitary origin[1]); for acromegaly (raised plasma growth hormone with lack of suppression by glucose or even a paradoxical rise during a glucose tolerance test); for hypothyroidism (low T4, high TSH) and for islet cell tumour (fasting hypoglycaemia with inappropriately raised plasma insulin level, C-peptide suppression test[2]).'

3. **'A 60-year-old man has been referred with a 6-month-long history of low back pain. What are your initial thoughts?'**

Remember that the examiner is experienced and well aware of the fact that investigating low back pain is often not a rewarding exercise. What is required here is not a long list of the causes you find in a textbook, but a realistic approach to this referral problem which will suggest to the examiner that you are an experienced, sound and capable physician:

■ 'Despite the frequent occurrence of low back pain, the aetiological diagnosis is often elusive and imprecise. However, there is a group of conditions which must receive serious consideration in a 60-year-old man who has had *persistent* low back pain.

A good history[3] and a proper physical examination, including that of the spine and lower limbs, should enable one to suspect whether this patient has **degenerative disease** (restricted flexion and extension of the spine with adequate lateral flexion, may have radicular pains, reduced disc spaces and spurring on the X-ray); **osteoporosis**[4] (incidence of 1 in 20 men over the age of 60; may have previous history of fracture or severe back pain) with or without compression fracture (may be on corticosteroids, kyphosis, compressed fracture resulting from sudden exercise, localised tenderness and radicular pain or poorly localised if there is no fracture, reduced bone density on the X-ray); **osteomalacia** (there may be evidence of malabsorption, liver disease, renal osteodystrophy, history of drugs such as phenytoin, proximal muscular weakness, waddling gait, low serum calcium and increased alkaline phosphatase, Looser's zones, pseudofractures – Milkman's lines – and wide osteoid seams on bone biopsy); **Paget's disease** (enlarged cranium, deafness, bowed legs, osteolytic lesions with sclerotic margins – 'picture frame' appearance on the X-ray, raised serum alkaline phosphatase); **malignant lesion** such as **myeloma** and **lymphoma,** or **secondaries** from breast, bronchus, prostate, kidney and thyroid, and neural tumours (pain worse at night and unresponsive to analgesics, localised

---

[1] Most cases of Cushing's syndrome are iatrogenic due to prednisolone therapy for asthma or rheumatoid arthritis.

[2] The plasma C-peptide levels measured after the administration of insulin (0.1 unit/kg body weight) do not show a fall in patients with insulinomas.

tenderness, progressive neural signs, systemic symptoms, characteristic bone scan); **spinal canal stenosis** (claudication type pain on sustained walking, radiates to thighs not readily relieved by standing but reduced by sitting); **referred pain** from an aortic aneurysm (throbbing pain, ultrasound evidence), and from **tumours** of the upper gastrointestinal tract, pancreas and the kidney; **infection** (osteomyelitis, tuberculosis of the spine, etc.); or "**compensation pain**" (history of traffic or industrial accident, resistant to analgesics, evasive answers to all specific questions).'

4. **'A girl of 16 has been referred with short stature. Both her mother and doctor are anxious that she may have some abnormality. How would you proceed?'**

This may be a case of delayed puberty and growth spurt (height throughout childhood below average and retarded epiphyseal development). Other causes must be considered:

1. **Familial short stature**: a child's height will tend to relate to the mean height of both parents
2. **Low birth weight**: intrauterine infections, genetic anomaly, abnormal pregnancy
3. **Nutritional**: ill health, poor social background, malabsorption syndrome, familial diabetes insipidus (poor intake), glycogen storage disease, kwashiorkor, delayed weaning (anything up to 8 years of age in third world countries), cystinuria (poor absorption and excessive loss), etc.
4. **Major system disease**[5]: cyanotic heart disease, chronic renal failure (e.g. Fanconi syndrome), chronic pulmonary disease (e.g. cystic fibrosis), chronic hepatic disease, anaemia, etc.
5. **Sex chromosome abnormalities**: Turner's syndrome (webbed neck, cubitus valgus, lymphoedema, karyotype 45/XO, impaired sexual development, rounding of the medial femoral condyle on X-ray, short 4th metacarpal, etc.)
6. **Skeletal disease**: achondroplasia, Hurler's syndrome, Laurence-Moon-Biedl syndrome, pseudo- and pseudo-pseudo-hypoparathyroidism, vitamin D-resistant rickets
7. **Endocrine disorders**: pituitary dwarfism, hypothyroidism, Cushing's syndrome, congenital adrenal hyperplasia
8. **Emotional deprivation**: may lead to temporary hypothalamic disturbance with impaired release of growth hormone.

Particular attention should be paid to a family history of growth and development, birth weight and length, the pattern of height and epiphyseal development, facial features – as a guide to skeletal maturity – secondary sexual characteristics or the presence of a 'syndrome', dental

---

[3]   Bear in mind that the back pain in lumbar spondylosis and the pain from vertebral collapse in osteoporosis rarely last more than a week or two at a time

[4]   Osteoporosis would come at the top of the list in a female (1 in 4 over the age of 60), osteochondritis (Scheuermann's disease) in adolescents and ankylosing spondylitis in young adults

[5]   Usually obvious clinically

development, appetite and pattern of weight gain, history and clinical features of infections. A physical examination should test the integrity of all systems and include an assessment of skeletal and body configuration – height, lower segment span, skull circumference, neck webbing, cubitus valgus, length of metacarpals and sexual development.

5. **'A 60-year-old man has been referred with dizziness. How would you proceed?'**

The evaluation of dizziness is made difficult in many cases by psychological factors which are either wholly responsible or alter the symptomatology. A penetrating history is one of the four steps that forms the cornerstone of the diagnostic strategy (see also p. 65).

1. **History**: depression, anxiety and hyperventilation are by far the commonest causes, relation of dizziness with stress situations, precipitating factors with position (positional vertigo), cough (cough syncope), and effort (hypertrophic obstructive cardiomyopathy), associated symptoms such as tinnitus (Ménière's disease, labyrinthitis, post-traumatic), hearing loss (Ménière's disease, cerebellopontine angle tumour), and visual disturbances such as diplopia.
2. **Examine the nervous system**: test cerebellar function (multiple sclerosis, infarction or tumour of the brain stem or cerebellum) and check for posterior column signs (subacute combined degeneration, tabes dorsalis).
3. **Test vestibular function** (viral labyrinthitis, vascular and infiltrative disease) – perform Hallpike procedure (see p. 66).
4. **Examine the cardiovascular system**:
   a. **Pulse** (arrhythmias, complete heart block, severe aortic stenosis, hypertrophic obstructive cardiomyopathy, etc.)
   b. **Carotid massage**[6] (vasovagal attacks due to hypersensitive carotid sinus)
   c. **Auscultation** (aortic stenosis, mitral stenosis, left atrial myxoma). Echocardiography would help establish the diagnosis
   d. **Blood pressure** (sitting and standing for postural hypotension)
   e. **ECG** (arrhythmias, sinoatrial disease, etc.). A 24-hour ambulatory monitoring study may have to be undertaken if arrhythmias are suspected as the cause of dizziness.

6. **'A 21-year-old law student has been referred to you "just feeling lousy". Discuss how you would manage him.'**

In practice, such a complaint in a young person usually turns out to be psychological (anger, isolation, bad performance in examinations, homesickness, etc.). A probing interview may reveal social isolation, low

---

[6]   This procedure should be attempted only if a cardiac monitor and resuscitation equipment are available, since the massage may trigger a cardiac arrest in a sensitive patient. It should be avoided if the patient has a carotid bruit, as cases where the procedure has precipitated cerebral emboli have been reported.

[7]   Often such patients are labelled as having the myalgic encephalitis syndrome, for which there are no strict diagnostic signs (see also pp. 24, 87).

self-esteem, chronic conflict, apathy, insomnia, withdrawal, anorexia, weight loss, etc.[7]

In assessing such a patient, there are a few organic conditions which must be borne in mind,[8] and one may have to undertake a few relevant investigations. When it is clear from the history and physical examination that there is no organic explanation then he should be reassured. If there is a social or psychological problem then he should be offered appropriate help.

Other examples from survey

1. **'A young, healthy woman is referred with a late systolic murmur. What would you do?'**

Presumably she has been seen by her GP for palpitations or for some unconnected reason. One should listen carefully for a late ejection click, and a cardiac echo should be arranged to look for prolapse of the posterior cusp of the mitral valve. Reassure, but advise antibiotic prophylaxis before dental and surgical procedures.

2. **'A 40-year-old man has been referred with his first grand mal fit. How do you manage him?'**

History and examination should explore the features of post-traumatic, infective, vascular and metabolic causes. A space-occupying lesion (or other focus, such as the scar of a previous CVA) may present with Jacksonian (focal) epilepsy, and evidence of this should be sought if a witness can be found. Investigations should include blood glucose, serum urea, electrolytes and calcium. An EEG may indicate the site of an epileptic focus, and slow-wave activity should raise the suspicion of a tumour. However, the CAT scan is the definitive investigation to exclude a space-occupying lesion. No treatment is recommended for a single unexplained fit, but driving is not advised for one year in accordance with the Driving Vehicles and Licensing Authority guidelines.[9]

3. **'An executive has been referred with hypertension. What do you do?'**

Obtain a family history, look for a primary cause and other risk factors; treat with a first-line drug such as a calcium antagonist.[10]

---

[8] **Organic causes of ill health**
1. *Chronic infection*: TB, brucellosis, toxoplasmosis, AIDS, etc.
2. *Endocrine*: hypothyroidism, hypopituitarism, Addison's disease
3. *Blood*: anaemia
4. *Liver*: chronic persistent hepatitis, chronic active hepatitis
5. *Neoplasm*: carcinoma, lymphoma
6. *Multisystem disease*: collagen diseases
7. *Viral*: postviral asthenia, myalgic encephalitis
8. *Neuromuscular*: myasthenia gravis, McArdle's disease
9. *Drug abuse*: heroin, marihuana, tranquillisers, etc.

[9] Raffle A (ed) 1985, Medical aspects of fitness to drive. The Medical Commission on Accident Prevention, HMSO, London

[10] A beta blocker will reduce sympathetic drive, which may be detrimental to an executive's work.

b. Referrals from nonmedical wards

This should be familiar territory for almost all candidates taking the membership examination. Most of you will have dealt with calls from colleagues on nonmedical wards for advice about medical problems. However, candidates with no recent 'on-call' experience may find these questions more difficult to tackle. It is important to remind yourself that anything less than a competent performance with these questions is going to weigh heavily against you. After all they are 'bread-and-butter' clinical situations. From the responses of candidates in our survey, it seems that a common mistake is one of skipping and a lack of attention to detail. For example, many candidates were asked how they would sort out the problem of a middle-aged man admitted for minor surgery (haemorrhoids, herniorrhaphy, etc.), who was found to have a raised blood pressure by an anaesthetist, who then initiated the referral to a medical registrar on call. Many said that they would assess the patient clinically and then go back the next day to re-check the blood pressure. They said nothing about the impending operation and what they would have said to the anaesthetist and the surgeon.

It is important to remember that in all referral questions there has to be an answer for the person referring the problem. Thus, when asked a question about a referral from a GP or from a colleague from another ward, you have to state what you would do about the problem, what you would say to the patient and, above all, what you would say to the person who referred the problem to you.

Since hypertension is asymptomatic, and the blood pressure rises with stress, it is not unusual for an anaesthetist to discover a new hypertensive now and again on the preoperative round. Rather than give a 'shorthand' answer using terms like 'clinical assessment', you would do well to be specific and reassuring:

■ 'I would obtain a complete history from the patient, questioning him about any family and previous history of hypertension, or any record of blood pressure measurements at a previous medical examination (for insurance, etc.). I would obtain a drug history asking especially whether the patient has been on nasal sprays, steroids or amphetamines. I would record the BP in the sitting and standing positions and check for radiofemoral delay to rule out coarctation of the aorta, and look for any features of Cushing's syndrome. My systemic examination would include fundoscopy for hypertensive changes, examination of the cardiovascular system, and auscultation over the abdomen (bruits over renal arteries). If the BP is elevated I would come back after a couple of hours to check again. If there is sustained elevation in the blood pressure or/and if it has been previously documented, then hypertension is probably established. Initial investigation would include urinalysis, serum urea and electrolytes (low K^+ suspicious of Conn's syndrome), ECG, chest X-ray for left ventricular enlargement and fasting serum lipids. In most such cases the raised BP is the only abnormality. If so, I would reassure the patient and the anaesthetist. If the BP is no higher than 160/100 mmHg then surgery can be undertaken and the patient should be followed up for attention to weight, smoking, alcohol, exercise and drug treatment. If the BP before surgery remains above 160/100, then I would start with a first-line drug to bring it down, since a higher BP is associated with higher perioperative morbidity (strokes, myocardial infarction, etc.).'

Other examples from survey

1. **'You have been asked to see a hypotensive patient on a surgical ward. What thoughts go through your mind?'**

   Look for evidence of septic, haemorrhagic or cardiogenic shock, pulmonary embolism, and arrhythmias. Inadvertent or overuse of drugs before surgery may be the problem, e.g. chlorpromazine, antihypertensive drugs, cardiodepressants, etc.

2. **'As a duty medical officer you have been called to a gynaecology ward to assess a patient's fitness for operation.'**

   A nonspecific question but it happens in real life! A complete clinical assessment is required – history, examination, urinalysis (and, if clinically indicated, FBC, U&E, CXR, ECG), looking to exclude respiratory (chronic obstructive airways disease), cardiac (ischaemic heart disease, hypertension) and renal diseases. It would obviously help if you can find out the specific reason why a medical opinion has been requested!

3. **'You have been called to see a pregnant woman with a DVT. What do you advise?'**

   Diagnosis and the teratogenicity of anticoagulant drugs are the main concerns. Diagnosis can be made clinically, but in doubtful cases one may have to resort to venography with the abdomen shielded by a lead apron. (Doppler ultrasound scanning, thermography and ultrasound imaging of the clot are helpful only in a few specialised centres.) Investigations should also include a check for 'lupus anticoagulant'. Heparin is the safest treatment as it does not cross the placenta, and on a long-term basis it can be given subcutaneously.

2. TOPICAL ISSUES

Examiners ask questions about topical issues discussed in the recent editorials of medical journals and also topics of interest that appear in the lay press. There is a general impression that the examiners read something on their way to the examination centre and then ask about it! This uncharitable view may sometimes be close to the truth, but usually these questions are asked deliberately by examiners to test your reading spectrum and social conscience. After all, what sort of a caring doctor would have no views on a major atomic reactor disaster, and its possible consequences on the environment and the health of people around it. Even if you are not an ardent reader of journals, you should develop the habit of leafing through the major journals, particularly reading their leading articles, and also know about recent national and international events of medical importance from the national newspapers, such as the aftereffects of a flood, earthquake or an oil leak at sea.

Topical issues can be subdivided into the following four subgroups:

a. public concern
b. recent publications
c. specialists' concern
d. colleges' concern.

By definition, these subjects are changeable and depend very much on what has happened around the world just before the examination, and on articles published that may have attracted the attention of the examiners. For example, soon after the outbreak of fire in the atomic reactor at Chernobyl, many candidates were asked questions about the hazards of radiation and the possible treatment for exposure. Without that incident, it is difficult to imagine that any examiner would have asked a question about what should be done for a person who has ingested meat from a lamb accidentally exposed to radiation, or what might be the health hazards of living close to the Sellafield plant! Let us look at a few examples in each group:

a. Public concern

1. **'These days, some insurance companies are asking for human immunodeficiency virus (HIV) testing before accepting any proposals. What would you do if you were a general practitioner of a patient who turned up a positive test?'**

   ■ 'I would hope that the patient had received proper and detailed counselling before his blood sample was sent for HIV testing. As his GP, I would hope to have been fully involved in the discussions before the test was done. The news about the positive test must come as a great blow, and there will be psychological, social, financial and medical implications. The patient is unlikely to be accepted for life assurance but a positive test is no bar to continued employment. I would reassure the patient very strongly about confidentiality; his peers and employers will not be told and every possible care will be taken against unnecessary dissemination of this information. The patient should be given psychological, social and emotional support through his family and trusted friends. The patient may wish to discuss the finding with his spouse but, if required, I would be happy to talk to them both. I would emphasise that having a positive test does not mean having the disease (AIDS), which develops in about half the cases after several years. He should be advised to tell his dentist and surgeon if he requires surgery. He should be referred to an appropriate specialist and seen and examined every 3 months, and at each visit his weight, blood count and ESR should be recorded. Particular attention should be paid to symptoms relating to the skin, and respiratory (dyspnoea, cough), gastrointestinal (dysphagia, diarrhoea, etc.) and nervous systems.'

2. **'A boy of 12 years is admitted with photophobia and neck stiffness. What are your initial thoughts?'[1]**

This is like one of those deceptive parliamentary questions which look very simple to answer but lead to hazardous supplementary questions (e.g. the place of steroids, the causes for a geographical spread of meningitis, etc.).

In this instance, the discussion revolved around the 1987/88 outbreak of meningococcal meningitis, its possible causes and geographical distribution, and the reasons for the previous postwar outbreaks.[2]

Other examples from survey

1. **'What are the likely diseases to be found at the seaside?'**

This topic received a great deal of publicity in the national press during 1987/88, and there was a leading article in the *British Medical Journal* in 1988 (296:1484). A high degree of pollution is found at some beaches, particularly on the southwest coast of England. Ailments associated with swimming include gastroenteritis, diarrhoea, conjunctivitis, oral ulcers, etc. Used needles carelessly scattered on some beaches present the potential hazards of hepatitis B and AIDS.

---

[1] The most likely diagnosis is one or other variety of benign lymphocytic meningitis.

[2] Outbreaks of meningococcal meningitis occur during wartime when there is large-scale mobilisation, overcrowding and scarcity of resources. Major epidemics caused by group A meningococci tend to occur in cyclical manner every 10 to 20 years. In recent years in the UK, group C meningococcus has emerged as the predominant organism. Although clusters of cases occur in schools and barracks, person-to-person infection is not predictable. In sub-Saharan Africa epidemics occur in the dry season, whereas in the UK infections are common in the winter and early spring. Sporadic cases caused by group B meningococcus tend to have a much worse prognosis.

2. 'What do you think about epidemic myalgic encephalitis?'[3]

Some articles in the Sunday papers (1988/89) concerning patients with myalgic encephalitis generated a public perception of misdiagnosis by doctors. The examiners may have seen patients who felt that their symptoms of chronic fatigue[4] were wrongly attributed to psychiatric illnesses. The syndrome is a prolonged and debilitating illness characterised by severe fatigue, fluctuations of mood, tiredness, muscular weakness and sometimes by neurological disorders.

The disorder begins insidiously with myalgia, fatigue on slight exertion, headache and a variety of other nonspecific symptoms. Laboratory investigations, including the results of cerebrospinal fluid examination, are invariably normal. The aetiological agents have been thought to be enteroviruses, but there is no definite scientific evidence for this. It is now thought that myalgic encephalitis is an example of 'the abnormal illness behaviour syndrome'.[5]

---

[3] Also known as Iceland disease or the Royal Free Hospital disease (see p. 87)

[4] Because of its subjective nature, fatigue is difficult to define, quantitate and disentangle from a variety of psychiatric illnesses such as depression. Even when an identifiable cause can be found (e.g. myasthenia gravis, Addison's disease, hypothyroidism, diabetes mellitus, chronic infection, neoplastic disorder, etc.) the contribution of other factors cannot be ruled out. Some patients tire easily after a minor illness which does not cause fatigue in many others. In view of the nonspecific nature of the symptoms, and the considerable overlap between various incriminating conditions, a careful and probing history should be obtained and a thorough physical examination carried out. Laboratory investigations are largely noncontributory in establishing the diagnosis of myalgic encephalitis, but new methods of analysing muscle action metabolically may provide objective evidence in patients with organic fatigue. For example, the use of ^{31}P nuclear magnetic resonance may show an abnormal decrease in muscle phosphocreatine and an increase of inorganic phosphate, during muscle fatigue in patients with McArdle's disease. Fatigue may be considered 'central' when there is difficulty in concentrating and thinking clearly, or when there is reduced motivation for voluntary motor activity. 'Peripheral' fatigue results from failure at or beyond the neuromuscular junction, as in myasthenia gravis, inborn errors of metabolism (e.g. myophosphorylase deficiency), congestive cardiac failure and in mitochondrial myopathies. Persistent and excessive fatigue has been associated with postviral asthenia, chronic brucellosis and recurrent episodes of infectious mononucleosis. In all of these conditions there is usually a psychological component.

[5] The concept of 'abnormal illness behaviour' was proposed by Pilowsky (Br J Med Psychol 1969; 42: 347) for patients with a wide variety of physical symptoms for which no organic explanation can be found. The behaviour of such patients is conditioned by their own perception of their symptoms and by the reaction of those with whom they have dealings (e.g. relatives, colleagues and doctors).

3. **'What would you tell a patient who refuses blood transfusion for fear of contracting AIDS?'**

A Government-sponsored advertising campaign and various press reports of AIDS occurring in haemophiliacs were probably the reasons behind this question. Transfusion-related AIDS represents a small proportion of cases. Some haemophiliac patients seroconverted as long ago as 1981/82, suggesting that the disease in these patients has a long incubation period. The danger of transmission has been minimised since 1988 as all blood donors are now screened for HIV antibodies.[6] Plasma products are now treated with heat or chemicals to decrease viral contamination. These procedures prevent HIV transmission, and the concern for young haemophiliacs is now much less. Continued vigilance over the safety of the blood supply will keep the risk of HIV transmission by transfusion very low, and such risks should be kept in perspective. According to one pessimistic estimate (N Engl J Med 1988; 318: 473) the risk of contracting AIDS from potentially infected blood is 1 in 40 000, compared with the higher odds of death from influenza (1 in 5000), or being killed in a road traffic accident (1 in 5000).[7]

b. Recent publications

1. **'Where is Lyme and what is it famous for?'**

Articles on this subject appeared in the national and medical press (N Engl J Med 1989; 321: 586)in 1989.

■ 'Lyme is a small town on the east bank of the Connecticut River. People here no longer walk on their lawns for fear of getting an illness called Lyme disease caused by the spirochaete *Borrelia burdorferi* and transmitted by the young adult deer tick, *Ixodes dammini*.[8] The disease is not confined to Lyme; cases have been reported from other parts of the USA, from Europe, including the UK (New Forest area of Hampshire), and from Australia. Like many other spirochaetal conditions, the disease occurs in three stages. The initial stage is characterised by fever, headache, muscle pains and weight loss. In over 60% of cases, patients

---

6   The main risk of transmission of the HIV virus through blood transfusions is in the period between the time a donor has been infected and the time he has a positive blood test for HIV antibodies. During this so-called 'window- period' of 6 to 8 weeks, the currently used screening procedures do not detect IgG antibody to HIV. The HIV-antigen assay has been found to show a positive result as early as 6 days after infection, but this test needs to be evaluated on a wider scale. Additional laboratory tests based on recombinant-DNA technology, synthetic peptides and gene-amplification techniques need to be developed. In the meantime a sharp focus must remain on improving donor education and screening. The risk of undetected infection can be reduced by transfusing fewer units, and units from fewer donors, recruiting more women and encouraging frequent donations from donors who have been tested recently and found to be safe.

7   The experts we have contacted say that the odds of contracting AIDS from a single blood transfusion are one in one million.

8   In Europe *erythema chronicum migrans* has been associated with the bite of the sheep tick, *Ixodes ricinus*.

develop a pink rash, surrounded by a dark ring (*erythema chronicum migrans*), often on the site of the tick bite but it may also occur elsewhere. The rash develops 2 – 30 days after a tick bite. It has an expanding edge spreading outwards gradually over a period of weeks. *Erythema migrans* is a self-limiting rash but in 10 – 15% of patients arthritis, neurological and cardiac complications develop. Early Lyme disease is curable (tetracycline or penicillin) but difficult to diagnose as the antibody level is too low to be assayed. Late-stage symptoms are associated with **multisystem involvement** (e.g. meningitis, cranial neuritis, radiculoneuritis, encephalitis, cardiomegaly, atrioventricular block, arthritis, etc.).'

2. 'What have recent trials taught us about the benefit of treatment in mild hypertension?'

This question was inspired by the recent publication of the MRC trial (Br Med J 1988; 296: 1565) on mild hypertension. Although some knowledge of this and other recent trials is necessary, a detailed analysis of the results is not required. The questioner's aim is to find out whether you have evolved a strategy from recent trials to deal with this common problem:

■ 'It is difficult to generalise the results of various trials with differing populations, entry criteria and drugs. Treatment of mild hypertension reduces the risk of stroke, but there is no convincing evidence to suggest that the incidence of coronary events is reduced. **Smoking** is a major risk factor for vascular disease, and particular attention should be directed at persuading patients to give this up. Patients should also be advised to reduce excessive consumption of **alcohol**, and lose weight if **overweight**, and **hyperlipidaemia** should be looked for and treated.[9] A persistently raised blood pressure (160/100 mmHg or more)[10] should be treated, but drug treatment should be weighed against side effects and metabolic changes. Where treatment is not recommended, follow-up should be continued to detect later rises in blood pressure.'

3. 'What are the recent developments in hormone replacement therapy in postmenopausal women?'

A plethora of publications[11] on this subject coincided with MRCP examinations when many candidates were asked some variation of this

---

[9] Although there is a clear association between hypercholesterolaemia and ischaemic heart disease, the subject does raise controversy and the examiner may take issue with it. (See also p. 32.)

[10] In diabetes mellitus, a lower threshold for starting treatment may be preferable. In patients with insulin-dependent diabetes mellitus who have microalbuminuria, reducing the BP below 150/90 mmHg may reverse renal damage. A strict control of hypertension may slow down the progression of renal damage even in established diabetic kidney disease.

[11] Lancet 1988; 2: 1243
Adverse Drug Reaction Bulletin 1987; 126
Drug and Therapeutics Bulletin 1989; 27: 24
British Journal of Hospital Medicine 1989; 41: 42
British Medical Journal 1989; 298: 1467
New England Journal of Medicine 1989; 321: 319

question. The question was open-ended in most cases, but the examiners' concern soon became obvious as they tackled the specific issues of **osteoporosis**, **ischaemic heart disease**, the contraindications of hormone replacement therapy and its link with **endometrial** and **breast cancer**.

■ 'The gradual cessation of ovarian function at the menopause, with the fall in ovarian hormones and a rise in gonadotrophins, is accompanied by some disabling symptoms (e.g. flushing, palpitations, sweating, irritability, joint and bone pains, etc.). Various studies have shown that severe **menopausal symptoms** are often relieved by hormone replacement therapy. **Atheroma** and **bone loss** accelerate after the menopause. Large studies (Lancet 1981; 1: 858; N Engl J Med 1985; 313: 1044) have shown that oestrogen treatment protects postmenopausal women from **ischaemic heart disease**. Hormone replacement therapy also helps to prevent or delay the development of osteoporosis and protects against **fractures** of the wrist, spine and hip. Ideally, prevention ought to be aimed at those most likely to develop osteoporosis.[12] Unfortunately, bone density measurements by single or dual photon absorptiometry and dual energy X-ray technology are expensive, and a single measurement is no predictor of the future rate of bone loss. As about 50% of women will sustain an osteoporotic fracture, it could be argued that in the absence of specific contraindications (hypertension, endometrial and breast cancer, fibroids and endometriosis[13]) all women at the menopause should be offered hormone replacement therapy. Oestrogens are the mainstay of such treatment but should not be given alone if the uterus has not been removed; oestrogen given alone causes **endometrial hyperplasia** and increases the risk of **carcinoma** of the **endometrium**. The addition of **progestogen**, given for 10 to 12 days each month, reduces this risk. Although the oral route has been safely used widely, the introduction of oestrogen skin patches is welcome, but the progestogen still requires to be given by mouth. Currently, there is no convincing evidence that oestrogen replacement therapy causes an increased incidence of **breast cancer**.'[14]

---

[12] Numerous risk factors for osteoporosis include an early menopause, long periods of amenorrhoea, excessive dieting, treatment with corticosteroids, excessive alcohol consumption, rheumatoid arthritis, early oophorectomy, hyperparathyroidism, smoking, thin body build and a family history of late menarche.

[13] Endometriosis and fibroids are **oestrogen-dependent** conditions and may deteriorate with hormone replacement therapy, but these can be closely monitored by clinical and ultrasound pelvic examinations. In patients with a past history of, or predisposition to, hypertension, coagulation disorders or liver disease related to oestrogens, the oral route should be avoided, since orally given oestrogens may cause gastrointestinal side effects and induce hepatic production of coagulation factors. For those who have had a total hysterectomy and salpingo-oophorectomy for endometriosis, provided there is no residual endometriotic tissue, the risk of activation of the disease is minimal.

[14] This concern must be kept under review until the results of long-term studies (15 years or more) are available, to show that there is *no* risk of developing carcinoma of the breast, after prolonged oestrogen combined with intermittent progestogen therapy. You must also bear in mind that your examiner may be one of the sceptics; you may have to accommodate the alternative view that the strong protective effect of hormone replacement therapy against ischaemic heart disease, is based on the data almost exclusively derived from the studies of women taking *unopposed* oestrogens. As many women with intact uteri are now prescribed a combination of oestrogen and progestogen, we need to know whether a similar protective effect can be achieved.

Other examples from survey

1. 'What are the medical complications of long-distance running?'

The examiners tended to ask this question (or a variation of it) after a brief preamble about the London marathon, or injuries caused by sports such as rugby (Br Med J 1988; 296: 149). Among the complications are dehydration, exhaustion, joggers' heel, arthritis, joggers' nipple, anovulation in females, decreased fertility, bradycardia, heart block, syncope and even sudden death.

2. 'What is Reye's syndrome and what do you know about its aetiology?'

This was a popular subject in both the lay and medical press because of its relationship with aspirins which are readily available for purchase over the counter (Br Med J 1986; 292: 1543). It is an acute encephalopathic syndrome[15] of children, with fatty degeneration of viscera characteristically seen in the liver. Epidemiological studies have linked its onset with the administration of salicylates during an antecedent illness, particularly for chickenpox or influenza. When first described in Australia in 1963 by Reye, 17 of 21 children died. However, milder cases are known to occur.

3. 'What are the hazards of treating hyponatraemia?'

This question coincided with publications in the *New England Journal of Medicine* (1986; 314: 1529) and the *British Medical Journal* (1987; 294: 261). Rapid correction of hyponatraemia (correcting serum Na^+ concentration at a rate of >12 mmol/1/day) especially by intravenous infusion of hypertonic sodium chloride has been associated with **pontine myelinosis** due to cellular shrinkage.

4. 'How would you investigate a patient with postural hypotension?'

A good history is the single most important investigation.

The causes include:

1. *Volume depletion* – diuretic therapy, gastrointestinal or renal fluid loss, aldosterone deficiency, haemorrhage, Addison's disease
2. *Drugs* – levodopa, antihypertensive agents, particularly vasodilator drugs such as hydrallazine and prazosin
3. *Hypersensitive carotid sinus* – (easily demonstrable by carotid massage)[16]

---

[15] A toxic origin has been implicated for both the hepatic and the neurological dysfunction. The former appears to be the primary problem (as a result of a **mitochondrial impairment**) causing secondary metabolic disturbances including **high blood ammonia concentration**, **lactic acidosis** and **elevated** levels of serum **free fatty acids**. Diagnosis is made by the presence of nonicteric hepatic dysfunction with high arterial blood ammonia and serum transaminase levels. Liver biopsy shows accumulation of fat droplets in the liver cells and mitochondrial damage (on electron microscopy). In addition to proper hydration, the developing abnormalities such as hypoglycaemia must be corrected.

[16] p. 18

4. *Brain and spinal cord lesions* – vascular accident, encephalopathies, demyelinating disorders, syringomyelia, tumours, previous sympathectomies
5. *Secondary* – vascular disease, autonomic neuropathy in diabetes, amyloidosis and alcoholism
6. *Primary idiopathic orthostatic hypotension* – Shy-Drager syndrome, familial dysautonomia (Riley-Day syndrome).

5. **'What are your views on asymptomatic bacteriuria in nonpregnant subjects?'**

The urine may have been tested in a subject with no urinary symptoms because of other renal concerns (**diabetes mellitus**, **polycystic kidneys**, **anatomical** or **neurological disorders, immunocompromised**, etc.). Such patients with bacteriuria should be treated. Asymptomatic bacteriuria (with no pus cells in the urine) in nonpregnant females who have no underlying structural or neurological disorders should not be treated, since there is a likelihood of reinfection and emergence of resistant strains.

c. Specialists' concern

There are always issues relevant to some specialities that make the headlines in the lay press as well as the medical journals. Cardiology is a good example, but now and again other specialities also feature. The examiner may not be a specialist in the subject but he will have sufficient knowledge to assess the substance of your views. In most cases what is wanted is a resumé of the currently held views together with your opinion, and if you happen to have read the subject recently, then there should be no difficulty in presenting a coherent summary of the topic. If you have not read anything about the subject, you may still be able to give an answer if you can support it with good reasoning. On the other hand, if you know nothing it is preferable to confess your ignorance, which will be discovered anyway if you try to waffle your way through. There are usually no hard and fast correct answers. The examiner has asked for your opinion so he will accept your views if you can support them with sound arguments. As the following example with two contrasting answers illustrates, any firm opinion based on a sound understanding can be acceptable.

1. **'Do you think we should add the heart to the list of endocrine organs?'**

If you would like to say 'Yes'
■ 'The atrial natriuretic peptide is secreted by the atria (mostly the **right atrium**) in response to **volume overload**, and it causes **vasodilatation** and **natriuresis**. Since we accept that endocrine organs secrete hormones which exert their effects in other organs of the body to which they are taken by the bloodstream, the heart surely qualifies to be added to the list.'

If you would like to say 'No'

■ 'It is true that the heart produces a factor called atrial natriuretic peptide, and that this factor should qualify as a hormone[17] since it has effects on organs other than the heart (e.g. kidney, vessels). However, the heart is not an endocrine organ in the strict sense, since its secretory activity is related to its own needs – as it secretes the hormone in response to a developing problem within itself. Other endocrine glands, like the pituitary and thyroid, produce hormones not only for actions in other organs but also in response to the *needs* of other organs. The heart is an autocrine organ and produces a factor in the same way as some cells produce growth factors for their own proliferation.'

2. 'What are the uses of recombinant DNA in medicine?'

As all living processes are ultimately controlled by genes, an understanding of genetic structure leading to genetic engineering (recombinant-DNA) has had a major impact on four areas in clinical medicine:

a. Knowledge of the molecular basis of various diseases
The isolation of a gene provides an opportunity for better understanding of physiological processes, as has happened in the thalassaemias and haemoglobinopathies. Most of the genotypes that can produce beta thalassaemia have been sequenced yielding more insight into the thalassaemia syndromes, and prenatal diagnosis has now become possible.

b. Prenatal diagnosis
A number of genetic disorders can now be detected prenatally, e.g. spina bifida, anencephaly, Down's syndrome and various inborn errors of metabolism. Fetal DNA can be obtained from amniotic fluid cells in the second trimester, or by chorion villus sampling during the first trimester. Many single gene defects can be determined by DNA analysis of these samples. Fetal blood samples can be obtained after 18 weeks' gestation and used for the diagnosis of a variety of fetal disorders, e.g viral infections, platelet disorders, inherited immunodeficiencies, chromosomal aberrations, etc.

c. Production of biological products
Examples include insulin, growth hormone, alpha- and beta-interferon, erythropoietin, vaccines, blood components, neurohormones, etc.

---

[17] The status of atrial natriuretic factor as a 'true circulatory hormone' remains debatable. There is no evidence that the plasma concentrations achieved during a physiological stimulus (e.g. stretch of the left atrial wall) can evoke acute responses. No evidence has been provided to suggest a causative link between stimuli within the physiological range, a rise in the plasma concentration of the peptide and the response of natriuresis and diuresis.

d. Gene therapy

The insertion of a functional gene to counteract a defective one to cure or ameliorate the genetic defect should be feasible within a few years. The most promising candidates for this approach are the various haemo-globinopathies.

3. **'Summarise your views on the modern treatment of heart failure.'**

■ 'The first objective should be to identify and, if possible, correct the **underlying cause**, e.g. arrhythmias, ischaemic heart disease, valvular decompensation,[18] hypertension, etc. **Diuretics** are the drugs of choice for initial treatment, but overuse (> 80 mg/day frusemide or equivalent) should be avoided[19] and serum urea and electrolytes and body weight should be monitored. Digitalis is suitable in patients with atrial fibrillation, but may be useful even in sinus rhythm associated with cardiomegaly. Activation of the renin-angiotensin system may be further stimulated by diuretics causing salt and water retention. Moderately severe heart failure should be treated with the combination of a diuretic and an **angiotensin converting enzyme (ACE) inhibitor** such as captopril (12.5 mg), enalapril or lisinopril 2.5 mg/day, which can be increased if blood pressure and renal function remain satisfactory. The addition of an ACE inhibitor should be considered if 40 – 80 mg of frusemide a day (or its equivalent) proves insufficient. Intravenous infusion of **inotropes** such as dobutamine for 2 or 3 days often produces sustained improvement for several weeks. Drugs which have not been fully evaluated are the dopaminergic receptor agonist (dopexamine), selective dopamine receptor agonists (fenoldopan), and phospho-diesterase inhibitors (milrinone). However, in severe cases with very poor ventricular function, only **heart transplantation** is likely to offer any real hope of restoration to a reasonable life style.' (See also p. 64.)

4. **'What is the place of fibrinolytic therapy in acute myocardial infarction?'**

The rationale for fibrinolysis is based on the fact that a myocardial infarction is nearly always due to a coronary thrombosis, and that whatever irreversible damage occurs does so in the **first few hours** after the infarction. There is accumulating evidence that thrombolysis not only reopens vessels but also limits myocardial damage and improves long-term survival. Some studies have suggested that **tissue plasminogen activator**

---

[18] All cases of heart failure should have echocardiography to assess their left ventricular function, and to exclude a valvular lesion. Severe aortic stenosis may be missed sometimes on clinical examination because the murmur is either of minimal intensity or is altogether absent.

[19] In severe congestive cardiac failure, absorption of oral frusemide may be reduced so that greater doses are needed for the same therapeutic effect. Intravenous administration will overcome this problem. In severe cases, resistant to frusemide, the addition of a **thiazide** (bendrofluazide or metolazone) will usually have a marked *synergistic* effect. Such a combination of a loop diuretic and a thiazide may lead to severe **volume depletion**, and so should be used with great caution and only for a limited time, with careful monitoring of the serum urea and electrolytes.

is more effective than **streptokinase** in producing coronary patency but is no different regarding mortality. There is not enough evidence at the time of writing to be unequivocally in favour of any one of the five agents available (streptokinase, urokinase, tissue plasminogen activator, prourokinase and acylated plasminogen-streptokinase activator complex; APSAC).[20]

Left ventricular function, predischarge patency rates and mortality data do not suggest that any one of the agents is preferable to the others. Although cost should not be the primary consideration, streptokinase is much cheaper than tissue plasminogen activator. Many experts prefer to use streptokinase and aspirin to treat patients admitted with electrocardiographic evidence of an infarct within the first 6 hours of infarction.

5. 'What investigation and treatment would you plan for a patient recovering from an acute myocardial infarction?'

Investigations should be designed to identify patients at high risk from sudden death, reinfarction and angina. **Hyperlipidaemia**[21] can be detected in the blood samples during the first two days after infarction, and if familial hypercholesterolaemia is suspected, one should screen the family and give appropriate advice (low-fat diet, exercise, abstinence from smoking, etc.). Smokers with ischaemic heart disease should be urged strongly to give up smoking. If hypertension is present it should be treated. The **prognosis** after an acute myocardial infarction is related to the extent of **left ventricular damage** and the extent of coronary artery disease.

Clinical assessment, chest X-ray and ECG will suggest the extent of the damage, but more accurate information can be obtained from echocardiography (especially after exercise) and radionuclide assessment of left ventricular function.

Exercise testing is useful and should be carried out within 7 to 10 days (if no contraindications) after the infarction. ST depression of 2 mm or more and angina, failure of the BP to rise and ventricular ectopics are all poor prognostic signs. **Coronary angiography** with a view to bypass surgery should be undertaken in a patient who does poorly on the exercise test and in those who are young and have physically demanding jobs. Beta blockers should be prescribed to all patients if there are no contraindications (e.g. asthma).

---

[20] This subject is likely to remain in active debate for some time, and candidates are advised to update their knowledge before the viva examination.

[21] Although everyone agrees that familial hypercholesterolaemia should be sought and rigorously treated, the management of rather modest elevations of serum cholesterol, found in the majority of patients with a myocardial infarction, is controversial. Reducing cholesterol levels reduces the incidence of coronary events, but this strategy has not led to a fall in the overall mortality (Br Med J 1990; 301: 309). This is due to an increase in deaths from other causes (e.g. suicide, accidental or violent deaths), in patients treated for hypercholesterolaemia. Furthermore, the steady reduction in the incidence of ischaemic heart disease experienced by North Americans during the last decade cannot be attributed to any single factor, but to an overall change to a more healthy life style. It would seem that a reasonable approach might be to advise patients with a myocardial infarction and mild hypercholesterolaemia, to follow a prudent diet with less fat and a high fibre content, to increase their exercise output, and to give up smoking.

d. Colleges' concern

The three Royal Colleges in the UK regularly review the objectives of both postgraduate training and the examinations, together with their success in achieving these. The Colleges are constantly on the lookout to improve the examination in order to maintain a high standard of postgraduate medical training. The examination is adjusted from time to time to overcome any shortcomings revealed among postgraduates in previous examinations. For example, when it became clear that many junior doctors did not communicate adequately with patients and their relatives, the Colleges were sufficiently concerned to introduce questions into the viva about communication. The examiners were advised to ask searching questions in the viva about how doctors talk to their patients and relatives, how they convey information about a serious illness, and how they discuss problems with the relatives of the patient. Admittedly, the situations created by the examiners' questions are artificial[22] and it is often difficult to consider the examiner as a relative of a hypothetical patient. However, your anticipation and basic skills will help you to cope with this.

A regular look at the medical press will make you aware of the various current interests of the Colleges. Although these change, the Colleges are always concerned about ethical issues. For example, you may be asked for your views on the resuscitation of terminally ill patients, euthanasia, donation of organs by living donors and the use of newly deceased patients for teaching intubation technique.

Examples

1. **'A man known to you comes to your clinic. He has been found to be positive for human immunodeficiency virus (HIV). What do you tell him about the prognosis and what do you tell his wife and GP?'**

This complicated question not only tests your knowledge of the acquired immunodeficiency syndrome (AIDS), but is also designed to explore your reserves of compassion and decency, which doctors are expected to possess in abundance, and your use of these attributes and skill in communicating the information. The patient would have been counselled before his blood sample was taken, and these various counselling avenues should be reactivated. In a condition such as AIDS, which has attracted so much publicity and has a hopeless prognosis at present, it is important to emphasise areas of hope while conveying factual information. Thus, each piece of bad news could be introduced with an optimistic statement. For example, before telling the patient that AIDS develops slowly and can affect almost any organ of the body, one could say: 'Not all individuals positive for the HIV test develop AIDS. After up to 8 years of follow-up only about half the cases who started with a positive test develop the disease. So you have a one in two chance of *escaping* the disease altogether. Judging from the speed of research in these last few years, it may not be too long

---

[22] p. 141

before a cure is found.' After this introduction one can give the bad news: 'However, at present there is no cure for AIDS and one has to be watchful for the signs and symptoms that indicate the development of the disease. This means that you ought to come to my clinic regularly, say every 3 months, for a check up.' The patient should be allowed some time to digest the information and encouraged to ask questions. Similarly, before telling him about his infectiousness, we can say: 'AIDS is not communicated by talking, walking and eating with other people. One can live with other people without passing it on to them, but sexual contact without a sheath is dangerous.' The patient's GP should be brought into the picture and kept informed: 'I will ring your GP about it and I should like to have a further discussion with you and your wife, if you would like to bring her with you in a couple of weeks' time. By then you may have thought of a few more questions; if so, please do not hesitate to ask me.'

2. **'You have just completed the investigations on a 50-year-old patient who you find to have carcinoma of the bronchus with metastases. What do you tell his wife?'**

The preliminaries do not vary from person to person; whatever the psychological, social, physical and spiritual makeup of the wife, she should be spoken to in a private room – usually in the Ward Sister's or your own office – and any other close relatives, such as a son or a daughter, should be encouraged to accompany her. In fact, it is more honest, and sometimes preferable, to have the patient present as well and one should tone down the gloomy aspects. The actual manner in which the news is broken will vary from person to person, and one may have some idea how the news will be received from one's own earlier conversations, and from reports gathered from the junior medical and nursing staff. In most cases, a sensible conversation may proceed like this:

'Well, Mrs Layperson, we have completed our investigations. I'm afraid the news is bad.' A short pause should be allowed here for the information to sink in and for her reaction to develop. She may ask a question which will facilitate further discussion.

'Your husband has a new growth of the lung which has spread to some other parts of the body as well but fortunately not to the head and bones, which is a very good thing.' (Pause and allow her to talk.)

'There is a good chance that we should be able to control it with drugs and radiation, if necessary. There have been some remarkably successful results in some recently conducted studies.' (Chance to have some general chat.)

'The offending type in your husband's case is what we call "small cell", and this kind responds reasonably well to a combination of drugs.' (She may ask whether it is curable.)

'Unfortunately, because of the spread, surgical treatment is not possible and a total cure cannot be achieved. However, patients are surviving for longer now – up to 2 years, sometimes for 5 years. We will make every effort to ensure that the quality of his remaining days is as good as possible.' (Discuss how it will affect home circumstances, holidays, etc., and add more information only if the recipient is prepared and willing to have more.)

'Of course, there are newer and better drugs available now. As it happens, a colleague of mine, a chest physician, is an expert in this field. She has already conducted a trial and is currently processing another trial. I met her in the corridor this morning and we talked briefly about this. She is quite happy to treat your husband and, if you would agree, I will arrange this. She would discuss the various pros and cons further with you.' (Allow some time for her questions.)

'There are side effects but less so in the doses that are usually effective. I will discuss this further with my colleague.' (Explore if there are more questions and uncertainties. Either now or at a later stage discuss terminal care, the possible use of Macmillan nurses, and admission to a nearby hospice.)

3. **'Doctors have been generally accused of not knowing about cardio-pulmonary resuscitation.[23] Prove them wrong and tell me what you would do if you saw me collapse in the street.'**

   ■ 'First, I would ascertain that you *are* unconscious and then I would open the airway by a combined manoeuvre of head tilt and chin lift. If there is no spontaneous breathing, I would clear the airway and start mouth-to-mouth breathing. If you have no pulse, I would initially deliver a quick thump over the precordium.[24] If still no pulse, I would commence cardiac massage. If a nearby person happens to know the technique, I would coordinate with him/her so that 60-massages-to-12-breaths rhythm can be started. I would also have asked some one to ring for an ambulance fitted with resuscitation equipment and I would continue until help arrives.'

4. **'What is your view about the ethics of organ transplantation?'**

   Organ transplantation, both from cadaveric donors and living subjects, is now an accepted therapeutic option for many life-threatening conditions (e.g. **end-stage renal failure**, **intractable heart failure**, **liver failure**, etc.). Renal transplantation has been established as the best treatment of irreversible kidney failure, but there is an increasing and serious shortage of donor kidneys. This shortage should be countered by increasing public awareness and education. However, importing 'kidneys for money' from the Third World should be strictly discouraged. Such malpractice has given a bad name to a worthwhile procedure which has restored many patients to a healthy and useful lifestyle. Doctors should themselves carry, and encourage the public in favour of carrying, **donor cards**. In the case of

---

[23]   Guidelines for cardiopulmonary resuscitation. Br Med J 1989; 299: 442; British National Formulary 1990; 19: 109

[24]   The use of the precordial thump is advised for witnessed or monitored arrest as it may be effective in pulseless ventricular tachycardia or ventricular fibrillation of recent onset.

cadaveric donors, every effort should be made, and be seen to be made, to save the life of the prospective donor *before* the subject of organ donation is discussed with the relatives, which should be done with compassion and sensitivity.

There is little doubt that cardiac transplantation is a life-saving treatment since there is a 95% mortality among the patients waiting for more than six months for a heart transplant. Like intractable heart failure, and unlike endstage renal failure, there is no effective alternative treatment for patients suffering from liver failure. Liver transplantation involving only a small portion of a liver from a cadaveric donor has been performed in several major centres. However, transplantation of a liver lobe from a living donor (e.g. the parent of the recipient), though technically feasible, raises major ethical issues such as the balance of risks to the donor and benefits for the recipient, the selection of donor and recipient, informed consent and the uncertainty of long-term results. Public evaluation and discussion of such issues should be encouraged. Clinicians should be willing to analyse and discuss ethical issues not only in their institutional ethical committees but also in wider public forums (e.g. in the press and on television).

Careful consideration is necessary before advising a transplant for a nonfatal condition, for those where the benefit is not yet proven, and for those associated with a high failure rate, e.g. pancreatic transplantation in diabetes mellitus. **Pancreas** and **kidney transplantation** for **diabetics with endstage renal failure** may be recommended when experienced surgeons are available.

Other examples from survey

1. **'What would you do if you found yourself to be positive for HIV at an insurance examination?'**

   ■ 'I would be surprised since I am not gay, do not inject myself with drugs and have not had any sexual contact or received a blood transfusion in Africa. I know that Health Service workers are at increased risk from accidental contact with the blood of infected individuals, but I take extra care when venesecting patients. However, if I am found to be positive for HIV, I would discuss it with my wife and have her tested too. If she is negative I would have no sex or use a sheath. I would monitor my health and hope for the best.'

2. **'A medical student was referred with a node in her neck. Your investigations (biopsy) showed that it is neoplastic in origin. Do you tell her outright?'**

   ■ 'No, I would not need to. Medical students are notorious neurotics who often exaggerate their trivial complaints into major syndromes. The possibility that the palpable node may be malignant will have occurred to her long before the biopsy is taken, and it will be further strengthened by the fact that I was going to talk to her. Far from breaking the news outright, I would have to reassure her. During a long conversation, I would let her do the talking and convey the news that the node is malignant. Above all, I would dwell on the possible positive aspects, such as the favourable response to therapy.'

3. **'I am a 40-year-old man with disseminated lung cancer. How would you break the news?'**

■ 'I would have some idea from previous chats as to what you suspect, and how much you want to know. Again, it would be better as a discussion with both you and your wife and allow you to talk as much as possible. I would lead gently by saying "bad news but", and would say a lot on how much could be done and how you can enjoy life in spite of it.'

Although questions on the audit of medical practice, the White Paper on the National Health Service (Working for Patients), the Griffith's Report on Community Care (Caring for Patients) have been asked only occasionally in the viva examinations, these topics are of current interest and will continue to occupy the attention of many fellows of the Colleges.

3. EMERGENCY MEDICINE

Testing your knowledge and your ability to cope with emergency situations is one of the most important roles of the viva. In no other part of the examination can you be assessed on how you would manage such problems as a patient with status asthmaticus, status epilepticus, or in diabetic coma, and how you would cope with rapidly evolving 'life-and-death' situations. In fact, the retention of the viva as a part of the membership examination has been discussed by the Board of Examiners on several occasions, and the consideration that emergency medicine cannot be tested except in the viva has weighed heavily in favour of its retention. It is clear that viva questions on emergency medicine are extremely important and that you cannot afford to fail in these.

The examiner usually introduces the question by describing a scenario, in which you will either be a medical registrar called by a casualty medical officer for advice, or be witnessing an acutely developing situation on one of the wards. In most cases, the examiner will have a particular diagnosis in mind (see *Detective* Stories). However, he is not only concerned with your diagnostic ability but also wishes to know how you would cope with the acute situation, and whether you would carry out the appropriate clinical and laboratory procedures needed to save the patient's life. The examiner is testing your clinical reflexes and thereby your soundness in coping successfully with an emergency situation.

It cannot be overemphasised that failure to satisfy the examiners in this category of questions can have serious consequences and may result in failure of the whole examination.

Examples

1. **'You are asked to see an acutely dyspnoeic patient in casualty. Clinically, how would you differentiate between cardiac and respiratory causes in this acute situation?'**[1]

The examiner was probably exploring the candidate's ability to distinguish between cardiac 'asthma' (acute left ventricular failure from any cause) and bronchial asthma, as sometimes (rarely in our view) the two may be difficult to distinguish. However, in answering this question it is important quickly to review the principal causes on each side. The main respiratory causes of dyspnoea of sudden onset are:

a. **Bronchial asthma**: family history, often a young patient, past history of attacks, history of atopy, prolonged expiratory phase and wheeze (though in severe cases of airways obstruction there may be no wheeze), improvement following bronchodilators, i.e. aminophylline and salbutamol.
b. **Pneumonia**: pleuritic pain, fever, cough, signs of consolidation.
c. **Pulmonary embolism**: history of recent surgery or immobility, pleuritic pain, fever, haemoptysis, there may be evidence of deep venous

---

[1]   The candidate asked this question reported that he found it difficult to answer, and that he was saved by the bell!

thrombosis, syncope, neck vein distension, a loud P_2, in severe cases the ECG may show an $S_1Q_3T_3$ pattern,[2] a right axis deviation or a right bundle branch block, PO_2 usually less than 85 mmHg with a concomitant decrease in PCO_2, CXR signs.[3]

d. **Pneumothorax**: sudden onset with pleuritic pain, in a young patient the habitus may be tall and lean, some have a past history of pneumothorax, there may be associated chronic lung disease, there is classically a loud resonant note over an area where breath sounds are absent or diminished.

Of the cardiac causes, the most important conditions requiring urgent treatment are:

a. **Acute left ventricular failure**: history of orthopnoea and paroxysmal nocturnal dyspnoea, usually in an older patient with an underlying cardiac disorder, i.e. ischaemic or valvular heart disease, hypertension, cardiomyopathy, etc., cardiomegaly and other features of associated disease (though in severe aortic stenosis there may be no murmurs), a gallop of S_3, inspiratory crackles over lung bases.

b. **Cardiac tamponade**: history of antecedent pericardial disease, there may be hypotension and oliguria, a monophasic rise in the jugular venous pressure with a prominent x descent, pulsus paradoxus and an early S3, clear lung fields, pericardial friction rub, sometimes ankle oedema; a cardiac echo would provide evidence.

If the question is interrupted by the bell, then the answer should be abbreviated to: 'The past history, history of paroxysmal nocturnal dyspnoea and orthopnoea, the presence of underlying conditions, and a purposeful physical examination looking for the gallop of S3 and inspiratory crackles at the bases will all help to differentiate cardiac from respiratory causes. An urgent cardiogram and chest X-ray would both help to resolve the issue. Cardiac cases are often associated with cardiomegaly and evidence of pulmonary venous congestion.'

2. **'You are asked to see a collapsed patient in the Accident and Emergency room who has a myasthenic crisis. What do you do?'**

The way this question has been phrased suggests two things: firstly, the patient is very ill with considerable muscular weakness, and has difficulty with respiration and feeding; and secondly, she may have been overtreated with anticholinesterases. The examiner invites you to demonstrate that you

---

[2]   A deep S wave in lead II, a q wave and an inverted T wave in lead III are electro-cardiographic signs of acute cor pulmonale and may be seen in a rapidly developing major pulmonary embolism. However, in most cases the electrocardiographic changes are highly variable and nondiagnostic. In patients whose ECGs are diagnostic, the clinical picture is often gross enough to be suggestive of a major cardiopulmonary catastrophe. In such cases the typical ECG changes of $S_1Q_3T_3$ are useful in distinguishing a pulmonary embolism from an acute myocardial infarction.

[3]   Although these signs are mostly nonspecific (e.g. elevation of one of the hemidiaphragms, basilar atelectasis, infiltrates, unilateral pleural effusion, cardiac dilatation, dilatation of the main pulmonary arteries, triangular densities, etc.), a normal chest X-ray is un-common in acute pulmonary embolism.

know the differences between **myasthenic** and **cholinergic crises** that may have been overlooked by the doctor in the Emergency room. Although overtreatment with cholinergic drugs – the so-called 'cholinergic crisis' – may be expected to be associated with muscarinic effects (e.g. abdominal cramps, nausea, vomiting, diarrhoea, lacrimation, sweating, miosis and bradycardia), occasionally it is difficult to distinguish it from a myasthenic crisis in a patient who is collapsed and in need of resuscitative measures. As the patient may need ventilatory support, your first action should be to send for an anaesthetist while you evaluate the situation. Edrophonium (2 mg intravenously) will improve the weakness in a myasthenic, but not in a cholinergic, crisis. In either event, the patient will require assisted positive pressure respiration with respiratory support and nasogastric or parenteral feeding. In cases of doubt as to the cause of respiratory failure, tracheal intubation allows the drugs to be withdrawn; they can be reintroduced gradually after the patient has improved. High doses of corticosteroids induce a remission in more than half the cases of myasthenic crisis, and in severe cases plasmapheresis may be worth trying.

3. **'What emergency investigations and treatment would you undertake on an acutely dyspnoeic patient with a pleural effusion?'**

   ■ 'A chest X-ray should not only confirm the clinical diagnosis of a pleural effusion but can also show its extent and whether it is the main reason for the dyspnoea. It can also help to exclude the presence of a tension pneumothorax. My next step would be a **thoracocentesis**, since the removal of fluid will serve both a **diagnostic** and a **therapeutic** function. A biochemical, microscopic, bacteriological and immunological evaluation of the aspirated fluid should help to provide the diagnosis of the underlying condition. A pleural biopsy obtained at the time of aspiration may provide a specific tissue diagnosis in malignancy. If the pleural effusion is an associated feature of an underlying condition causing the acute dyspnoea (e.g. acute left ventricular failure), then the treatment should be directed to the basic problem.'

4. **'You are awoken by your houseman at 2 a.m. asking for advice about a patient with chronic obstructive airways disease who had been stable but suddenly became much more breathless at 1.30 a.m. As you change and walk towards the ward, what things go through your mind?'**

   Take a long breath and think carefully before you say anything. This sort of acute situation presents to physicians in many guises, and your competence to deal with it is under examination. The scenario seems, by its elaborate description, to be familiar to the examiner and he has an answer in mind (see *Detective* Stories). Under such charged circumstances, it is a good ploy to start with general, noncontroversial, but highly pertinent remarks.

   ■ 'The story suggests a sudden decompensation in either the cardiac or respiratory system. An episode of acute pulmonary embolism or myocardial infarction and/or arrhythmia could make him breathless; in fact, while the houseman is on the phone I will ask him whether he suspects cardiac trouble and what the heart rate and blood pressure are, whether there is any evidence of a DVT or pulmonary embolism, and whether he has obtained an electrocardiogram. However, given the basic condition of chronic airways disease, I will be wondering whether this patient has a **pneumothorax** which has compromised his respiratory equilibrium. A small pneumothorax is easy to miss clinically but can be of critical importance in a patient with chronic respiratory disease, so I will ask the houseman to obtain an X-ray of the chest while I am on my way.'

5. 'A surgical registrar calls you to the Emergency room to see an 18-year-old female patient who was sent in with a suspected diagnosis of acute appendicitis. He found nothing abnormal on examination of the abdomen but as the patient was an established diabetic he checked the blood sugar level, which was 32 mmol/l. Enumerate your immediate steps of management.'

■ 'I can summarise my actions in six steps:

1. I would quickly go over the **clinical details** with the registrar and the doctor on duty in the Emergency room who may already have assessed this patient. In particular, I would ask whether they have ascertained any precipitating causes of her **diabetic ketoacidosis**, e.g. an infection (which is often the problem), her usual daily insulin dose and whether she has missed a dose,[4] any past history of admissions and her usual diabetic control. I would also talk to the patient and her relatives to get as much information as possible, particularly about any preceding symptoms, e.g. vomiting, diarrhoea, etc.

2. I would **examine** the patient, assess her state of **hydration**, and look for any evidence of infection (upper respiratory tract infection, pneumonia and urinary infection). I would check the urine for ketones, take a venous blood sample for full blood count, serum urea, electrolytes, and bicarbonate,[5] unless these samples have already been taken.

3. I would set up an **intravenous infusion** of normal saline (1 litre during the first hour) and administer a bolus dose of 10 units of **soluble insulin** intravenously. With the saline infusion *in situ*, I would transfer the patient to a medical ward where I would set up an infusion of soluble insulin using a pump to deliver 6 units/h.

4. Once on the ward, we would maintain a **flow chart** showing details of the treatment, laboratory investigations and urine output. **Adequate fluid replacement** is essential and she may need 6–8 litres over 24 hours.

---

[4] Some diabetic patients who miss a meal or have vomiting due to gastroenteritis, infection or ketoacidosis itself, stop insulin because of the misapprehension that insulin is not required when food is not taken. This common, but preventable, cause of ketoacidosis can be avoided by good patient education.

[5] The degree of acidosis can be gauged adequately from the serum bicarbonate level.

5. Within the first hour, the results of the investigations should be available. Bicarbonate replacement should not be necessary if the pH is 7 or more.[6] However, **potassium** (20 mmol/l) should be added in the second hour. The blood sugar level should be monitored hourly, and as the level falls the rate of insulin infusion may have to be adjusted downwards to 2–4 units/h.

   The serum K[+] level will also tend to fall, and potassium supplementation can be increased if necessary to 40 mmol/l as the phosphate salt, particularly if the serum phosphate level is low.

6. I would maintain **constant supervision** and frequently monitor the **biochemical profile** to normalise diabetic control and prevent complications such as *hypokalaemia*, late *hypoglycaemia* and *rebound CNS acidosis*.'[7]

6. **'You are called to see a 20-year-old female patient who is reported to have ingested 20 tablets of paracetamol. How do you plan your management?'**

■ 'I would carry out **gastric lavage** if she has been admitted within four hours of the overdose. If the time of ingestion of paracetamol is uncertain but near enough to 4–6 hours, the lavage may still be worth considering. I would set up an **intravenous infusion** line and collect blood samples for **prothrombin time**, plasma **paracetamol concentration**, serum urea, electrolytes and liver function tests. As the reported

---

[6] As bicarbonate concentrations equilibrate slowly across the cell membranes compared with dissolved CO_2 which diffuses quickly, the hypocapnia due to hyperventilation in these patients *lowers the intracellular acidity* thereby maintaining a near normal pH within the cells. Changes in intracellular pH lag behind systemic changes in diabetic ketoacidosis, which accounts for the relatively well-maintained CNS function. When fluid replacement with insulin and without additional bicarbonate is started, the *systemic pH gradually increases* within the next 6–10 hours. Bicarbonate is not necessary unless the systemic pH is less than 7, or there are associated complicating neurological, renal or cardiac problems with poor cardiac output and tissue perfusion, and even then it should be given very cautiously. There is a danger that bicarbonate given quickly will *worsen intracellular acidosis*: if the CO_2 generated from the infused bicarbonate is greater than can be excreted by ventilation (especially if the patient is very ill and ventilation is failing) and it diffuses into the cells, it increases intracellular CO_2, thereby pushing the intracellular bicarbonate equilibrium towards the generation of hydrogen ions. These changes of bicarbonate apply to its use in all types of metabolic acidosis (Diabetes Care 1984; 7: 99).

[7] Since dissolved CO_2 in plasma rapidly equilibrates with that in the CSF and the interstitial compartment of the brain (while bicarbonate does not), the pH of the CSF is initially normal or slightly *increased*. After the acidosis has been well established, CSF pH falls, and medullary centres are recruited to increase ventilation and maintain respiratory compensation. The administration of bicarbonate under these circumstances corrects the systemic acidosis, with a resultant decrease in peripheral chemoreceptor stimulus to hyperventilation. Retention of the CO_2 generated from the administered bicarbonate, and its equilibration across the blood – brain barrier, in the presence of fixed CSF bicarbonate concentration, results in a decreasing CSF pH at a time when systemic pH is *improving*. When the CSF pH falls to 7.2 or below, CNS functions suffer and unconsciousness supervenes. This is the main reason why many diabetologists never use bicarbonate therapy in diabetic ketoacidosis.

overdose amounts to 10 g, I would start an **acetylcysteine infusion**[8] (a 20% solution in 200 ml of 5% dextrose to be given over 15 minutes as an initial dose of 150 mg/kg) while waiting for the results of the initial investigations. I would follow the first loading dose of acetylcysteine by an infusion of 50 mg/kg in 5% dextrose over 4 hours. At this stage the infusion can then be stopped, if the plasma paracetamol concentration is below a line on a semilogarithmic plot joining 200 μg/ml at 4 hours after ingestion and 30 μg/ml at 15 hours. If the plasma level is above this line, then the acetylcysteine treatment should be continued (100 mg/kg in 1 litre of 5% dextrose during the next 16 hours).

Should the time of ingestion of paracetamol be uncertain, then I would err on the side of continuing the acetylcysteine infusion longer. Since excessive paracetamol overdosage can cause a variety of problems, including **liver** and **renal failure**, **hypoglycaemia** and **lactic acidosis**. I would monitor prothrombin time, liver enzymes (both 12-hourly) blood sugar level (hourly if the blood sugar level shows a fall despite initial 5% dextrose administration) and serum creatinine level (daily). I would take corrective procedures and obtain specialist advice if any of these serious complications occur. Early and effective treatment with acetylcysteine should prevent liver and renal failure. If the prothrombin time is normal 48 hours after admission, the patient can be discharged after a psychiatric assessment and appropriate advice.'

Other examples from survey

1. 'Your house physician calls you to see a 60-year-old man in the Accident and Emergency room where he was brought in after a sudden onset of severe low back pain. You find the patient is writhing with pain despite an intravenous injection of diamorphine. Apart from the pain he complains of numbness in the right leg. What do you do?'

The sudden onset and severity of the pain suggest a vascular cause, e.g. **dissecting aortic aneurysm**, haemorrhage in an **epidural** or **extradural tumour**, **epidural haemorrhage** or a massive **central disc herniation**. A careful physical examination should include a neurological assessment and the palpation of the carotid, femoral and other peripheral pulses, together with auscultation for evidence of aortic incompetence. Computed tomography and magnetic resonance imaging are the preferred investigative techniques. Aortography is the definitive investigation if a dissecting aneurysm is suspected.[9]

---

[8] Paracetamol is partially transformed in the liver to a toxic metabolite which is detoxified by intracellular glutathione. After an excessive overdose, tissue glutathione is used up faster than it can be synthesised, and the reactive metabolite forms irreversible complexes with intracellular macromolecules, enzymes and membrane lipids, leading to liver cell necrosis. Acetylcysteine and methionine replete glutathione and probably also increase paracetamol sulphation and prevent liver damage. Although treatment with acetyl-cysteine or methionine 15 hours after paracetamol ingestion is thought to be useless, a recent study (N Engl J Med 1988; 319: 1557) has shown that the treatment can be effective even if given as late as 24 hours after the ingestion.

[9] The examiner guided the candidate to the diagnosis of dissecting aortic aneurysm.

2. **'A young woman aged 16 years has been brought in with an alleged overdose of 100 aspirin tablets. How do you manage her?'**

Gastric lavage should be undertaken irrespective of the time of ingestion. This should be followed by terminal instillation of **activated charcoal**. Blood samples should be obtained for a serum salicylate level, serum urea, electrolytes, liver enzymes and a blood sugar level, and these should be monitored frequently. **Hydration** with **alkalinisation** of the urine is recommended (unless the urinary pH is 8 or more) for salicylate levels of 300–700 μg/ml (1.9–4.4 mmol/l). Use forced alkaline diuresis if the serum salicylate level is >700 μg/ml. Charcoal haemoperfusion or haemodialysis may be necessary if the serum salicylate level is 1000 μg/ml (6.2 mmol/l), if there is metabolic acidosis, or if the clinical condition deteriorates.

3. **'You have been asked to see a man with bradycardia (heart rate 45 beats/min) who was sent in after he had taken 6 tablets of digoxin.'**

The patient should be monitored in a coronary care unit. Insertion of a temporary pacing wire will be necessary if the bradycardia becomes symptomatic. Serum urea and electrolytes should be checked and hypokalaemia looked for, as the patient, having access to digoxin, may also have been on diuretics.

4. DATA INTERPRETATION

The ability of candidates to interpret data is tested in the written part of the Part II MRCP examination, and examiners are not generally expected to bring laboratory data to the viva table. However, some candidates are asked about these during the viva examination.[1] Examiners usually do this for two main reasons: firstly, they wish to test the candidates' reasoning ability and justification of their conclusion when shown some results of routine investigations; secondly, the examiners are exploring the clinical judgement of the candidates and assessing whether they have the soundness and maturity to disregard the 'bits of paper' if the clinical features do not justify their validity. This is an important issue in clinical practice, since every clinician has at times been faced with laboratory results which conflict with information gained at the bedside, and has had to reconcile the two by discarding or repeating the laboratory investigation.

Candidates have been shown laboratory reports such as a full blood count, urea and electrolytes, liver function tests or a graph, and asked to comment. It was not unusual for one of the examiners to start the viva by showing some data and asking for an opinion. Candidates were expected to behave as if they were in a ward looking at the results and giving a few comments for the benefit of their house physician. Unless the findings are very specific for a diagnosis (e.g. an ECG showing unequivocal features of an acute myocardial infarction), the examiners do not expect a single accurate diagnosis; they would prefer to hear your reasoned analysis of the report. In recent examinations, examiners have offered more and more graphs to test the knowledge of candidates on statistical interpretation. Depending on the depth of your knowledge and your manipulative skills, such questions may lead the discussion to *significance, probability,* setting up of trials, *randomisation,* double-blindness and so on. On the other hand, if you are completely blank you can still pass in the viva as long as you score better in other, more specifically 'bread-and-butter' clinical questions (e.g. emergency medicine and *Biblical* stories). Here we briefly present some examples from various viva experiences together with the answers the examiners were aiming at.

Examples from survey

1. **'Urea and electrolytes results with a low sodium level from an oedematous patient with severe congestive cardiac failure on high doses of frusemide.'** *(Dilutional hyponatraemia.)*

   The candidate was expected to give the possible clinical scenario and the reasons why this picture suggested dilutional hyponatraemia. As the patient is oedematous, he must be **salt-overloaded** and the hyponatraemia is not a reflection of a low-salt state. The loop diuretics such as frusemide inhibit chloride and sodium reabsorption at the ascending limb of the loop of Henle, thereby impairing urinary dilution and stimulating renin activity. The consequent increase in thirst and fluid intake presumably exceeded

---

[1]   pp. 124, 131, 153, 201, 225, 230, 238

the renal excretory capacity. **Water restriction** with **demeclocycline** (if necessary) will increase water excretion, reduce the oedema and improve the hyponatraemia.

2. **'Raised urea and creatinine levels and a full blood count which showed a normocytic, normochromic anaemia.'** *(Chronic renal failure.)*

The candidate was asked to discuss the mechanisms of anaemia in chronic renal failure (marrow suppression, shortened red cell survival, haemorrhage, etc.).

3. **'Urea and electrolyte results: urea 2.5 mmol/l, Na$^+$ 109 mmol/l, K$^+$ 2.9 mmol/l.'** *(Syndrome of inappropriate secretion of antidiuretic hormone; SIADH.)*

The candidate was asked about the possible causes, clinical features and management.[2]

The chief characteristic of the SIADH is an **inability** of the kidney to excrete **osmotically free water** with the resultant **volume expansion** without oedema. The urine osmolality is higher than that of the plasma. There is an increased glomerular filtration rate with reduced tubular reabsorption of osmotically active electrolytes, creatinine, urea and urate, producing low serum levels of Na$^+$, K$^+$ urea, urate and creatinine. The symptoms of **water intoxication** range from weakness, nausea, confusion and muscle twitching to fits and coma. Treatment includes water restriction to about one litre/day, daily weighing, demeclocycline and, in severe cases, a slow infusion of hypertonic saline to raise the serum Na$^+$ concentration by around 12 mmol/day.

4. **'A blood count showing a high RBC count, low MCV and MCHC, high WCC and platelet counts.'** *(Polycythaemia rubra vera.)*

This is a malignant proliferative disorder and the overproduction of erythrocytes creates iron deficiency.

---

[2] **Causes of SIADH**
   1. **Malignant conditions:**
      a. Carcinoma – bronchogenic, pancreatic, urinary tract, prostate, colon, etc.
      b. Lymphoma and leukaemia
      c. Thymoma and mesothelioma.
   2. **Pulmonary disorders**: tuberculosis, Legionnaires' disease, pneumonia, positive pressure ventilation, abscess, etc.
   3. **Nervous system**: trauma, infection, tumours, porphyria, haemorrhage, vasculitis
   4. **Psychiatric disorders**: schizophrenia
   5. **Endocrine causes**: hypothyroidism
   6. **Drugs**: chlorpropamide, carbamazepine, amitriptyline, fluphenazine, indomethacin, cyclophosphamide, vincristine, barbiturates.

5. **'When do you use *parametric* and *nonparametric* tests?'**[3]

The candidate was shown a graph on which the distribution of data was skewed, and the discussion led into the appropriateness of *nonparametric* tests.

6. **'Lung function tests suggestive of emphysema.'**

The **residual volume** was greater than the volume predicted for the age of the patient, and its ratio with the **total lung capacity** was 60%.

7. **'Blood gas results.'** *(Acute/chronic respiratory failure.)*

The discussion revolved around the renal compensatory changes to account for the alkaline pH associated with respiratory acidosis.

8. **'Electrocardiograms.'** *(Acute myocardial infarction with arrhythmias.)*

Our suggestion for tackling the questions in this section is that you should keep your comments clinical. It is important to emphasise to the examiner, without stating it too bluntly, that you do not entirely depend on the 'bits of paper', and that you use investigations in support of your clinical impression.

---

[3] A **parametric** statistical test is valid when certain conditions about the parameters of the population are satisfied. These conditions are:

a. The observations must be drawn from *normally distributed* populations. Since the most commonly used parametric test, the Student's *t*-test, is based on a normal distribution, the research sample to be tested must have a normal distribution. However, the *t*-test, being a robust statistical test, can be applied as an initial procedure to samples in which there is some skewness.

b. The observations must be *independent*, i.e. the selection of any one case from the population must not bias the chances of any other case for inclusion.

c. The variables involved must be capable of being subjected to simple arithmetic operations such as adding, dividing, finding *means*, etc. **At least the *mean* must be a good reflection of the samples.**

A *nonparametric* test is appropriate when the model does not specify any particular distribution for the population from which the sample is drawn (e.g. when the data are skewed).

5. BASIC SCIENCES

Occasionally, examiners ask questions which are aimed at testing the candidates' grasp of fundamental scientific concepts underlying important clinical situations. To cope with these questions you will need to have some basic knowledge of the preclinical subjects of anatomy, physiology and biochemistry.

None of these questions is unfair, and a postgraduate student of medicine ought to be able to deal with them. Try to give simple, straightforward, free-from-waffle answers. In general, the more distant the question is from clinical practice, the less likely you are to fail if you are unable to answer it. On the other hand, the more relevant the question is to a common clinical condition (e.g. diabetes mellitus, renal failure, etc.), the more likely the examiner is to expect a comprehensive answer. So, judge the situation and do the best you can. If you do not know, confess as nicely as you can, 'I am afraid I don't know this subject well!'

Examples

1. **'You must have performed the Valsalva 1 manoeuvre many times. Give me some details of its principle, the procedure and its uses. How can it be helpful in distinguishing between various cardiac problems?'**

The standard test consists of asking the patient to blow into a sphygmomanometer and to maintain a pressure of 40 mmHg for 15–30 seconds.

The ensuing changes in the heart rate and blood pressure give an idea of the **integrity** of the **heart** and its **reflexes**. As the patient blows into the tube of the sphygmomanometer, there is a marked increase in the intrathoracic pressure and a reduction in the venous return to the heart and hence in its stroke output. The arterial pressure tracing shows four phases:

1. An **initial rise** in the **arterial pressure** which is a reflection of the increased intrathoracic pressure.
2. With a continuation of the *strain* and accompanying decrease in the venous return, there is a **fall** in **systolic, diastolic** and **pulse pressures** producing a **reflex tachycardia.**
3. On release of the *strain*, there is a sudden drop of arterial pressure equivalent to the fall in the intrathoracic pressure.
4. Next, there is an *overshoot* of arterial pressure with a wide pulse pressure and **bradycardia** due to an increased venous return released from the venous bed.

In *myocardial failure*, there is no *overshoot* upon release of the *strain*, as the reduction in venous return does not affect stroke volume (the heart being on the flat portion of its Starling's curve).

In *mitral valve prolapse*, as the left ventricular volume decreases during the *strain* phase, the click will occur early and the duration and the intensity of the systolic murmur will be increased. Conversely, the click will be delayed and the intensity of the murmur will be decreased during the *overshoot* phase.

---

[1]   See Appendix II

In *hypertrophic obstructive cardiomyopathy*, during the *strain* phase there is an increase in the intensity of the systolic murmur, due to an increase in the gradient, associated with a fall in the venous return and arterial pressure. During the *overshoot* phase there is a decrease in the intensity of the murmur, associated with a reduction in the gradient due to an increase in the preload and afterload.

The Valsalva manoeuvre is also used to diagnose autonomic neuropathy by testing the integrity of cardiovascular autonomic nervous reflexes.

2. 'What are the functions of the atria?'

The atria receive and propel blood, provide the ground for transmission of electrical impulses from the sinus node, and support the ventricles in emptying. Cardiac output falls considerably in the absence of atrial contractions (e.g. atrial fibrillation). An additional function, not yet fully proven, is the hormonal regulation of blood volume, in which the atria participate by releasing a natriuretic factor.

3. 'What are the functions of the spleen?'

1. Blood formation in fetal life; it can resume this function in adult life in certain forms of marrow failure, such as myelofibrosis.
2. Blood destruction: erythrocytes, platelets and probably leucocytes.
3. Defence mechanism: the spleen is the largest lymphoid organ in the body and plays an important role in the cellular and immune responses to infection. Circulating antigens and opsonised microorganisms are phagocytosed by macrophages in the spleen and antibody production is stimulated. The spleen is a major source of IgM production in the body.

4. 'What is the physiological basis for the electrocardiographic changes in SVT?'

Supraventricular arrhythmias either arise from an irritable ectopic focus in the atrium or A-V junction (enhanced automaticity), or are due to a circulating wavefront involving the atria or A-V junction or both (reciprocating or circus-movement tachycardias). They are characterised by abnormal P waves and (unless they are complicated by coincident intraventricular block) by normal QRS duration.

For many years, the circus-movement theory was regarded as the mechanism underlying atrial flutter and fibrillation; whereas tachycardia was thought to be due to enhanced automaticity (repetitive firing) of a pacemaking focus in the atrium. On the other hand, some investigators propose that enhanced automaticity accounts for all atrial tachyarrhythmias (the 'unitary nature' of the atrial arrhythmias). Recently, the electrophysiologists have suggested that most supraventricular tachycardias – including 'atrial' tachycardia – are circus-movement or reciprocating or 're-entry' tachycardias, and that they are the product of a circulating wave that gives off 'branches' to the atria and ventricles. Though the universality of this reciprocating mechanism is not established, there is no doubt that there are numerous mechanisms which produce similar and even indistinguishable electrocardiographic patterns. The re-entry circuit that encompasses the circulating wavefront may involve the sinus node, the atria, the A-V node – separately or collectively – and perhaps the His bundle.

True ectopic atrial tachycardia – due to rapid firing (enhanced automaticity) of a pacemaking centre in the atrium – undoubtedly also occurs, and may sometimes be differentiated in the ECG tracing. The ectopic tachycardia 'warms up' (accelerates), all P' waves, if identifiable, are similar to the initiating P', and premature atrial stimuli will reset but usually not terminate the tachycardia. In a reciprocating tachycardia, on the other hand, subsequent P' waves differ from the initial P', there is no warm-up, and premature stimuli often terminate the tachycardia (Practical Electrocardiography, 6th ed. H J L Marriott. The Williams and Wilkins Co., Baltimore, MD, USA). For re-entry to occur there are three requirements: an available circuit, a difference in refractoriness in two limbs of the circuit, and slow enough conduction through the less refractory limb for the more refractory limb to recover by the time the impulse approaches it again.

Other examples from survey

1. **'What factors are important for the maintenance of blood sugar levels within normal limits?'**

   It is prudent to keep your answer simple to enable you to handle the ensuing discussion – food intake, digestion, metabolism and the regulatory role of various hormones. In the case from the survey, the discussion led to the role of counter-regulatory hormones[2], hypoglycaemia[2], and the 'dawn phenomenon'[3] in diabetics.

---

[2] Some insulin-dependent diabetics fail to produce adequate amounts of the counter-regulatory hormones – glucagon and adrenaline – during hypoglycaemia, and these patients are particularly at risk of **neuroglycopaenia** leading to coma without adrenergic warning symptoms. The mechanism for the **inadequate counter-regulatory response** is uncertain. The failure of glucagon release during hypoglycaemia (which happens in most insulin-dependent patients after 5 years) is selective to the hypoglycaemia, and not related to the loss of beta cell function or to autonomic neuropathy. It is not improved even after several months of intensive therapy. The failure of adrenaline release during hypoglycaemia occurs less often, and is probably related to the blunted responsiveness of hypothalamic centres to hypoglycaemia (Br Med J 1990; 301: 783).

[3] **Morning hyperglycaemia** may be the result of activation of counter-regulatory mechanisms in response to nocturnal hypoglycaemia (*Somogyi phenomenon*), or due to the waning of previously injected insulin. The term *'dawn phenomenon'* is used to describe morning hyperglycaemia which is not attributable to either of the above-mentioned mechanisms, since it may occur in normal subjects, noninsulin-dependent diabetics and even in association with a continuous infusion of exogenous insulin. Management of the dawn phenomenon and early morning insulin waning consists of adjusting upwards or/and delaying the evening dose of intermediate or long-acting insulin. On the other hand, management of the Somogyi effect consists of reducing the evening dose of insulin, or providing additional late-evening carbohydrate, or both.

2. 'What is the role of urinary specific gravity in the diagnosis of renal failure and in the syndrome of inappropriate ADH secretion?'

It reflects urinary osmolality which can be measured and used as a part of the overall diagnostic approach in acute renal failure. In prerenal failure due to extracellular fluid volume contraction, urinary osmolality is more than 500 mosm/kgH$_2$0, whereas in acute renal failure it would be less than 300 mosm/kgH$_2$0. In the syndrome of inappropriate ADH secretion, the kidney is unable to excrete osmotically free water, and the urinary osmolality is, paradoxically, higher than that of plasma.

3. 'What is meant by osmolarity and osmolality?'

Osmolarity is the concentration of osmoles per litre and osmolality is expressed per kg.

4. 'What are lymphocyte subsets?'

The maturation pathways and surface properties of lymphocytes differentiate them into two major subpopulations, T and B cells. Both of these have functionally distinct subdivisions:

1. **T cell subsets**: T cells and B cells working together can produce an antibody response which neither is capable of bringing about on its own. T cells which promote antibody response by stimulating B cells are called *helper T cells*. Their opponents *suppressor T cells* reduce their activity in B cells to produce antibodies.
2. **B cell subsets**: B cells can make antibodies to most antigens with the help of *helper T cells*. B1 subsets produce antibodies to T-dependent antigens, whereas B2 subsets are stimulated by T-independent antigens.

A minority of circulating lymphoid cells originate in the bone marrow and do not carry the phenotype markers of T or B cells. Some of these appear to be 'killer' cells with cytotoxic properties, while others may be 'natural killer' cells with lytic properties.

5. 'What are the ECG criteria for left ventricular hypertrophy?'

Unfortunately, there are no internationally agreed criteria for left ventricular hypertrophy. However, the eight criteria given below would meet general acceptance. It has to be remembered that left ventricular hypertrophy is a graded abnormality, and the greater the number of criteria fulfilled, the more likely the diagnosis becomes. The voltage criteria 1–5 are generally sensitive indices. Alternatively, a point score system can be used (as given below). A score of 6 points suggests left ventricular hypertrophy and a score of 5 points is suggestive of probable left ventricular hypertrophy.

Criteria for left ventricular hypertrophy

1. The R waves in any one or more of leads V_4, V_5 or V_6 exceed 27 mm
2. The tallest R waves in any of leads V_4, V_5 or V_6 plus the deepest S waves in any of leads V_1, V_2 or V_3 exceed 40 mm
3. The S waves in one or more of leads V_1, V_2 or V_3 exceed 30 mm
4. R wave in aVl exceeds 13 mm
5. R in aVl exceeds 20 mm
6. The ventricular activation time (intrinsicoid deflection time, i.e. from the start to the peak of the R wave) exceeds 0.04 s (i.e. equals or exceeds 0.05 s)
7. Abnormal S-T segment depression (i.e. more than 1 mm below the isoelectric line in any lead facing the left ventricle (e.g. in V_4, V_5 or V_6 and in lead I and aVL when the heart is *horizontal,* or in II and aVF when the heart is *vertical*)
8. T wave inversion in the leads facing the left ventricle (as outlined in 7 above).

Electrocardiographic criteria (Point system for diagnosis)[4]

1. **Negative component of P in V_1 ⩾ 1 mm and 0.04 s** (3 points).
2. **QRS amplitude**
   a. Largest limb lead R or S ⩾ 20 mm or largest chest lead S before transition or R after transition ⩾ 30 mm
      OR
      Largest S before transition *plus* largest R after transition = 45 mm (3 points).
   b. Frontal plane axis ⩾ −30° (2 points).
   c. Duration in limb lead ⩾ 0.09 s (1 point).
   d. Intrinsicoid deflection ⩾ 0.05 s (1 point).
3. **ST-T**. In general, opposite QRS:
   Without digitalis (3 points).
   With digitalis (1 point).

---

[4]   Braunwald E (ed) 1980 Heart disease. A textbook of cardiovascular medicine. W B Saunders, London

6. SPECIALISTS' QUESTIONS

As may be expected, specialists always feel at home with their own subject and are likely to ask questions in the field they know best. Unlike the short cases, where specialists cannot contrive to have cases in their own field, in the viva they can choose the questions they ask. So beware, if you are asked a question which probes deep into a special topic, then be certain of your ground. If you do not know, say so. Some candidates have a relaxed view about this, based on the (inaccurate) rumours that specialist questions are not asked by those who possess a deep knowledge of the subject themselves.[1] This attitude is dangerous and can cause trouble. In the words of a famous teacher: 'If the examiner is an expert in the subject, he will expose your weakness in one minute, if he is not he will confuse you in 60 seconds!' If you are unprepared you are likely to lose either way, so it is safer practice to avoid 'stabbing in the dark'. You should only proceed to answer the question if you have a reasonable grasp of the subject.

Examples

1. **'A nurse shows you a patient with a foot ulcer. Tell her what to do.'**
    (Examiner: a diabetologist)

    If you have had no worthwhile experience of managing leg ulcers, this may be your Achilles' heel, and you may soon find yourself in a maze of the numerous available applications and dressings. If that is the case, you should dwell more on the medical aspects of leg ulcers – e.g. clinical assessment, including the pathogenesis of the ulcer (neuropathic, arterial, venous, etc.), and the diagnosis of the underlying condition (diabetes mellitus, atherosclerosis, etc.) which in any case should form the introduction to your answer. On the other hand, you may be an expert and can afford to spend time on the basics of ulcer management (cleansing and debriding applications with good supportive therapy).[2]

2. **'What do you know about drug interactions?'**[3]
    (Examiner: a clinical pharmacologist)

    Drug interactions may occur outside or inside the body; the former are called **pharmaceutical** incompatibilities (e.g. denaturation or precipitation from mixing of incompatible solutions). The latter result either from a drug-induced alteration in the delivery of the drug to its site of action

---

[1]   The experience of many candidates is contrary to this view. See pp. 103, 138, 150, 153, 203, 231, 237, 243

[2]   A diabetologist may also lead the discussion on to the management of diabetic foot care in general, i.e. education of the patient regarding the prevention of foot problems, the need to look after their feet, regular chiropody, wearing extra-depth, well-fitting shoes for those at risk, extra-depth shoes for those with deformed feet, and special soft insoles to redistribute weight for feet where ulcers have occurred at pressure points.

[3]   Also see p. 55

(**pharmacokinetic** interactions) or from a drug-induced alteration in the receptor or organ response to another drug (**pharmacodynamic** interactions).

Pharmacokinetic interactions may occur due to a drug-induced change in the rate or extent of absorption of another drug caused by a change in drug distribution, metabolism or excretion. The most important of these mechanisms is the effect of one drug on the metabolism of another due to **enzyme induction** (e.g. by barbiturates, phenytoin, carbamazepine or rifampicin) or **enzyme inhibition** (e.g. by cimetidine, erythromycin or fluconazole).

Pharmacodynamic interactions may occur due to direct antagonism at the same receptor (e.g. morphine and naloxone) or when drugs act at separate sites to cause **summation, potentiation** or **antagonism** of their actions (e.g. the potentiation of digoxin toxicity by diuretic-induced hypokalaemia).

3. **'What is the use of a yellow card?'**
   (Examiner: a clinical pharmacologist)

Yellow cards are used to report adverse clinical phenomena appearing with the use of a therapeutic agent. The use of yellow cards can accumulate evidence and help to distinguish between coincidence, and a definite relation between a side effect and a drug effect (e.g. thrombosis and the contraceptive 'pill').

4. **'Tell me all you know about trace elements.'**
   (Examiner: a physician with an interest in nutrition)

Trace elements were originally defined as elements essential for normal metabolism that occurred in amounts too small to be measured accurately. With the advance of technology, these elements can be measured in milli-, micro- and nanogram amounts, or their SI equivalents. The majority of trace elements are either essential components of **metalloenzymes** (e.g. zinc in carbonic anhydrase) or are essential **cofactors** for normal enzyme action. Essential trace elements are usually considered separately from the toxic elements such as lead, mercury and cadmium, but lines can become blurred as most essential elements can become toxic if present in sufficient amounts or under certain circumstances.

Trace element status depends on the **balanced intake, absorption** and **excretion** of the element. Absorption can be impaired by dietary factors such as phytate, fibre and other elements competing for the same binding sites, and by abnormalities of the gastrointestinal system. Excretion can be accelerated by catabolic states, renal disease and diarrhoea. Trace element status can be difficult to determine, as measurements of the elements in body fluids can give misleading information, due to either instability of the element (e.g. selenium and chromium), or binding of the element to a plasma protein (zinc), or compartmental shifts within the body. In some cases, estimation of the relevant metalloenzyme can be the best measure available (e.g. glutathione peroxidase as an indicator of selenium status).

Dietary deficiencies are uncommon in developed countries, except in infants and the elderly, those on unusual diets and those with intestinal malabsorption or fistulae. The most **common deficiencies** encountered are those of **iron**, **zinc** and **copper**. In areas of endemic goitre **iodine** is lacking, and in large areas of China a cardiomyopathy associated with **selenium deficiency** (Keshan disease) has been reported. When possible, dietary deficiencies should be treated by correcting the diet, and oral supplements should be given for as short a time as possible.

Trace element deficiencies are seen most commonly in clinical practice in patients on total **parenteral nutrition**; the elements recommended as supplements are iron, zinc, copper, selenium, chromium and molybdenum.

Clinical manifestations of deficiency include anaemia for both iron and copper; **skin lesions**, **impaired taste**, **anorexia** and **abnormal T cell function** for zinc deficiency; muscle pains and weakness and **cardiomyopathy** in selenium deficiency; **glucose intolerance** and **peripheral neuropathy** in chromium deficiency and **amino acid intolerance**, tachycardia and tachypnoea in molybdenum deficiency.

5. **'Tell me something about the cutaneous manifestations of nutritional deficiencies.'**
(Examiner: a dermatologist)

1. **Protein and energy**: kwashiorkor – hyperpigmentation, thinning and fissuring of the skin (*mosaic* skin), follicular hyperkeratosis, folliculosis, thinning and premature greying of hair, oedema.
2. **Vitamins**
   a. *Vitamin A*: dermatomalacia, follicular hyperkeratosis (*toad* skin)
   b. *B-complex*: rough, hard and cracked skin (*goose* skin)
   c. *Niacin*: pellagra – lesions on the face, neck and dorsal surfaces
   d. *Riboflavin*: oro-oculo-genital lesions
   e. B_6: seborrhoea
   f. B_{12}: hyperpigmentation
   g. *Biotin*: scaly eczematoid lesions
   h. *Vitamin C*: haemorrhagic lesions, keratosis of the hair follicles
   i. *Vitamin K*: bleeding tendency
3. **Metals**
   a. *Iron*: pallor, koilonychia
   b. *Zinc*: eczematoid lesions
   c. *Copper*: pallor, depigmentation of hair and skin
   d. *Selenium*: white nail beds

6. **'What are the common types of drug interactions?'**
(Examiner: a clinical pharmacologist)

1. **Extracorporeal**. If PZI is mixed with soluble insulin, it converts it to PZI.
2. **Intracorporeal**
   a. *Chelation*: cholestyramine will delay absorption of other drugs
   b. *Protein binding*: warfarin, tolbutamide and phenytoin are displaced by phenylbutazone
   c. *Metabolism*: inducers or accelerators stimulate their own metabolism

and that of other drugs, thereby decreasing the plasma levels –
barbiturates, phenylbutazone, phenytoin, meprobamate and
chronic ethanol consumption will increase the metabolism of
anticoagulants, tolbutamide, tricyclic antidepressants, etc.

d. *Monoamine oxidase*: inhibition of this enzyme by drugs such as
phenelzine and iproniazid will decrease the oxidation of natural
amines like noradrenaline and histamine, and ingested ones such as
tyramine. Severe hypertensive reactions can occur in patients on
oxidase inhibitors if they ingest tyramine-containing foodstuff, e.g.
cheese, bovril, marmite and red wine

e. *Alcohol dehydrogenase inhibitors* (disulfiram; antabuse) produce
unpleasant symptoms if alcohol is ingested because of acetaldehyde
accumulation

f. *Miscellaneous*: bacteriostatic agents reduce the activity of bactericidal
drugs.

Other examples from survey

1. 'How many people in England have psoriasis?'
   1–2%

2. 'What is the modern treatment of psoriasis?'
   PUVA, retinoids[4]

3. 'What is the criterion for cardiac transplantation?'
   Endstage cardiac failure

4. 'How do you distinguish homocystinuria from Marfan's syndrome?'
   Autosomal recessive *vs* dominant inheritance, tight-jointedness *vs*
   hyperextensibility, thromboembolism *vs* aortic dissection, and the
   presence of homocystine in the urine.

5. 'What do you know about the biological markers of depression?'
   Sodium transport abnormalities in the red cell have been reported in
   various depressive illnesses, but these findings lack specificity. Cortisol
   levels are raised in the CSF, plasma and urine. In some patients,
   particularly in those with a family history of endogenous depression, the

---

[4]   **Methotrexate**, a folate antagonist which blocks purine synthesis, is indicated as
maintenance treatment for chronic plaque psoriasis, which relapses quickly or is resistant
to topical treatment. Alcoholics, diabetics or patients with significant liver disease are
excluded from treatment with methotrexate.

   PUVA (interaction of psoralen and long-wave ultraviolet radiation, known as UVA) may
be considered for chronic discoid psoriasis in the over-60s or for those under 60 in whom
treatment with **dithranol** has failed. It may increase the risk of developing skin cancer, and
long-term surveillance should be maintained.

   The introduction of **retinoids**, particularly etretinate (only available in hospitals) has
been a major innovation in the treatment of severe psoriasis. However, remissions are not
always complete and well-sustained.

   Hydroxyurea is another antimetabolite which is helpful in psoriasis, but causes
marrow suppression.

   Small doses of **cyclosporin** (3 mg/kg) have been shown to clear resistant psoriasis.
Hepatic and renal function should be monitored during therapy. Recently, there have been
some anecdotal reports of success with haemodialysis and peritoneal dialysis.

circadian rhythm of cortisol is lost and there is an abnormal response to the dexamethasone suppression test.[5]

6. 'What is first-pass metabolism?'

A number of drugs,[6] when orally administered, undergo systemic elimination, as they are metabolised on the first-pass through the gut wall or/and liver. The rate-limiting factor in their elimination is liver blood flow. Under normal circumstances, the mean bioavailability of these drugs varies from 10–40%.

7. 'What are cheese reactions?'

A severe hypertensive reaction due to the release of increased amounts of noradrenaline following the ingestion of cheese by patients taking monoamine oxidase inhibitors.[7]

As may be seen from these questions, you can get by even if you know very little as long as you know it well. Do not try to bluff, because physicians do not like to see their favourite subjects mocked.

---

[5]   Used as a diagnostic test for depression (a plasma cortisol level of >100 nmol/l, after the oral administration of 1 mg dexamethasone the previous evening, indicates nonsuppression) but has proved to be unreliable.

[6]   Among the drugs that undergo substantial presystemic elimination are aspirin, chlormethiazole, chlorpromazine, dextropropoxyphene, glyceryl trinitrate, isosorbide dinitrate, labetolol, lignocaine, morphine, oral contraceptives, paracetamol, pethidine and propranolol.

[7]   p. 56

7. STRAIGHTFORWARD FACTUAL QUESTIONS

As stated previously, examiners are advised by the Colleges to avoid asking questions on factual recall and data interpretation, since these are tested in the written section of the examination. However, examiners use their discretion and ask questions which on the surface appear a straightforward test of factual recall, but also test the candidates' powers of reasoning, intellectual ability and clinical discrimination. Like their parliamentary counterparts during Question Time (e.g. Is the Prime Minister going to have Sunday luncheon with the family? When did the Home Secretary last visit Bristol?), these 'straightforward factual' questions appear simple but the sting follows in the supplementary tail.[1]

Unpleasant supplementary questions can be avoided by keeping the answers simple, straightforward, brief and succinct. This is no place to bring in long personal reminiscences.

Examples

1. 'Discuss allergic alveolitis.'

2. 'How do you determine the severity of the disease in bronchial asthma?'[2]

3. 'Describe the histology of the liver in alcoholic cirrhosis.'

4. 'How do you stage the lymphomas?'

5. 'What is the treatment of Parkinson's disease?'

6. 'How do you diagnose giant cell arteritis?'

7. 'What are the side effects of diuretics?'

8. 'What are the actions of aldosterone?'

9. 'How does a phaeochromocytoma present?'

10. 'Discuss malaria prophylaxis and the treatment of malaria.'

11. 'Classify acute pancreatitis.'

---

[1]   pp. 106, 108, 110, 130, 137

[2]   Five p's – pulse (tachycardia), pulsus paradoxus, falling PEFR (peak expiratory flow rate), falling PO_2 and rising PCO_2

8. CLINICAL STORIES

Questions in this group are always presented in the form of a clinical story, in which the examiners describe a scenario, usually from their own experience, comprising a brief history with or without some relevant physical signs and investigations. Almost every candidate is asked to comment on one or more clinical stories. The examiner is probing your comprehension and ability to pick up critical clues and to assess a clinical situation. Your alertness, clinical acumen, reactivity and medical knowledge are all on trial. In most cases the examiners do not expect or welcome supplementary questions from you. Apart from a few situations (e.g. *Detective* Stories) where it may be imperative to ask one or two direct or rhetorical questions to clarify the clinical setting, you should avoid engaging in verbal ping-pong! Clinical stories usually fall into various subgroups (see below) and you may find it helpful to try to work out which particular group a given question belongs to. Your response, and thereby your fate in the examination, will depend on your handling of the question. For example, it would be fatal to make a blunder in a 'bread-and-butter' scenario such as the management of diabetic coma (*Biblical* Story), whereas you will have almost a free hand in tackling a 'small print' case history about a snake-bite (*Wild* Story). The subgroups are:

a. **Biblical** (well established and everyday clinical practice)
b. **Detective** ('*what dunnit*' diagnostic problems)
c. **Ghost** (usually the real diagnosis lurks like a ghost behind the somewhat facile possibility)
d. **Bedtime** (mostly open-ended or differential diagnosis)
e. **Wild** (exotic or small print)
f. **Historical**

In most cases it is obvious, but if not we would suggest that you do not waste too much time in seeking an exact classification of the examiner's narrative. These subgroups are to guide you in formulating your response; it should not be regarded as vital to assign a story to its correct pigeonhole!

a. Biblical stories

As we have already emphasised, you cannot afford to make many mistakes in responding to a straightforward *Biblical* Story question. If you are facing an MRCP viva examination, it can be safely assumed that you have the required knowledge and skills to cope with any story. The trick is to assess quickly what the examiner is getting at, and therefore what to say. Many of the questions in this section are referral problems (see Referrals Section), but the key element in each of them is that there is a well-defined clinical approach which all clinicians are expected to use. All candidates know that the orthodox approach of a good history and physical examination are required, but many present stereotyped verbiage without saying anything specific, e.g. 'I will take a complete history and then carry out a comprehensive examination!' This is done partly to reassure the examiner that nothing important will be missed, but words like 'complete' and 'comprehensive' are no substitute for getting down to the problem, and indicating the **relevant parts of the history and examination** that would be looked for. Obviously, it is important to guard your flanks and to keep various possibilities under consideration, but you must identify and address the main purpose of the story and attempt to solve the problem.

Examples

1. **'The Accident and Emergency room doctor calls you to see a 50-year-old unconscious man. The patient was found unconscious in bed by a neighbour who had not seen him since the previous evening. He called the police, for help, who had to force the front door open to gain entry. The referring doctor tells you that the patient is pyrexial (38°C), deeply comatose without any lateralising neurological signs, and that the blood sugar level is 10 mmol/l. As you come near the patient, you find that his breathing is regular and deep, and that he is covered with sweat. What would be your strategy?'**

The elaborate scenario described by the examiner suggests that he expects you to guess the diagnosis. The management of an unconscious patient is one of the most important *Biblical* Stories, and any candidate who does not satisfy the examiner is likely to fail. So, even if the probable diagnosis of this case has become obvious to you (salicylate poisoning), we would suggest that you start by outlining your overall approach to the patient in coma. Any such approach must include an immediate assessment, maintenance of vital functions and setting up an intravenous infusion.

■ 'I would quickly check that the airway is clear, and set up an infusion if this has not been done already. As the patient has been *sweating profusely* (emphasises to the examiner that you have been listening carefully for important clues), he is probably **dehydrated** and it would be very helpful to set up a central venous pressure line. This procedure presents an opportunity to take a few blood samples for serum urea and electrolytes, liver function tests, a full blood count, pH and blood gas tensions, and for a **drug screen** (e.g. salicylates and narcotics). While these procedures are in progress, I would ask the referring doctor whether he has any further information about the circumstances of this patient's unconsciousness; namely, any antecedent illnesses, recent prescriptions and whether any labelled bottles were found by his bedside. It may become necessary to get a colleague to ring the patient's relatives, doctor and his local chemist to get as much information as possible about the patient's recent medical and drug history.

I would carry out a systematic general, systemic and neurological examination with *three* objectives in mind: firstly to look for **any signs** (e.g. petechiae, bruises, scratch marks, colour of the skin, pattern of breathing, spider naevi, clubbing, cardiac murmurs, abdominal masses, etc.) to suggest a possible cause of the coma. Secondly, I would assess the **depth of the coma** (response to painful stimuli, ocular movements, pupillary size and reaction to light, fundi for papilloedema, oculocephalic or doll's head reflex,[1] and conjugate eye movements).[2] The third important objective would be to **examine the nervous system** in detail, starting with the skull which should be inspected for any swelling and blood stains[3] and palpated for any oedema which usually overlies fresh fracture lines. I would check for neck stiffness (meningitis, cerebellar tonsillar herniation) and the reflexes to look for localising signs.'

We have dealt with this subject in some detail and deliberately strayed a little away from the examiner's given scenario, because in subjects like this the examiners do want to satisfy themselves about the candidates' general approach. During your presentation, the examiner may interrupt and lead you to the specific problem, or you may wish to conclude by saying:

■ 'There are six groups of disorders which can cause coma:

1. *Traumatic*: closed head injury
2. *Neurovascular*: brain stem infarction or haemorrhage, subarachnoid haemorrhage, haematoma in the hemisphere pressing on the brain stem, decreased cerebral blood flow (multiple emboli, severe aortic stenosis, polycythaemia, cryo- and macroglobulinaemia, hypertensive encephalopathy, etc.)
3. *Inflammatory diseases*: encephalitis, meningitis, cerebral malaria
4. *Space-occupying lesion*: tumours, brain abscess
5. *Metabolic*[4]
6. *Exogenous poisons*: salicylates, psychotropic drugs, alcohol (methyl and ethyl), anticonvulsants, etc.

The patient with coma you described who had profuse sweating and hyperglycaemia, I believe may have had **salicylate poisoning**. The diagnosis would be confirmed by obtaining a serum salicylate level, which in his case would be in excess of 1000 μg/ml. At that deep stage of coma, it

---

[1] Passive head rotation causes conjugate ocular deviation in the opposite direction to the induced head movement. This reflex is not present in conscious subjects, appears in coma, and disappears in deep coma, brain stem lesions and in brain death.

[2] Sustained conjugate lateral gaze towards the lesion ('looking towards the *normal limbs*') occurs in association with damage to supranuclear pathways. In brain stem lesions, sustained conjugate lateral gaze occurs towards the *paralysed limbs*.

[3] In basal skull fractures, there may be bleeding through the ears, or blood pigment stains behind the ears (Battle's sign) and/or about the orbit (*racoon* eyes).

[4] **Metabolic causes of coma**
   1. *Hypoxia*: pulmonary disease, alveolar hypoventilation, anaemia, methaemoglobulinaemia, CO poisoning
   2. *Hypoglycaemia*: spontaneous or from exogenous insulin
   3. *Vitamin deficiency*: thiamin (Wernicke's encephalopathy), B_{12}, folate, pyridoxine, etc.
   4. *Acid-base and ionic disturbances*: hyper- and hypo-osmolality, hyper- and hyponatraemia, acidosis, alkalosis, hypokalaemia, hyper- and hypocalcaemia, hyper- and hypomagnesaemia
   5. *Diseases of organs other than brain*:
      a. Endocrine – hyper- or hypofunction of the pituitary, thyroid, adrenals and parathyroid
      b. *Nonendocrine* – hepatic encephalopathy, uraemic coma, CO_2 narcosis, porphyria, diabetes mellitus, septicaemia
   6. *Miscellaneous diseases*: postictal states, postoperative delirium.

is likely that he had a metabolic acidosis. The management would have to address the elimination of salicylates by haemodialysis and correction of the acidosis by infusion of fluids with bicarbonate.'

2. **'A 30-year-old female has been referred to your clinic. She has been having recurrent headaches which mostly start on one side, often wake her up in the morning and during which she feels very unwell. What would you do?'**

This examiner has provided sufficient information to indicate the possible diagnosis (**migraine**), and seems to want to know your approach to establishing it. Success in achieving that objective will lead straight to a discussion of the management of this particular condition, and hence an easy passage through the viva. On the other hand, a general historical review of all the possible causes of headaches is likely to slow the tempo and plant a seed of doubt in the examiner's mind. Coming up with the probable diagnosis straightaway may not please the examiner either; you may appear a little impetuous, and your narrative will certainly lose its impact. The preferred introduction would seem to be a statement which represents a universal truth:

■ 'The diagnosis can be established by a careful history. I would enquire whether the patient had been diagnosed as having migraine previously, or had a family history of migraine, if there are any precipitating factors such as coffee, chocolates, alcohol, stress, etc., or any **prodromal symptoms** (alteration of mood, any preceding symptoms such as flashing lights or loss of part of the peripheral field of vision). You mentioned (in an effort to keep the examiner's concentration and to avoid a dry monologue) that the headaches mostly start on one side and that she is unwell during these. I would probe further to find out whether this unilateral start is strictly one-sided or sometimes goes to the opposite side, since unilateral headaches that *never* occur on the opposite side suggest a nonmigrainous aetiology (a further pointer to the diagnosis). I would enquire about the accompanying symptoms, i.e whether she suffers from nausea, vomiting, diarrhoea, phonophobia (noise-intolerance), and about the duration. A perfectionist personality, a positive family history and relationship to menstruation would be additionally helpful to suggest the diagnosis of migraine.'

3. **'A 40-year-old woman has been sent to your outpatient clinic with anxiety and palpitations. What are your thoughts to get to the bottom of this?'**

It is clear from the wording of this story that the examiner wishes to explore whether the candidate can distinguish between anxiety and thyrotoxicosis. However, in one survey many candidates asked this type of question are known to have given a long account of a history that would establish the nature of the palpitations. In order to give an impression that the palpitations are not being ignored, and that an attempt is being made to get to the diagnosis to provide definitive treatment, one may start by saying:

■ 'I think that the clinical assessment of this patient should be directed at answering the question whether she has thyrotoxicosis or simple anxiety. I would check her intake of coffee and ask her about any weight loss, increased appetite, heat-intolerance, and personal or family worries. During the examination, particular attention should be paid to whether she is fidgety, whether the hands are cold or warm and moist, any tremor, pulse rate, whether the thyroid gland is enlarged and if there is a bruit audible over it. As regards her palpitations, I would ask her about any factors that precipitate or terminate the episodes, their duration and whether she has any associated symptoms (e.g. breathlessness, dizziness, etc.). However, the main concern in this case would be to establish whether the underlying problem is anxiety or thyrotoxicosis so that appropriate treatment can be given.'

4. **'A 40-year-old obese woman has been sent with a label of Cushing's syndrome. How do you proceed?'**

The examiner's concern is obvious and should be addressed promptly without waffle:

■ 'Most patients sent with a label of Cushing's syndrome turn out to be examples of simple obesity (emphasises that you have come across such problems before, as most clinicians do!). Unfortunately, many clinical features such as hypertension, hirsutism, excessive bruising, menstrual disturbances, striae, hyperglycaemia and, of course, obesity are common to both. However, there are differences, and a careful scrutiny of various clinical features can help to differentiate between the two. In Cushing's syndrome, the obesity is mainly of proximal distribution (e.g. 'orange on matchsticks', supraclavicular fat pads, buffalo hump, moon facies), the striae tend to be purple and can be distinguished from the paler pink ones found in simple obesity, there is *thinning of the skin*, *proximal muscle wasting* and *weakness* (patients with Cushing's syndrome can seldom stand up from the squatting position without assistance). Obese subjects may have a slightly raised cortisol production rate, even when this is corrected for weight and surface area. The 24-hour urinary free cortisol levels are high in Cushing's syndrome. Obese subjects retain the normal hypothalamic control of ACTH production and, unlike patients with Cushing's syndrome, show a normal circadian pattern of plasma cortisol levels. Patients with Cushing's syndrome show resistance to the suppression of blood and urine corticosteroid.[5]'

5. **'A 60-year-old man has been admitted with increasing frequency and severity of angina pectoris. His doctor has been treating him with nitrates, beta blockers and calcium antagonists. How do you manage such a patient?'**

■ 'The story is suggestive of unstable angina and it would be wise to admit such a patient to a coronary care unit. The initial clinical assessment should rule out various possible precipitating or aggravating causes

---

[5] *Short dexamethasone screening test*
Dexamethasone (2 mg orally) is given at 2200 hours and the plasma cortisol is checked at 0900 hours the following day. Normal subjects show suppression of cortisol to <100 nmol/l.

such as anaemia, arrhythmias, infection and thyrotoxicosis (*de novo* or overtreatment in a hypothyroid patient). Cardiac enzymes and an ECG should be obtained to rule out an acute myocardial infarction. A transient deviation of the ST segment is suggestive, but its absence does not rule out unstable angina. While these investigations are in progress, the patient should be given complete bed rest, sedation, relief from pain with opiates, oxygen, nitrates by infusion and a beta blocker. In centres with full cardiac facilities, aortic balloon counterpulsation should be used in such patients with intractable angina. Coronary angiography is advisable for three reasons: firstly, it can identify patients with left main stem stenosis in whom urgent bypass graft surgery is mandatory. Secondly, a small proportion of patients have normal coronary arteries, and they can be reassured about a good prognosis. Thirdly, a knowledge of the state of the coronary vessels is essential for the proper management of these patients, since a good proportion of them will require surgery.'

6. **'A GP refers to you a man with congestive cardiac failure who has been resistant to large doses of diuretics. How do you proceed?'**

The examiner seems to have the limited objective of probing your knowledge about the role of digitalis, vasodilators and the angiotensin-converting enzyme inhibitors in cardiac failure. However, from the details of various viva encounters, it is clear that you need to be prepared to take up the challenge of managing *refractory* (persistent failure despite intensive therapy) and *intractable* (resistant to adequate treatment) heart failure. There are five principles which can help one to explore the reasons for the failure of apparently adequate treatment, and lead to a satisfactory management of intractable heart failure (see also p. 31).

1. **Exclude underlying reversible causes of failure**, e.g. arrhythmias, decompensating valvular lesions, alcoholic cardiomyopathy, left ventricular aneurysm, cardiac tumours, constrictive cardiomyopathy without calcification, etc.
2. **Check compliance**. The patient may be cheating on sodium or unwittingly eating high-salt foods (bacon, treated ham, beef, etc.). He may have forgotten to take the prescribed drugs or may have deliberately reduced the dose of diuretics. Elderly patients often fail to take the full dose of diuretics for fear of incontinence.
3. **Assess therapeutic status**. It is easy to check whether the patient is on optimal doses of the prescribed drugs, but overtreatment may be the cause of the symptoms which cannot be detected without a complete clinical assessment. Thus, lethargy and weakness may be due to digitalis toxicity, to excessive volume depletion, or to electrolyte disturbances resulting from high doses of diuretics.
4. **Look for associated disorders**. These may masquerade, as well as aggravate, the failure, e.g. unrecognised pulmonary embolism, pulmonary infection, infective endocarditis, hyperthyroidism, etc.
5. **Give proper treatment**. Taking into consideration the above factors, decide upon the appropriate treatment tailored to the circumstances of the individual patient. In addition to bed rest, oxygen and diuretics,

consider stepwise introduction of angiotensin-converting enzyme inhibitors (after a test dose to observe for any hypotensive response) and intravenous inotropes.

7. **'A 65-year-old man has been sent to you with fainting attacks. What clinical methods would you use to assess this patient?'**

A specific history is the key to the diagnosis. As far as possible, an exact description of the attacks should be obtained: rotational and vertiginous; whether on standing or on turning to one side; loss of balance on walking; their duration and onset – abrupt without warning or preceded by lightheadedness; their frequency; precipitating causes; and about any accompanying symptoms (tinnitus, nausea, sweating, palpitations, etc.). A full examination should include careful attention to the following:

1. **Neck vessels** for any bruits
2. **Pulse**: bradycardia (complete heart block), tachycardia, atrial fibrillation
3. **Auscultation of the heart** in various positions (aortic stenosis, atrial myxoma, etc.)
4. **Neck twist**: walking and turning of the neck to look to one side (vertebrobasilar insufficiency)
5. **Carotid sinus massage**: (hypersensitive carotid sinus—only massage one side at a time). This procedure should be accompanied by ECG monitoring in the elderly, and should not be carried out in patients with known heart disease[6]
6. **Potentiated Valsalva manoeuvre**: (patient asked to squat for 30 s and then stand and blow in a mercury sphygmomanometer to raise the level of mercury to 40 mmHg). Syncope and/or hypotension may be precipitated in patients with orthostatic hypotension and in hypertrophic obstructive cardiomyopathy
7. **Orthostatic hypotension**[7]
8. **Cerebellar function**: dysarthria, nystagmus, incoordination with eyes open
9. **Hallpike manoeuvre**: patient's head bent backwards from a seated position so that it hangs 45° below the horizontal and 45° to one side, vertigo and/or nystagmus suggests **positional vertigo**. The nystagmus is usually transient and fatiguable.

---

[6] See also p. 18

8. **'A woman with jaundice seems reasonably well and has been referred to you by her GP for investigation. How do you establish the cause?'**

■ 'A detailed history and physical examination are an absolute pre-requisite to narrowing down the number of possibilities from a wide array of disorders. A particular note should be made of the occupation (**alcohol**), *drugs* (e.g. chlorpromazine), exposure to a jaundiced person (**viral hepatitis**), ingestion of shell fish (**hepatitis A**), travel, transfusion (**hepatitis B** or **hepatitis C**), pale stools (**biliary obstruction**), skin pigmentation and xanthelasma (**primary biliary cirrhosis**), pruritus (**chronic cholestasis**), recurrent abdominal pain (**gallstone disease**) and weight loss (**malignant diseases**, especially carcinoma of the head of pancreas). Routine laboratory investigations are helpful but additional investigations (mitochondrial, smooth muscle and antinuclear antibodies, ultrasound, liver biopsy, cholangiography, etc.) may have to be undertaken. If a raised serum bilirubin is the only abnormality then **Gilbert's disease** is a likely diagnosis, especially if precipitated by fasting, dieting or infection, though a **compensated haemolytic** state should be excluded.'

---

[7]   **Causes of orthostatic hypotension**

Primary

1. *Primary autonomic dysfunction*
   a. Type 1: chronic idiopathic hypotension. This syndrome (the *Bradbury-Eggleston syndrome*) often occurs in older men and is characterised by postural hypotension *without* a compensatory tachycardia, decreased sweating, impotence and disturbed sphincter control. The treatment is symptomatic and involves a high-salt diet, judicious use of mineralocorticoids, a monoamine oxidase inhibitor (combined with tyramine or cheddar cheese) and mechanical support by elastic stockings
   b. Type 2: chronic idiopathic hypotension with neurological deficit (*Shy-Drager syndrome*)
2. *Familial dysautonomia (Riley-Day syndrome)*

Secondary

1. *Vasoactive drugs*: antihypertensive drugs (particularly if accompanied by dehydration and hypovolaemia), nitroglycerine, antidepressants, bromocriptine, hypnotics, tranquillisers, etc.
2. *Volume depletion*: haemorrhage, severe chronic anaemia, sodium depletion, glucocorticoid deficiency, pregnancy
3. *Disorders of the peripheral and central nervous systems*: diabetes mellitus, alcoholism, amyloidosis, pyridoxine deficiency, uraemia, Parkinson's disease, tabes dorsalis, pernicious anaemia, multiple sclerosis, Wernicke's encephalopathy, syringomyelia and porphyria
4. *Cardiovascular deconditioning*: after prolonged recumbency due to illness, especially in the elderly
5. *The supine hypotensive syndrome of pregnancy*: obstruction of the inferior vena cava with reduction in venous return
6. *Surgically induced sympathectomy*

9. **'A 70-year-old man has sharp pains in various parts of his body. He has had night sweats and on examination you find that he has an aortic systolic murmur. What do you do?'**

■ 'Sharp pains may be a manifestation of embolic phenomena, with infective endocarditis being the underlying disorder. A diligent search should be made for other stigmata, e.g. petechiae, splinter haemorrhages, *Roth's spots, Osler's nodes, Janeways's lesions,* clubbing, *splenomegaly, haematuria, heart failure, positive blood cultures,* and an ultrasound looking for *vegetations'.*

10. **'How do you establish the diagnosis of the Zollinger-Ellison syndrome?'**

Emphasis on *establish* calls for restraint, and any urge to shout 'abnormally high serum gastrin level' should be resisted. A methodological approach should be adopted:

■ 'This syndrome should be suspected in patients with peptic ulcers in unusual places and which are *resistant* to medical treatment, where there is a family history of ulcer disease, when the patients also have diarrhoea or large gastric folds seen on barium meal or at endoscopy, recurrent ulcers after surgery or when there are manifestations of *other endocrine tumours* (MEN type 1)[8]. If the serum gastrin level is high, a pentagastrin and secretin stimulation test should be performed. Computerised axial tomography (CAT scan), angiography and laparotomy may all have to be carried out'.

Other examples from survey

1. **'How would you manage a newly diagnosed diabetic patient?'**

The question is of a rather general nature and invites a general answer covering both types of diabetes and including general education about diabetes, dietary advice, restoration of normoglycaemia, self-monitoring, self-injecting of insulin, care of the eyes and feet, etc. The examiner will lead the discussion into more specific areas.

---

[8]   In multiple endocrine neoplasia (MEN) type I, there is a familial (autosomal dominant) occurrence of tumours of the anterior pituitary, parathyroid glands, pancreas and adrenal cortex. MEN type IIa is characterised by medullary carcinoma of the thyroid gland (or C-cell hyperplasia), phaeochromocytoma (>20% of adrenal medullary hyperplasia) and parathyroid hyperplasia (20–30%). It is inherited as an autosomal dominant trait. The phaeochromocytomas are frequently bilateral (occasionally extra-adrenal), and a constant feature of the medullary thyroid carcinomas is the hypersecretion of calcitonin, which serves as a useful marker for the presence of this neoplasm. In multiple endocrine neoplasia type IIb, mucosal adenomas of the tongue and eyelids are present and there is a characteristic facial appearance with thick lips.

2. **'A 28-year-old man with one child admits to previous homosexual contact and wants to be tested for HIV. What would you do?'**

'I would initiate a full discussion and counselling regarding the implications of a positive test.'

Examiner: 'Would you tell his wife?'

'I would offer my presence during the discussion with his wife.'

3. **'A 70-year-old man has been referred to you with a history of blackouts. How do you proceed?'**

Consider transient ischaemic attacks, epilepsy, space-occupying lesion, Stokes-Adams attacks, sinoatrial disease, postural hypotension, hypotensive drugs, etc.

4. **'A 45-year-old man has been brought into the Accident and Emergency room with a central chest pain of sudden onset. What would be your immediate plans?'**

A more specific history is needed about the site, nature and radiation of the pain, factors precipitating or aggravating the pain, and any past history of myocardial infarction or angina; clinical examination, particularly of the cardiovascular system; ECG and cardiac enzymes. Relieve pain with opiates, and if a myocardial infarction is confirmed or suspected, transfer to the coronary care unit for thrombolytic and other appropriate treatment.

These examples illustrate that all questions in this subgroup are of the 'bread and butter' type, and you are expected to have a plan of action in each case. None requires additional information or supplementary questions from you. You can state your assumptions and proceed from there. If the examiners want to alter any of the assumptions they will say so, and you can take up their lead. Whatever happens you are expected to know the answers because these represent day-to-day clinical situations that all general physicians have to cope with.

b. Detective stories

When presenting these stories the examiner usually has a specific diagnosis (*what dunnit?*) in mind, and gives what he thinks is enough information for you to find your way to the diagnosis. Sometimes the details may appear scanty and it is usually acceptable to ask the examiner a few more questions, or state some assumptions, in order to clarify the clinical scenario so that a diagnosis is possible. Indeed, sometimes the examiner may enjoy the game, and release information progressively in response to each purposeful question! One of the hallmarks of these case histories tends to be that a diagnosis is always possible and is usually very obvious to the examiner! Your approach in tackling these questions should be more or less the same as suggested for *Biblical* Stories (history, examination and investigations), and the possible diagnosis should be developed logically to a probable one. No matter how transparent the diagnosis appears to you as the examiner presents the story, you should resist the temptation to shout it out without a proper supportive clinical assessment. Even if you turn out to be right, the examiner will think that you guessed it and will not give you as much credit. In the examples below, we indicate the diagnosis which was in the examiner's mind in each case.

Examples

1. **'On your routine ward round, you find an elderly patient with a painful inflamed joint. What is your differential diagnosis and how will you manage him or her?'**

   Although the examiner has asked for a differential diagnosis (as is usual for *ghost* stories; p. 74), a clinical development apparently unrelated to the primary condition for which the patient was admitted is a typical *Detective* scenario. Astute clinicians who are also good teachers make the most of such situations with their students and junior staff. The important points in the history and examination should be pointedly presented; statements like 'I will take a complete history' may invite the reprimand that you should have done that when you had admitted the patient. The fact that the examiner has asked for a differential diagnosis suggests that not only does he have a definite diagnosis in mind (*what dunnit?*), he is also concerned that the candidate should not miss a serious possibility. Before taking the examiner's cue and embarking on presenting your differential diagnosis, you should endeavour to resolve this problem. In this clinical setting septic arthritis would seem to be the possibility that should not be missed along the way, while an attack of acute gout is confirmed and treated.

   ■ 'I would consider gout, pseudogout, infection, trauma and haemarthrosis (if the patient is a haemophiliac). As the patient is already on the ward, I would have the benefit of the critical background information necessary to narrow down the diagnostic possibilities. You did not specify the sex of the patient; if the patient is female (assuming the examiner remains silent!) then haemophiliac haemarthrosis would be unlikely and acute gout less likely. I would know whether there has been any past history of gout, any conditions associated with secondary gout (e.g. polycythaemia, myeloid metaplasia, chronic myeloid leukaemia, chronic haemolytic anaemia, etc.) or with pseudogout (e.g. hyperparathyroidism, haemochromatosis, myxoedema, ochronosis, hypophosphatasia, acromegaly, etc.), whether the patient has been on diuretics or whether there has been any trauma. The uncertainty between gout, pseudogout, infective arthritis and traumatic haemarthrosis can be resolved by needle aspiration. The aspiration of pus would suggest an infective cause, and blood would point to haemarthrosis though the procedure would not be necessary or desirable in a haemophiliac. If the fluid is clear then it should be examined for the presence of the negatively birefringent, needle-shaped urate crystals of gout, and the weakly positively birefringent calcium pyrophosphate crystals of pseudogout.'

2. **'A young female in the puerperium becomes confused and pyrexial with pains in the fingers and abdomen. In the recent past she has had a urinary tract infection for which she was treated with nitrofurantoin and metronidazole.'**

This is one of the most typical *Detective* Stories presented in the MRCP viva examination. The clinical scenario is brilliantly worded and must have rung like music in the ears of any knowledgeable candidate. The examiner has not wasted any words and has packed his two sentences with six clues, conjuring up a single diagnosis in the mind of the listener. The mention of confusion, pyrexia, pains in the abdomen *and fingers* suggests that the disorder has multisystem manifestations, and discourages any thoughts of an acute abdomen as the underlying diagnosis. Even though the diagnosis is obvious (the examiner knows this), it should not be stated at the outset: the examiner has left a few blank areas on the canvas, which should be painted in to develop a complete picture of the disorder:

■ 'The development of a wide spectrum of symptomatology after a urinary infection suggests that the infection or/and the drugs used for its treatment have precipitated an attack of a condition with multisystem manifestations. I would go over the history paying particular attention to any past or family history of a similar disorder, whether the patient had been exposed to these drugs in the past, and whether any other drugs had ever precipitated a similar attack. A wide variety of drugs, especially barbiturates, alcohol, oestrogens, chlordiazepoxide, imipramine, hydantoin, sulphonamides and nitrofurantoin precipitate an attack of **acute intermittent porphyria** in sensitive patients, by stimulating ALA synthetase and thereby increasing the flow of haem precursors. The attacks occur more often in young females, particularly in the last trimester of pregnancy and in the puerperium. I would examine this patient for the presence of *tachycardia*, for rigidity and rebound tenderness in the abdomen (which are usually absent) and for any sensory or motor deficit. Pyrexia is unusual in acute porphyria but in this patient it may have been due to the antecedent urinary infection. Routine laboratory investigations are generally unhelpful but she may have *hyponatraemia*, which is sometimes quite severe and may reflect an inappropriate secretion of antidiuretic hormone. The diagnosis can be confirmed by the demonstration of a large concentration of porphobilinogen in the urine. This may be readily accomplished by using Ehrlich's reagent (dimethylaminobenzaldehyde in HCl) which reacts with porphobilinogen in the urine to form a *red* complex.'

In the next example, the story was given in stages and a diagnosis demanded at each step.

3. **'A 61-year-old heavy drinker has not passed urine or opened his bowels for 5 days. He is hypotensive'.** *(Acute renal failure)* **'There are bilateral basal crackles and absent bowel sounds. He is pyrexial and has rigors'.** *(Septicaemia)* **'You note spontaneous bruising and bleeding at venepuncture sites.'** *(Alcoholic cirrhosis – septicaemia, pancreatitis, shock and disseminated intravascular coagulation)*

4. **'You see an ill child in casualty with purpuric spots. What would you think?'**

Acute meningococcal meningitis: explore the particular features of the illness (e.g. headache, vomiting, pyrexia, etc.) and examine the child. Exclude a blood dyscrasia. If no papilloedema, proceed to urgent lumbar puncture and CSF examination.

5. **'A dusky looking man has been sent in with phlebothrombosis. What might be the underlying disease?'**

Polycythaemia rubra vera: check for splenomegaly, do full blood count looking for raised WBC, RBC and platelets and low MCV.

6. **'A 52-year-old man with weight loss and mild anaemia has an elevated ESR. What would you be thinking of?'[9]**

Polymyalgia rheumatica, collagen disease, neoplasia, etc.

Examiner: He has difficulty in getting out of his chair.

Polymyalgia rheumatica.

7. **'I am a 20-year-old girl with a two-week history of headaches. Ask me some questions.'**

Are you on the contraceptive pill?

8. **'You see a man in your clinic with impotence and a headache of recent onset.'**

Prolactinoma.[10]

9. **'An Indian girl has difficulty in walking. What would you suspect?'**

Osteomalacia.[11]

10. **'A 55-year-old hypertensive man was admitted with severe back pain of abrupt onset. What would you think?'**

Dissecting aortic aneurysm.

---

[9]   As presented, this scenario has features of a *Biblical* Story and the candidate should (as did happen in this case) start with the history and clinical examination, and then discuss the differential diagnosis. During the discussion the examiner converted it into a *Ghost* Story by providing the *ghost-link* (see next section).

[10] A prolactinoma must be considered (which was the examiner's diagnosis), though a psychiatric cause is often more likely.

[11] An Indian *Muslim* girl would have constituted a more helpful hint, as females of other religions from the Indian subcontinent are not obliged to cover their face, arms and legs. Presented in this way it is permissible to ask the examiner a question or two in order to define the walking difficulty.

11. **'A pale, elderly lady with systemic venous congestion was admitted with a haemoglobin level of 4.2 g/dl. What is the most probable diagnosis?'**

Pernicious anaemia.[12]

12. **'A healthy young woman is seen in the outpatients with recent weight loss. What questions would you ask and why?'**

Bowel habits, eating habits, pyrexia and abdominal pain. All the supplementary questions were asked to lead the candidate to *Crohn's disease.*

13. **'A young female with a recent painful swelling of the thyroid was referred to you. You find that she is euthyroid but has a raised T4 level. What diagnosis would you suspect and how would you confirm it?'**

Subacute viral thyroiditis: this should be confirmed by a low thyroid radio-iodine uptake.[13]

14. **'An elderly man had difficulty changing gears in his car followed by increasing difficulty in walking. On the day of presentation he had developed incontinence. What is the diagnosis you must think of?'**

Cord compression: this presentation is suggestive of a *rapidly developing lesion* such as an **epidural haematoma, midline herniation** of a disc or a **metastatic tumour.** Obtain a more comprehensive history of any previous pains and paraesthesiae, and examine neurologically to assess the extent of spinal cord dysfunction and to get an idea of the level of the lesion. X-ray of the spine followed by CT scanning with contrast and magnetic resonance imaging are the preferred investigations.[14]

---

[12]   Even though pernicious anaemia seems to be the probable diagnosis, blood loss and acute myeloid leukaemia should be excluded.

[13]   Painful swelling of the thyroid was a *ghost-link* the examiner was looking for: de Quervain's thyroiditis (also known as viral or granulomatous thyroiditis) which is an acute or subacute self-limiting condition and can be distinguished from subacute lymphadenoid goitre by a *low thyroid uptake of radioiodine* and *low or absent titre of thyroid antibodies*, both of which tend to be raised in the latter condition.

[14]   When cord compression is suspected from a patient's clinical presentation, a neurological examination and plain X-rays of the spine often suggest the area of impingement. Traditionally, **myelography** has been used for the diagnosis and accurate localisation of the compression. **Computed tomography** (CT) can detect erosions of vertebral bodies and paravertebral masses, but its use without contrast media is only advisable below L3, where the adjacent fat can provide the contrast against which the abnormalities can be seen. Recently, **magnetic resonance imaging** (MRI) has been suggested to be superior to myelography as a test for the detection of spinal cord compression (Radiology 1986; 161: 377). MRI has the advantage of being noninvasive and can reveal paraspinous masses that are not seen on myelography. However, myelography allows the examination of the entire spine, and if **metastases** are suspected to be the cause of the compression, the *entire spine* should be examined with either myelography or MRI, since there may be more than one area of compression distant from the suspected lesion. Although MRI is a sensitive method for detecting spinal cord metastases, imaging of the entire spine is time-consuming and may take up to 2 hours.

15. 'A young girl with a weak voice complains of tiredness. On physical examination you find nothing abnormal except that she is thin and looks somewhat droopy-eyed. What diagnosis would go through your mind and what bedside test would you use?'

Myasthenia gravis: demonstrate fatiguability by asking her to count up to 100 and use the anticholinesterase test.[15]

16. 'A 70-year-old man collapsed in a chair. His wife said that he had had a few dizzy spells during the last year.'

Sinoatrial disease: obtain a full history of the dizzy spells, and of any palpitations, their onset, duration and the appearance of the patient during these attacks. Examine the patient (see also p. 65) and obtain an ECG to look for instability of sinus node firing, i.e. variable PR intervals and P wave morphology, sinoatrial block, bradycardia, A–V junctional beats, etc. A 24-hour ambulatory monitoring study may be necessary to establish the diagnosis. Recurrent dizzy spells is an indication for a pacemaker in a patient with sinoatrial disease.

17. 'A 50-year-old man is found to have a raised MCV on the blood count during an incidental[16] examination.'

Alcoholism.

We would suggest that the best way to make the most of these questions is to play the game and give the examiners a little bit of their own medicine by keeping up the suspense. If you suspect the diagnosis, you should present a few more features of history/examination and gradually narrow down to the diagnosis. For example, in the case of the Indian girl you may say that you would obtain the dietary history and examine her gait. Similarly, in the patient with sudden back pain you may proceed to examine the patient to consider the possible clinical signs that might distinguish a dissecting aneurysm from the prolapsed intervertebral disc syndrome. Playing the game like this provides a safety margin; if you get the diagnosis right it shows that you have the confidence of a mature physician, and that you are able to fill in the important details leading up to a diagnosis. On the other hand, if your diagnosis happens to be wrong, the examiner will feel that at least you have the right approach which is often likely to be successful in making a diagnosis.

---

[15] The 'weak voice' and 'droopy-eyed' were *ghost-links* (see *Ghost* Stories) for myasthenia gravis. The anticholinesterase test can be performed at the bedside by giving 2 mg of edrophonium intravenously and watching the improvement in the patient's ptosis and voice over the next 30 seconds. If there is no response, an additional 8 mg should be injected to see if it reduces the degree of ptosis and improves the pitch of her voice.

[16] There may have been some reason other than for insurance purposes that the doctor had asked for a full blood count, and one would need to explore further any history of weakness, lassitude, spontaneous bruising, etc. The question implies that the other haematological indices were normal but this needs to be confirmed. All the other major causes of a high MCV (e.g. megaloblastic, haemolytic, sideroblastic and aplastic anaemias, hypothyroidism) may be asymptomatic in the early stages.

c. Ghost stories

The chief distinction between the *Ghost* and the *'what dunnit?'* Detective Story is that in the former there are usually two or more immediately obvious diagnoses that could fit the clinical picture, and the actual one (or the eventual one, as may have been the case in the examiner's own experience) lurks like a shadow linked by some unusual but *specific* event in the story (the *ghost-link*).

Examples

1. **'A patient in a psychiatric ward develops polyuria and polydipsia and was transferred to your ward. What are your thoughts?'**

   This story suggests a number of possibilities, particularly **overuse of lithium**[17], **psychogenic diabetes insipidus**, **diabetes mellitus** and **hypercalcaemia**, all of which should be mentioned. In this case, all of these diagnoses will hover like ghosts during the discussion, but the significant link with the real diagnosis (**primary hyperparathyroidism**) is the fact that the patient had been admitted to a psychiatric ward before the present problem developed. Thus, after presenting these possibilities, it should be stressed that the psychiatric history points to psychogenic polydipsia, lithium and primary hyperparathyroidism as the initial favourites, which can be further explored by going into the history of the primary referral to a psychiatrist and the details of the treatment. At this stage, the examiner may participate in the discussion and offer a further clue (see below) or/and you may have to suggest a few investigations such as serum calcium, PTH, X-ray of the hands and skull, and so on. Sometimes, the *ghost-link* may emerge in the subsequent discussion, and it is important to bear this in mind and not burn your boats by giving a definitive single diagnosis at the outset.

2. **'A 60-year-old man has difficulty in walking, and his friends have been chiding him for his peculiar gait.'**

   This story suggests that the patient is capable of his usual daily activities and looks reasonably well, since his friends are unlikely to be so insensitive as to tease him if he were seriously handicapped. The candidate may find it prudent to state this assumption:

   ■ 'It would seem that this patient has an abnormal gait and is otherwise well enough to be tolerating the chiding by his friends. He may have an **ataxic gait** and his friends may be accusing him of drunkenness, or he may have a **spastic gait** and his colleagues are calling him clumsy and stiff. Other possibilities are a **prolapsed disc**, **osteoarthrosis** or **trauma** causing him to limp while walking.'

   Examiner: 'There is no history of trauma but he did have an operation for his obesity.'

---

[17] Other drugs known to cause nephrogenic diabetes insipidus are demeclocycline, amphotericin B, propoxyphene, glibenclamide, outdated tetracycline and gentamicin.

You may be lucky or astute enough to spot the *link*. It would seem that the patient has developed **osteomalacia** after his ileojejunal bypass operation, and the peculiarity in his walk is the **waddling gait**. Even if you miss the *link*, the examiner has opened up an area for fresh discussions and you may be led to *the* diagnosis.

The principal aim of the examiners in presenting *Ghost* Stories is to test your astuteness and the depth of your contemplation, in assessing a medical history which has many diagnostic possibilities. The examiners also enjoy this game because *Ghost* Stories present them with an opportunity to test your response to the key features in these stories. For your own and the examiners' enjoyment,[18] and for getting extra marks, you should make an attempt to recognise that the story belongs to this group and look for the *ghost–link*. After giving the initial differential diagnosis, you should attempt to assemble a few more details about the clinical scenario by asking the examiners some additional questions or by stating some well-measured assumptions. The examiner may accept the challenge and good progress can be made in reaching the real diagnosis. If the examiner declines to answer any more questions then, assuming that you have not missed the *ghost–link*, you must make the most of it by painting the clinical picture of each possibility.

Remember, the real diagnosis in each case is a *ghost* which may hover over the story and over the ensuing discussion like a shadow.

We present some more examples below, and the final diagnosis is indicated in italics. We have briefly outlined our approach of dissecting out the *ghost-link(s)* in reaching the *actual* diagnosis and presentation to the examiner. Weigh carefully the words used by the examiner which could easily fit more than one diagnosis.

3. **'A 50-year-old man with a shuffling gait had become increasingly forgetful over about a year. He developed incontinence which alarmed his wife, who had him referred to you. What would be your most likely diagnosis?'**

Normal pressure hydrocephalus, Alzheimer's disease, Jacob-Creutzfeldt disease.[19]

This interesting scenario reveals the intricate complexities of a *Ghost* Story and was presented as a stiff challenge, because not only would the candidate need to have a precise clinical knowledge of the various possible diagnoses, but she would also need to have a fine discriminating ability to reach the *actual* diagnosis. The story is typical of an ideal *Ghost* Story as it possesses all three characteristics: firstly, it brings to mind at least three conditions that could fit the story; secondly, the real diagnosis (**normal pressure hydrocephalus**) would not seem to be the first preference since **Alzheimer's disease** is much commoner than the others; thirdly, there is

---

[18] We accept that many of you will not be in the mood for seeking enjoyment at this critical time!

[19] The full differential diagnosis is extensive (e.g. neurosyphilis, tuberculosis, lymphomatous or carcinomatous meningitis, granulomatous angiitis, multiple infarcts, etc.), but the mention of the triad without any focal events suggests that the examiner had a limited list of conditions in mind.

a *ghost-link* that only an astute clinician who has some experience of these conditions is likely to recognise. Any knowledgeable candidate would find this story intellectually stimulating, as surely did the examiner!

The triad of **dementia**, **gait disorder** and **urinary incontinence** associated with ventricular dilatation and with no evidence of increased intracranial pressure (normal pressure hydrocephalus), was presented as a clinical entity by Adams and colleagues (N Engl J Med 1965; 273: 117). Early reports emphasised dementia as an important diagnostic feature, but it has turned out to be less reliable than the *abnormal gait*. In the early stages, as in this case of one year's duration, the abnormal gait is useful in differentiating normal pressure hydrocephalus from Alzheimer's disease. A patient with the latter disease of one year's duration would be expected to walk briskly despite a major impairment of intellect. On the other hand, the gait disorder is often the initial, and a more striking, feature than the coexisting mild mental impairment in normal pressure hydrocephalus. The small-step gait disorder has been described as *marche à petits pas*, gait apraxia, a frontal gait disorder, or a magnetic gait; it is not specific to normal pressure hydrocephalus and is also associated with Alzheimer's disease. However, the early appearance of this gait disorder, and its constant association with normal pressure hydrocephalus, makes it an important discriminating clinical feature.

The abnormal gait and its appearance during the first year of illness as described by the examiner in this story were the two mutually related *ghost-links* suggesting that normal pressure hydrocephalus was the actual diagnosis.

4. **'A young man has been referred with recurrent attacks of suddenly developing breathlessness. What might be the cause of it?'**

Asthma, left ventricular failure, *occupational exposure to toxic fumes.*

A subtle blend of carefully chosen words makes this clinical scenario a very challenging *Ghost* Story. There are three *ghost-links* in this brief story: firstly, a young man is unlikely to have recurrent attacks of left ventricular failure, and the word 'young' probably suggests an otherwise healthy subject. Secondly, although recurrent attacks of breathlessness occur in asthma the examiner has made a special mention of 'recurrent attacks in a young man', and one wonders whether the word 'recurrent' has a special connotation. One may have to ask the question, 'recurring with what?' Thirdly, 'cause' points to a possible agent rather than a diagnosis.

The *actual* diagnosis, **occupational asthma**, would accommodate the double meaning of 'recurrent', as in this condition attacks of breathlessness recur with exposure to the offending fumes or toxins at work, and the patients remain asymptomatic at weekends, when at home or on holiday.

Numerous causative agents have been recognised and the list continues to grow. One needs to have a high index of suspicion to identify the offending agent.

The common causes of occupational asthma (with occupational exposure) are:

1. *Low molecular weight chemicals*
   a. Isocyanates (plastics, spraying)
   b. Anhydrides (epoxy resins)

       c. Metals – platinum, chromium, nickel (metal plating, refining)
       d. Wood dust (carpentry)
   2. *Organic materials*
       a. Plant dust, grains (agricultural work)
       b. Laboratory animals (laboratory work, animal handling)
       c. Biological enzymes (detergents, chemical industry)
   3. *Gases*
       a. Chlorine (plastic industry, water purification)
       b. Ammonia (refrigeration)
       c. Sulphur dioxide (paper manufacturing, smelting)
       d. Nitrogen dioxide (corn silage)
       e. Phosgene (aniline dyes)

5. **'A 27-year-old man was brought in after an episode of sudden unconsciousness during a football match.'**

Head injury, subarachnoid haemorrhage, *hypertrophic obstructive cardiomyopathy.*

    A moment's reflection on this question shows that this is another of the cleverly worded *Ghost* Stories. Although a head injury during a football match seems to be the obvious answer, the loss of consciousness following a trauma to the head is hardly a diagnostic challenge. One need not stretch the word 'episode' too much to extract from it the special meaning that the event of unconsciousness was brief, that the patient had recovered, and that there possibly might have been a similar episode(s) in the past. Brief episodes of unconsciousness, particularly during heavy exercise, are not uncommon in patients with **hypertrophic obstructive cardiomyopathy.** Loss of consciousness may occur briefly in **subarachnoid haemorrhage,** but the examiners would probably have chosen *sudden headache* instead of unconsciousness. The *young* age, the *episode* of unconsciousness and the *athletic* ability are all *ghost-links* to suggest that the *actual* diagnosis was **hypertrophic obstructive cardiomyopathy.**

6. **'You have a man with rheumatoid arthritis whose serum urea level has risen to 28 mmol/l. You ask yourself why?'**

Toxic damage to the kidney by drugs (gold, penicillamine), interstitial nephritis from nonsteroidal anti-inflammatory drugs or antibiotics, glomerulonephritis, *amyloidosis.*[20]

    This interesting *Ghost* Story requires some lateral thinking on the part of the candidate to suspect what the examiner is getting at. Nephrotic syndrome with heavy proteinuria is a complication commonly found with toxic damage to the kidney by gold or penicillamine and from amyloidosis. The unexpected finding of uraemia ushering in amyloidosis must have been a surprising development for the physician who was carefully monitoring the patient for proteinuria and haematuria. During the discussion with the examiner, one would need to give equal importance to all the possibilities, as happened in this viva experience.

7. **'A young man presents with a pyrexia, sore throat, loss of appetite and swelling in the neck. What diagnostic possibilities would you consider?'**

Infectious mononucleosis, Hodgkin's disease, toxoplasmosis, subacute viral thyroiditis, *viral hepatitis.*

This clinical picture would seem to be the prodromal phase of hepatitis A, which emerged as the *actual* diagnosis during the discussion with the examiner. Loss of appetite was presumably the *ghost-link*.

8. **'A young man aged 20 developed septicaemia and shock 3 days after a trivial cut on his hand. On admission to hospital he had a blood sugar of 3 mmol/l.[20] What do you think is the underlying problem?'**

Insulinoma, *Addison's disease.*

As the examiner has singled out hypoglycaemia, one should consider **acute adrenocortical insufficiency** as the underlying disorder in this patient. Presumably, the stress of the septicaemia called for an increased requirement for glucocorticoids thereby leading to shock and hypoglycaemia. Frank Addisonian crises are rare in **hypopituitarism** (which is the other possibility) because some aldosterone secretion is maintained through the renin-angiotensin mechanism, which is independent of ACTH. Insulinomas occur more frequently in females, are uncommon in young adults, and produce episodes of a variety of symptoms such as palpitations, weakness, confusion or abnormal behaviour.

It is always important when answering these questions to consider the possibility that both you and the examiner may be chasing a *ghost* and that he may not know the real diagnosis. It is usually safer to define the clinical situation than to guess wildly. You may have to ask a question or two or attempt to set the scene yourself. The examiner will contribute now and again and the game can be played to everyone's satisfaction. Thus, when you are given a short story that a man presented with a sudden onset of chest pain and breathlessness (**pulmonary infarction, pneumothorax**), you may either ask the examiner about the character and abruptness of the pain and dyspnoea, or state your assumptions and give the possible diagnosis of **pneumothorax**. Sometimes the examiner may be narrating from his own experience where the diagnosis had remained undetermined. The questions must be purposeful and directed at a particular diagnostic target, rather than fired off haphazardly in all directions.

---

[20] **Causes of spontaneous hypoglycaemia**:
  a. Islet cell hyperfunction – hyperplasia, adenomatosis, benign or malignant neoplasm
  b. Leucine and fructose sensitivity
  c. Galactosaemia
  d. Liver disease
  e. Endocrine disease – hypopituitarism, Addison's disease, adrenogenital syndrome
  f. Glycogen storage disease
  g. Nonpancreatic neoplasm – retroperitoneal sarcoma, bronchogenic carcinoma, etc.
  h. Reactive to alcohol, fructose, etc.

d. Bedtime stories

The hallmark of these stories is the relaxed manner with which the examiner starts the question: 'Tell me something about . . .', 'What do you think about . . .?', 'How would you deal with . . .?', etc. These questions allow you some freedom in what you say. You can deviate from the line drawn by the examiner and you do not need to have the same views as him so long as your opinions are logical and well supported by scientific data.

Examples

1. **'Tell me about the use of laser treatment in medicine today.'[21]**

■ 'Laser (light amplification by stimulated emission of radiation) system consists essentially of a source of high energy, visible or infrared radiation, which can focus on a fraction-of-a-millimetre spot size, together with a delivery system that conveys this radiation to the target. After its introduction into medicine by a dermatologist in 1961, its use has spread into almost all areas of medicine and surgery.

The best-known application of lasers in medicine is the laser-induced *vessel closure* due to its high power radiation. Choosing optimal impulse duration, wavelength, and optional parameters such as spot size and power, a vessel of suitable length can be heated to shrinkage leading to vascular occlusion. This property is made use of during surgery to reduce haemorrhage, and on retinal neovascularisation in diabetes mellitus to prevent blindness. Other medical areas in which lasers have been particularly useful are:

1. *Dermatology.* The wavelength of ruby lasers (0.69 μm) and argon (0.5 μm) corresponds to that of visible red and green which makes it suitable for use in **removing tattoos**, **haemangiomata** and **port-wine stains**. The absorption of blue and green laser light by blood transforms light energy into thermal energy and causes coagulation of the capillary plexus, necrosis and thermal denaturation. This has not yet found wide acceptance, as some other tissues containing haemoglobin and melanin also suffer denaturation, but improvements in decreasing the target area and beam size should overcome this problem.

2. *Cardiovascular medicine.* Percutaneous **laser angioplasty** in conjunction with balloon angioplasty is now widely used to open up discrete vascular lesions, and laser angioplasty on its own is now under investigation in many centres. Purely thermal angioplasty has been used in many cases with only minor complications.

3. *Gastroenterology.* As noted above, laser treatment can be used for the management of **bleeding lesions**. The use of both the argon and Nd:YAG lasers has reduced mortality and morbidity from bleeding peptic ulcers. Lesions in both upper and lower gastrointestinal tract respond well to endoscopically delivered laser beams.

4. *Urology.* Because of its coagulative powers, the Nd:YAG laser is useful

---

[21] The candidate reported that he was allowed to talk for as long as he could without interruption.

in the endoscopic management of benign and malignant **urological tumours**. It can be used to remove small tumours and as a palliative measure to debulk large tumours with extravesical extension. Wavelengths that can be transmitted through fine fibres allow the use of lasers throughout the urinary tract.

5. *Oncology.* Nd:YAG lasers are most effective in causing **necrosis of tumours** and have been used to dissolve condylomata, spider naevi, haemangiomata, adenomata and penile carcinomas. Argon, CO_2 and Nd:YAG lasers can be used with effective parameters (focus, wavelength, pulse duration and power) to cause ablative effects externally and endoscopically in internal organs using flexible fibre instruments.

The lasers are being used in various laboratory procedures and for stimulating healing in tissues. Future attention to design and the development of newer accessory technologies are expected to expand the clinical scope of lasers.'

2. **'Sum up your views on the trials regarding the use of beta blockers in the management of acute myocardial infarction.'**

■ 'Clinical trials on the usefulness of beta blockers after myocardial infarction fall broadly into two groups. Firstly, there are those trials that examine the benefits of beta blockers immediately after the acute event (during approximately the first 72 hours), when correction of arrhythmias and limitation of infarct size are the important concerns. Secondly, there are those that address the prevention of reinfarction and sudden death, and are termed 'late intervention' trials, i.e. the administration of beta blockers after recovery from the acute event, when the early complications of arrhythmias and haemodynamic disturbances would have taken their toll.

Despite the potential benefits of beta blockers (i.e. abolition of sympathetic tone and prevention of arrhythmias) and the multiple trials, the results of *early-intervention* trials do not provide unambiguous conclusions. One trial (Lancet 1981; 2: 823) using metoprolol (15 mg intravenously followed by 200 mg orally) showed a 36% reduction in mortality, but since oral metoprolol was continued for 90 days it is debatable whether the benefits can be attributed to early or late intervention. Further, these results are in marked contrast with those of another large multinational and multicentre study (Eur Heart J 1985; 6: 199) in which metoprolol showed only 13% benefit compared with the placebo. The ISIS I study of over 1600 patients showed that intravenous, followed by oral, atenolol reduced mortality in the first 24 hours, mostly due to a reduction in deaths from cardiac rupture (Lancet 1988; 1: 921). As thrombolysis may result in an increased tendency to cardiac rupture in the first 24 hours (Lancet 1989; 2: 655), early beta blockade combined with thrombolytic therapy is probably the best therapeutic approach at present (N Engl J Med 1989; 320: 618), though further studies are needed to clarify the issue.

In an extensive statistical review of randomised trials of *late intervention* with beta blockers (Prog Cardiovasc Dis 1985; 27: 335), the reduction in mortality rates was found to be about 25%. This means that if the placebo-treated patients have a mortality of 8%, then a 25% improvement produced by beta blockers will give a mortality of 6%. The benefit derived from later intervention with beta blockers looks small, considering that all trials had excluded from active treatment patients with known contraindications to beta blockade (e.g. asthma, heart failure, heart block, intermittent claudication), and that there was a dropout rate of about 12% because of adverse reactions (e.g. lassitude, fatigue, reduced libido, etc.). This raised a pertinent question: should beta blockers be given to low-risk patients (i.e. young age, small infarct size, absence of complications during the early course after the infarct) at the expense of a reduction in their quality of life? This inevitably leads to a debate as to the cost-effectiveness of the routine use of beta blockers in low-risk patients.

In a survey of 100 British cardiologists, it appeared that about 70% of them advised routine use of beta blockers after myocardial infarction (Br Med J 1984; 289: 1431).) A recent study (N Engl J Med 1988; 319: 152) analysed the costs and effectiveness of routine beta blocker therapy in patients who survived an acute myocardial infarction, and concluded that beta blocker therapy had a favourable cost-effectiveness ratio, compared with coronary artery bypass graft surgery and the medical treatment of hypertension. As regards the choice of agent, convincing positive data have been obtained with the lipid-soluble beta blockers, propanolol and timolol, neither of which possesses partial agonist activity.

In summary, most physicians use beta blockers after acute myocardial infarction if there are no contraindications. This inclination is motivated forcibly if there are unfavourable circumstances, such as a large infarct size, angina or abnormal electrocardiographic changes after exercise two weeks after the infarct. The question about optimal duration of beta blocker therapy has not been addressed specifically by any of the studies. We know that continuing benefit was apparent for two years with beta blocker therapy and further continuation of the treatment must be left to clinical judgement.'

Both these questions represent typical examples of *Bedtime* Stories, and the candidate is invited to give a detailed answer as long as he can keep it relevant to the question. Any deviations are likely to invite interruptions from the examiners, and any unsupported or vague comments will be challenged. The following questions are similarly open-ended and call for detailed and informative answers.

3. **'What do you know about the medical problems of Asian immigrants?'**[22]

Numerous medical problems have been recognised in Asian immigrants which are broadly the results of a conflict between the two evolutionary processes. The various adaptive social, dietary and cultural responses of Asians to the environmental constraints in Asia are not necessarily suited to the European milieu, yet many Asians live and eat in this country as they

---

[22] The candidate mentioned infections, social and nutritional problems but forgot rickets!

would in their country of origin. This conflict of two cultures is compounded by the maladaptive responses of immigrants to the demands of the new circumstances; many years may be needed to adjust to this environment. Unless these basic principles are taken into account it is impossible to explain, let alone treat, the multiple **psychosomatic** disorders that tend to afflict all immigrants in their new environment. Thus, after the Second World War many Polish immigrants used to consult doctors in the East End of London with multiple aches and pains. A new syndrome was coined from the German 'Und hier' (and here) by the physicians at the receiving end. It was said that no matter where on the body you touched a Polish patient, he would complain of pain in that part, 'And here, doctor!'

In recent times the syndrome of 'Und hier' has appeared in Asian immigrants. Asian women and unemployed men, who were happy chatting with their friends and neighbours in their own country, are lonely and friendless in this country. This social deprivation leads to the development of multiple basic bodily ailments such as pains, dizziness, headaches, indigestion, etc. Women who were used to covering their bodies in black overalls (*purdah*) in a sunny country back home, now do the same here and so deprive themselves of even what little sunshine is available, and so develop **vitamin D deficiency** and **rickets**.

Stresses of unemployment, Western diets, difficulties in communication and a change from an agricultural to a wholly cash economy must be in part to blame for the high incidence of **hypertension** and **ischaemic heart disease** among Asian immigrants in this country. Even though fewer Asians smoke as much as Europeans do, about 40% develop ischaemic heart disease, and the atheromatous process involves the coronary arteries diffusely, which often renders them unsuitable for bypass graft surgery. Their dietary habits, and in particular their fat intake, which amounts to over 60% of the total calorie intake, may have some role in the high prevalence of **insulinaemia** and **diabetes mellitus** in Asian immigrants. Recent studies have shown that diabetes mellitus is ten times more common among Asians than in native Britons. Their change from a high fibre diet at home to refined carbohydrates and an unbalanced intake in this country would seem to be responsible for their multiple **gastrointestinal disorders** and many **deficiency states** including some **trace element deficiencies** that are still unrecognised.

4. **'What are the industrial, environmental and social causes of neoplasia?'**[23]

Despite decades of research, the aetiology of neoplasia has remained one of the most baffling problems confronting medical investigators. Strong associations have been suggested between various industrial, environ-

---

[23] The candidate discussed recent evidence of dust, toxins, etc.

mental, social, genetic and inflammatory provocative factors and cancer, but Koch's postulates[24] have seldom been fulfilled. Most of the evidence is based on a strong association between various agents and the high incidence of neoplasia. The principal industrial products and chemicals which have been incriminated are **aromatic hydrocarbons** (soots, coal tar, creosote, benzene), **aromatic amines** (benzidene and derivatives), **wood products** (sawdust), **plants** (senecio alkaloids), **radiation** (ionising, ultraviolet) and **organics** (vinyl chloride).

Exposure to the **ultraviolet light** in sunshine has been considered to be a major aetiological factor for skin cancers. The incidence of melanomas on the lower legs of females has increased since short skirts became fashionable. Similarly, there is a higher incidence of skin cancers in patients with albinism and a lower incidence in the darker races.

Racial and environmental factors operate together with different results: in African negroes there is a high incidence of hepatomas, Kaposi's sarcoma, Burkitt's lymphoma and carcinomas of the oesophagus, but this is not the case in American negroes. A high incidence of nasopharyngeal neoplasia occurs in Chinese people everywhere. There is a lower incidence of Ewing's sarcoma and testicular carcinomas in blacks than in whites.

Smoking clearly contributes to the aetiology of cancer and may be responsible for up to 40% of all neoplasias in Europe and the USA. Among smokers, an increased **alcohol** consumption has been associated with the head and neck and oesophageal cancers. Inhalation of **asbestos**, **radioactive minerals** and occupational exposure to **radiation** have all been strongly associated with various neoplasia.

5. **'Tell me something about genetic counselling.'**

During the last two decades there has been a vast increase in the precision of diagnosis achieved by the clinical application of recombinant DNA technology. There are now a number of conditions (adult polycystic kidney disease,[25] cystic fibrosis, Duchenne and Becker muscular dystrophy, haemochromatosis, haemophilia, Huntington's chorea, phenylketonuria, myotonic dystrophy, etc.), which can be diagnosed using gene probes. All prospective parents wonder if their offspring will be normal, and great distress is caused among parents as well as relatives following the birth of a child with a handicap. Even a distant family history of genetic disease

---

[24] *Koch's postulates:*
1. The aetiological agent should be found in every case of disease and not in normal subjects.
2. The incriminating agent should be cultured in pure form.
3. The disease should be reproduced in animals inoculated with pure culture.
4. The agent should be reisolated in pure culture from the experimental animal.

[25] p. 169

causes relatives lifelong anxiety. There is a great need of counselling for those participating in a screening programme, those found to be at high risk, and for their relatives.[26]

A **careful genetic history** is the most important prerequisite for counselling. Full details of any genetic illnesses should be obtained about parents, siblings, aunts, uncles and cousins, and a family tree should be constructed with affected relatives clearly marked.

An **accurate diagnosis** is very important, and every effort should be made thoroughly to examine and investigate the patients with a suspected disorder to establish the correct diagnosis. Help may be sought from the regional genetic centre which may have additional facilities for sophisticated tests and may hold a computerised data base of literature references. Such centres also maintain registers for many of the genetic disorders, and useful information may be available about either the patient or his relatives. Genetic heterogeneity may complicate the issue and may require special tests in the patient or family members.

For informative counselling it is imperative to estimate the **probability** of the event (e.g. the risk of recurrence) that concerns the person seeking advice. If the disease is known to have a *mendelian basis*, then the probability can be calculated according to the known mode of inheritance. For example, if a man's parent has Huntington's disease (which has a variable age of onset), then the man had a 50% chance of inheriting the gene at conception, but the longer he lives free of the disease, the greater the chance that he did not inherit the gene. Diseases that do not fit the mendelian rules of family segregation often fit the expectations for *multifactorial inheritance*, and the risk can be calculated according to the numbers of affected and unaffected relatives. Expert genetic counsellors, who have computer programmes based on the assumption of multifactorial inheritance, should be consulted in difficult cases.

Once an accurate diagnosis and probability have been established it is time for **informative**, **supportive** and **nondirective** counselling. The conversation must be kept simple and comprehensible, particularly when discussing the prognosis, probability of recurrence and reproductive options. Questions must be encouraged and answered with empathy, and the discussions must be tailored to the individual after having taken into account the patient's emotional state, religious and ethnic background. It is desirable to involve the patient's family practitioner in the discussions. Further sessions should be arranged and long-term follow-up should be ensured, preferably through a regional genetic centre.

---

[26] Some of the questions that often necessitate counselling are:
1. My child was born with a handicap (e.g. spina bifida). What caused it? Will it happen again? Should we avoid having any more children?
2. I am a 30-year-old woman. My uncle has haemophilia. What are my chances of passing it on to my children?
3. My grandfather has developed Huntington's disease. Might I get it?
4. I am 35 years old and I am pregnant. My friends say that I should have a test that will show that my baby will be normal. Should I? What happens if it turns out to be abnormal? What are the dangers of the test?

Other examples from survey

1. **'What do you think of the "blind" use of antibiotics? When and why would you use them?'**

   The 'blind' use of antibiotics is justifiable when a patient with a serious infection, such as meningitis, pneumonia or an unexplained high fever, is too sick to be left untreated until adequate bacteriological information is available. Under such circumstances, the antibiotic cover should be aimed at an appropriate broad-spectrum antibiotic, e.g. gentamicin, a broad-spectrum penicillin or a cephalosporin together with metronidazole to cover anaerobes. In the 'blind' treatment of pneumonia, many physicians would add erythromycin to cover the possibility of an atypical pneumonia, especially Legionnaires' disease. Chloramphenicol should be added to penicillin if meningitis is suspected.

2. **'How would you teach immunity to medical students?'**

   (1) Start by asking simple questions about immunity and fill in the gaps. (2) Develop the concept of host-defense mechanisms and give simple examples of local, cellular and humoral immune systems. (3) Give them some homework for the next session.

3. **'Tell me what you know about Legionnaires' disease.'**

4. **'What are your views on night sedation in the elderly?'**

5. **'Tell me about carbon monoxide poisoning.'**

6. **'Tell me something about opportunistic infections.'**

7. **'What do you know about the chemotherapy of Hodgkin's disease?'**

8. **'Tell me something about dementia.'**

9. **'How do you investigate weight loss?'**

10. **'Tell me about familial mediterranean fever.'**[27]

e. Wild stories

There are three characteristic features of *Wild* Stories: (1) the questions mainly refer to **uncommon** medical problems or practice, and the examiners usually have either personal or secondhand knowledge of these; (2) the examiner almost invariably knows the correct answer; (3) you need not necessarily know the answer as long as you can give a common-sense approach befitting a trained clinician and do not 'go to pieces'. Usually, questions in this group are asked as light relief, and so rather than panic you should try to share the fun. If you happen to know something about the subject then it will be your chance to score a high mark. There is

---

[27] The candidate discussed the genetics of the condition, the populations affected, geographic distribution, pathology, clinical features of amyloidosis, renal disease and drugs.

no shame in admitting that you know nothing about the topic, but in most cases you can salvage something by adhering to the basics of medical management.

Examples

1. **'You are in the Emergency Room of a hospital somewhere in a third world country. A patient is brought in with a snake bite and his colleague has killed the snake which he has brought with him. How do you proceed?'**

   Obviously, the dead snake has been brought into the discussion for a purpose, so the least you can do is to suggest that you would send for an expert to identify whether it is poisonous or not. If you do possess some knowledge about poisonous snakes then you will examine the snake yourself as soon as you have assessed the patient.

   ■ 'The dead snake presents an opportunity to determine whether or not it is poisonous. A coral snake is colourful with alternating black, yellow and red stripes with very short fangs and can be deadly. Noncoral poisonous snakes generally have elliptical pupils, well developed hinged fangs and a single row of posterior scales. The second important question is to determine whether **venom** has been injected. This is easy if the culprit belongs to the *Crotalidae* family, as these cause severe pain, rapid swelling with ecchymosis, and one can usually see 1 to 4 adjacent fang marks. Coral snakes may not cause any local injury but there may be evidence of **systemic toxicity** (nausea, vomiting, muscle weakness, dysphagia, etc.) and the patient should be observed carefully in hospital. Nonpoisonous bites should be treated with **antitetanus** prophylaxis, local cleansing, frequent wound checks, and prophylactic antibiotic therapy with a cephalosporin. Patients with poisonous bites should be admitted and observed for systemic symptoms. General supportive care should be given, and antivenom administered if there has been significant evenomation.'

2. **'How do you manage hymenoptera stings?'**

   ■ 'Most hymenoptera stings (honeybees, bumblebees, wasps, fire and harvester ants, and yellow jackets) cause immediate pain and local reaction (itching, erythema and oedema) which resolve over a few hours. Although most patients developing *anaphylaxis* give no past history, they should be questioned about it and observed for 1 to 2 hours. Patients with a prior history of angioedema, bronchospasm, urticaria and anaphylaxis should be given 1:1000 (0.5 ml) adrenaline (intramuscularly) prophylactically. The wound should be thoroughly *cleansed* and if a *stinger* is present it should be *removed*. Patients who remain asymptomatic for 2 hours after the injury can be discharged and asked to return if wheeze or pruritus occurs. Patients with a systemic reaction should be admitted for the appropriate treatment.'

3. **'Name the diseases that are more severe (not merely more common) in women than in men.'**

Despite being biologically superior to their male counterparts and hardy survivors, women are peculiarly prone to more severe forms of some common diseases (hypertension, thyrotoxicosis, bronchial asthma, etc.), during some of their milestones (pregnancy, puerperium, menstruation, premenstrual period and menopause). Apart from pregnancy, during which the usual diseases become problematical to manage, women tend to have more severe forms of some of the common diseases such as **diabetes mellitus** and **bronchial asthma**. Difficult-to-manage ('brittle') diabetes mellitus tends to occur much more frequently in women than in men. Some women have a characteristic pattern of asthma that is difficult to manage and is termed '**brittle asthma**'. Women may have sudden and quite unpredictable falls in lung function with no obvious precipitating factors. Sometimes there is a large fall in lung function 2 to 3 days before the menstrual period. These attacks of asthma may sometimes be so severe as to require ventilation.

Many epidemiological studies have reported an association between oral contraceptives, **myocardial infarction** and **sudden death** in women over 40. Studies on the outcome of coronary artery bypass grafting have suggested poorer results in women than in men. The association between **cigarette smoking** and **myocardial infarction** is particularly marked in women who are otherwise at low risk of ischaemic heart disease (e.g. normotensive, normal weight and nondiabetic). There is accumulating evidence to show that **impaired carbohydrate intolerance** may be of greater importance in women than in men. Mortality rates from ischaemic heart disease are higher in diabetic women compared with diabetic men.

Considerable epidemiological evidence indicates that women are more susceptible than men to the adverse effects of **alcohol**, particularly with regard to liver damage. The basis for this difference is uncertain, although it may be due to higher blood alcohol concentrations in women, resulting from a smaller volume distribution because of their lower body water content, their larger body lipid content and a relatively **lower rate of alcohol dehydrogenase** activity in the gastric mucosa. Women may also be more prone than men to have **neuropsychiatric illnesses** related to alcohol consumption. **Systemic lupus erythematosus** is not only more common but also **more severe** in women than in men.

There may be other diseases which affect women more adversely than they do men. There is some evidence that AIDS has a worse outcome in women than in men. More work is needed fully to elucidate the outcome of various common diseases in the two sexes.

Other examples from survey

1. **'What is the Royal Free Disease?'**[28]

In July 1955, a resident and a ward sister in the Royal Free Hospital (London) developed an obscure illness which has since been recognised as myalgic encephalomyelitis. Seventy more members of staff were affected,

---

[28] pp. 18, 24

and the hospital had to be closed until October 1955. For this reason, the condition was referred to as the Royal Free disease, even though it was first described in 1934 in the USA. *

2. **'What drugs would you take to a desert island?'[29]**

Simple analgesics, opiates for severe injuries, antimalarials, antihistamines, hydrocortisone for anaphylaxis, and a few antibiotics.

3. **'Why are there a number of elderly Caucasian men in the UK with a positive hepatitis B antigen?'[30]**

4. **'What do you know about feigned illnesses?'**

f. Historical stories

As the name suggests, questions under this heading are related to historical events or personalities. You may invite these questions by name-dropping and using eponyms instead of descriptive titles (Babinski's response for extensor plantar) or the examiners may have a 'bee in the bonnet'.

Examples

1. **'Which sign did Wilson[31] miss in the disease that goes by his name?'**

Golden-brown or greenish rings in Descemet's membrane at the limbus of the cornea described by two ophthalmologists, Kayser and Fleischer, in hepatolenticular degeneration. The ring cannot be seen easily without the use of a slit-lamp, which is why Wilson, an astute clinician, missed it.

2. **'When were nitrates first used in angina pectoris?'**

In 1867, Brauton discovered the benefit of amylnitrite in angina.

3. **'Who was Osler?'**

A Canadian physician (1849–1919) who practised and taught medicine in Canada, England and America, and published well over 1000 articles, lectures and books on all aspects of medicine.[32]

---

[29] This question was asked at the time when Roy Plumley, a BBC broadcaster and founder of the *Desert Island Discs* programme, had just died.

[30] Acquired in the course of their travels during the Second World War.

[31] Samuel Alexander Kinnier Wilson (1878–1937) described hepatolenticular degeneration in his MD thesis in 1912, which won him the gold medal in Edinburgh.

[32] See also Appendix II.

9. CONTROVERSIAL SUBJECTS

Controversies arise in medicine, as they do in other disciplines, when there is no conclusive or hard evidence on which to base a decision, or when there is no uniform view on the ethics of a particular practice. As new diseases, aetiological factors, and therapeutic stratagems emerge, controversies shadow these until major studies are carried out to throw definitive light on the outcome. Some subjects never emerge clearly out of the smoke and dust of debate, and this is when there is no adequate literature to guide us. Unfortunately, some practitioners tend to harden their views with the passage of time without any concrete evidence to support their opinions. Since all medical practitioners will come face to face with some of these prevailing controversies at some stage in their career, it is inevitable that you may be asked for your opinions in this examination.

These questions are asked to probe the width of your knowledge of a subject, your understanding of the problems and general concern about them, your ability to critically evaluate the available evidence and abstract it, and your competence to justify your opinions. Tackling these issues can be very difficult; taking a strong position and stating very clear, dogmatic opinions can be risky and may annoy the examiners. Some candidates use a skilful ploy of passing the buck: '*My boss believes in . . . and follows . . .*', or '*Where I work the practice is to give anticoagulants to patients with atrial fibrillation only if they have moderately severe mitral stenosis*'. This approach may get you out of a tricky situation but it does not say much for your own clinical opinions, and introduces a doubt about *your* commitment to important medical issues. Besides, it sounds more like a narrative and less like an opinion, which is what has been asked for. An alternative, and sometimes successful, approach is to please the examiner by offering a view which you may have known, by his reputation, agrees with his own, e.g. 'There is no evidence to suggest that salt intake has anything to do with hypertension, since most epidemiological studies have concentrated on salt alone and ignored other environmental factors'. Some candidates who were certain about the examiners' views, put their conclusions even more vigorously, e.g. 'If anticoagulants were to be of any benefit in acute myocardial infarction, we would not be arguing 25 years after they were first tried'.

The urge to be so assertive should be restrained because the examiner, even though reputed to have the same view, may have formed his opinion after an exhaustive review of the literature together with long personal experience. Such well-informed examiners may see through your efforts to please them and may decide to challenge you! Our suggestion is that you should avoid giving authoritative opinions; what is required is a rational debate and a logical conclusion. For example, you may present both sides in answering a question such as the following.

1. **'Are coronary care units a worthwhile investment?'**

   ■ 'The proponents of coronary care units (CCU) point to the enormous amount of useful research that has been conducted in these units, the early detection and treatment of lethal arrhythmias, the reduction of early mortality following acute myocardial infarction, and the treatment of other cardiovascular emergencies that require continuous monitoring and intensive nursing care. On the other hand, the opponents remind us about some studies which have shown that there is little difference in the mortality between patients treated at home, in a general ward and in a CCU. They point out that 'hi-tech' equipment can frighten patients and so hamper rather than help their progress. Even if we admit that CCU care is not superior to home care for many patients, we cannot ignore that we have learnt a lot about the management of arrhythmias as a result of all the studies that have been conducted in such units, that more research needs to be done, and that these units are now needed to provide modern treatment such as thrombolysis after an acute myocardial infarction, and the emergency treatment of life-threatening arrhythmias.'

Such a middle-of-the-road approach allows you to give your personal opinion and also leaves room for discussion of the opposite point of view. Even if you have not formed a definite opinion on a subject you can dispassionately summarise the current debate on a popular subject.

2. 'What are your views on the value of health screening?'

■ 'The popularity of health screening is an inevitable result of widespread health education. If we believe, as we do, in increasing health education, then we must accept a wider application of screening. Unfortunately, vested interests have marched in to capitalise on it with the result that indiscriminate health checks are used without regard to age, disease and the level of care available. For example, it is difficult to justify mammography in young women, when the money would be better spent in identifying those who have a high risk of having myocardial infarctions and strokes. Due regard should also be paid to the fear that can be generated among healthy people.'

Ethical issues raise even more intense controversy than do problems related to medical or surgical treatment. The debate is often clouded by the plethora of discordant views coming from various interested groups and by the lack of any scientific evidence. Although one can offer only a personal opinion it should be supported by the reasoned views and recommendations of recognised authorities. The subject of AIDS is of universal concern, so you will be expected to have a well-informed opinion on questions like the following.

3. 'What are your views regarding HIV testing of patients?'

■ 'On the question of the ethics of HIV testing, Sir Douglas Black (president of the Royal College of Physicians, London, 1977–1983) wrote,[1] 'The ethical considerations relating to HIV testing are in general

---

[1]   Black D 1989 Ethics of HIV testing. Journal of the Royal College of Physicians (London) 23: 19

terms governed by the requirements for informed consent; for confidentiality; for access to counselling; and for the maximising of good and for the minimising of harm to the individual and to the community'. Even if a patient asks for AIDS testing, and a doctor agrees on good evidence that such a test should be carried out, the need for expert counselling should never be ignored. On the other hand, a clinical situation may demand the need to rule out AIDS, and sound professional judgement should then be exercised in the best interests of the patient. As recommended by the Annual Representative Meeting of the British Medical Association,[2] 'HIV testing should be performed only on clinical grounds and with the specific consent of the patient. There may be individual clinical circumstances where a doctor believes that, in the best interests of a particular patient, it is necessary to depart from this general rule, but if the doctor does so he or she must be prepared to justify this action before the General Medical Council.'

4. **'What is your view about the ethics of using human fetal tissue for research or for transplantation into patients suffering from Parkinson's disease?'**

Recent advances in the use of fetal cells for research and transplantation have created a major ethical debate. The question is often considered in terms of the ethical justification of destroying a potential life to save an established one.[3] The rights of the unborn have always been a contentious issue, which needs to be debated on the widest possible platform if any progress is to be made in this potentially explosive field of major scientific endeavour. The issue needs to be looked at from the point of view of four parties: the fetus, the pregnant woman, the investigator and the recipient.

The belief that the fetus is a potential human being entitled to life and freedom, and that it cannot defend itself, is the chief concern underlying the public debate. The propounders of fetal tissue research and transplantation believe that the tissue will be obtained only from those women who have chosen elective abortion for personal reasons. The protesters regard this view as being naive, since an increase in elective abortions for the sole purpose of obtaining fetal tissue will occur, especially if the use of the fetal tissue for transplantation holds even a slight promise of cure in diseases not otherwise amenable to treatment at present. It may be argued that adults are not killed for their organs even though organ transplantation is both legal and beneficial. Recent revelations about organ trade from the third world belie this argument. Besides, whereas killing an adult is illegal, abortion has legal sanction. Although a pregnant woman may have her own reasons for terminating her pregnancy, the use of monetary gain may prove irresistible for many women, and a fetal tissue industry may emerge in due course. The investigators have essentially altruistic motives of widening the frontiers of knowledge, and they follow

[2]   Scrutator 1988 *The week in Norwich*. British Medical Journal 297: 206
[3]   Many doctors, including one of the authors (REJR), believe that from the time of conception the fetus, with its unique and individual genetic code, *is already an established life* and deserves the same consideration as the potential recipient of its tissue. Because of personal and deeply held convictions, doctors such as this author, are opposed to abortions for any reason and to the use of fetal tissue for research.

strict ethical and scientific protocols. However, the anticipation of fame and glory, together with the academic pressures of having to undertake some research, may induce some to cut corners in obtaining fetal tissue. The possibility cannot be ruled out that an obstetrician may perform an abortion to become a coauthor on a scientific paper rather than for strictly medical reasons. The potential recipients of fetal tissue transplantation—i.e. patients with Parkinson's disease or type 1 diabetes (the two diseases for which clinical trials have been started) – have a strong lobby of their own. Both diseases have an ominous outlook despite the current treatment.

In view of the above considerations, several committees have been set up both here and in the USA to consider the various issues surrounding fetal tissue research and transplantation, and to formulate codes of practice. The Ministers of Health for England, Scotland and Wales set up a committee chaired by the Reverend Dr John Polkinghorne. The main guidelines set down by the Polkinghorne Report[4] are that great care should be taken in separating the decisions relating to the abortion from those relating to the subsequent use of the fetal tissue. There should be a central organisation which separates the institution carrying out the termination from that using the tissue for research.

The mother should not be informed of the specific use to which the fetal tissue may be put, nor whether it will be used at all. The NIH director's Advisory Committee of the USA has recommended the development of this potentially important line of research and treatment only in 'centres of excellence' following very strict ethical and clinical protocols.

Although some controversial issues have remained unresolved for many years, new ones keep cropping up. Some of the other topics that have recently featured in the MRCP viva examination are as follows:

1. **Anticoagulants in atrial fibrillation.**

2. **Steroids in meningitis.**

3. **Digoxin in heart failure.**

4. **Early against late discharge after acute myocardial infarction.**

5. **The value of a CAT scanner in a district general hospital.**

6. **Salt and hypertension.**

7. **Euthanasia.**

---

[4] Polkinghorne J 1984 Review of the guidance in the research use of foetuses and foetal material. HMSO, London

10. OLD CHESTNUTS

There are some general questions which have been recurring for many years. Even the answers are well known. The examiner may perhaps just throw one in while he or she is thinking of something more specific to ask. We present a few examples here and leave you to think of some more, and to ponder the answers along the lines outlined in earlier sections.

Examples

1. 'What is the value of the ESR in clinical practice?'

2. 'What are your views on night sedation in the elderly?'

3. 'How useful is an ECG machine in the casualty department?'

4. 'Tell me about the important problems in contemporary cardiology.'

11. BEES UNDER THE BONNET

It is one thing to show a man that he is in an error, and another to put him in possession of truth[1]

All examiners are clinical teachers, and over the years some of them become interested in a few unusual and eccentric subjects and questions, which are often an unorthodox variation of the normal repertory. Clinical demonstrations, being ever elastic and accommodating, allow bizarre theatricals, and clinical 'actors' enjoy stunning their students by asking them clever and off-beat questions. A distinguished American teacher used to enjoy asking students about the progress of a bolus of barium swallowed by a man standing on his head! Some students were inquisitive enough to subject themselves to the experiment to confirm that the barium would reach the stomach irrespective of the position of the subject. On one occasion, a contemporary teacher, who was well-known among his students for his idiosyncrasies, had finished a teaching session by the bedside of a patient with a massive pleural effusion. Instead of dismissing the well-satisfied students he took them to the side room and addressed them in sombre tones, 'Well, friends! I am left with a serious question which troubles me, and I hope you can help me with it. My houseman aspirated 3 litres of bloodstained fluid from this patient's right pleural cavity, it still contains at least a litre of fluid and a large part of the right lung can be seen on the X-ray. How is it that so much can be accommodated in one half of the rib cage when a fully expanded lung can at most contain only 2.5 litres of air?'[2] The tired students suddenly got a 'second wind' and started firing possible explanations which were rejected one by one on logical grounds. The same teacher, after demonstrating the apex beat on a patient with severe aortic incompetence asked, 'The left ventricle contracts during systole, in other words, becomes smaller towards the aortic root. How does it contrive to hit the chest wall?' In the ensuing discussion, students felt compelled to suggest that the apex beat is a diastolic event when the left ventricle is full of blood and more likely to hit the chest wall. To which the teacher softly retorted, 'Unless of course the left ventricle is obeying Newton's Third Law of Motion during systole!'

Another distinguished teacher, now retired, would start his session by a gentle enquiry, 'Before I discuss hypertension with you, maybe you could tell me something. How does a patient with hypertension present?' After hearing a galaxy of symptoms he would say triumphantly, 'It is asymptomatic, don't you know? Mostly discovered on an incidental medical examination'.

---

[1]   John Locke (1632–1704)

[2]   The rib cage expands to accommodate the extra fluid in massive pleural effusion, and contracts on aspiration of the effusion.

No doubt you have similar experiences and can add many more to those presented here. Our purpose was to present the background to some of the idiosyncratic and individualistic questions that find their way into the viva section of the MRCP examination. It should be pointed out, in fairness to such eccentric teachers, that the underlying purpose of their distinctive and unorthodox style of teaching is to make students think for themselves. Anyone can teach but very few can train, and still fewer can teach their students, or some of them at any rate, how to think and learn. The MRCP examination is not only a test of competence but it can be, and often is, an educational experience which induces students to think about the subjects they had previously taken for granted. It is with this understanding that such off-beat questions, and examiners asking them, should be approached. What is required is sensitivity and consideration and not a brash dismissal of what may appear to be an examiner's pet bee under his or her bonnet!

Thus, in answer to the question, '**What is the noblest invasive procedure of them all?**', you may not know the examiner's own answer (**manual removal of faeces**), and he may not get a chance to discuss the subject of constipation with you, but you can attempt to think on your feet and suggest one of your own, such as 'mouth-to-mouth respiration', and play the game as an equal.

Candidates have to be aware of two problems which bedevil questions in this group: (1) answers are as personal to the examiner as his questions; and (2) it can be very difficult to guess the right ones. However, if the examiners' eccentricity is a true manifestation of their intellectual rigour, then they will accept any honest attempt and enjoy the ensuing discussion. For example, in the following questions, we believe that any of the answers given could lead to a fruitful discussion. Our suggested answers are given in italics, and the examiners' answers, where known, are marked in bold print.

1. **'What is the most important discovery made by human beings on the earth?'**

   Cultivation of food, wine, music, fire.

2. **'What is the most important scientific discovery of the last three centuries?'**

   Sewage disposal, electricity, telecommunication.

3. **'What are the most important new advances in endocrinology?'**

   Growth hormone-releasing hormone, somatostatin analogues, growth of neuroendocrinology.

4. **'If you were the Queen of the United Kingdom, what would be your ideal diet that you would like to prescribe for everyone?'**

   A balanced diet that is based on the recommendations from a National Advisory Body such as COMA[3] or NACNE[3], or the one that was

---

[3]   COMA – Committee on Medical Aspects of Food Policy
       NACNE – National Advisory Committee on Nutrition Education.

constrained by rationing during the Second World War, *based entirely on natural foods* – undercooked vegetables, fruit including skins, even lemons and oranges, etc.

5. **'What is the most important pharmacological advance of the last decade?'**

Bromocriptine, **angiotensin-converting enzyme inhibitor, cyclosporin**.

6. **'Which is the worst drug ever produced?'**

Digitalis, thalidomide.

The other problem that candidates must take into consideration is that the examiner may have formed an extreme or unusual view coloured by his or her own experience. In answering a question where it seems that the examiner may not be in agreement with you or, for that matter, with common practice, you should address his concern and tread gently.

Other examples from survey

1. **'Give me an example of a nondrug.'** (metformin)[4]

2. **'Name an unacceptably dangerous drug.'** (indomethacin)[5]

3. **'Tell me about screening and treatment for hypercholesterolaemia.'** (expensive and not cost-effective)

A candidate can disagree with the examiner, but he should concede that the contrary opinion has been based on some genuine grounds which are worth taking issue with.

There is a small group of clinicians who like taking up unpopular causes. Such an examiner may ask a question because he or she has an opinion (e.g. aggressive use of parenteral nutrition in sick patients) which is not universally accepted or followed, or because the subject is unfairly neglected (e.g. zinc deficiency, malnutrition in hospitals, magnesium deficiency, etc.).

These examiners usually ask a question about an uncommon subject because they think it ought to be asked, or ask a question about a common subject because they have a different opinion. It is prudent to go prepared to discuss some of these subjects and make a positive contribution in the discussion with the examiners.

4. **'How do you diagnose zinc deficiency?'**

5. **'What are the clinical features of aluminium toxicity?'**

6. **'Does malnutrition occur in hospitals?'**

---

4 Considered to be useful in obese patients with diabetes mellitus, as it may help in weight reduction. The examiner presumably had had a disappointing experience with his/her obese patients.

5 A very effective nonsteroidal anti-inflammatory drug, but the examiner's view must have been coloured by a series of side effects in his patients.

7. 'We know that there is tachyphylaxis of headache; does the same apply to the beneficial effects of nitrates?'

8. 'How do you diagnose magnesium deficiency?'

9. 'What is the link between haemochromatosis and DVT?'[6]

10. 'Is oesophageal reflux an overworked diagnosis?'[7]

11. 'Is renal transplantation a cost-effective means of treatment in end-stage renal failure compared with chronic ambulatory peritoneal dialysis and haemodialysis?'

New opinions are always suspected, and usually opposed, without any other reason but because they are not already common.[8]

---

[6] The examiner's answer was polycythaemia.

[7] It is certainly a common problem and, like all common conditions, it is sometimes diagnosed on insufficient evidence by a busy clinician.

[8] John Locke (1633–1704) Essay Concerning Human Understanding.

Section 3
Viva experiences

The most vivid fiction yields far fewer lessons than the dullest true story!

The overall key seemed to be ensuring that I was safe rather than omniscient.[1]

---

[1] p. 103

The examiner asked me to pretend that he was the mother of a diabetic adolescent and to give her advice on the management of her daughter. I found it extremely difficult to treat him as anything other than an examiner.[2]

The other examiner mouthed 'phrenic nerve' and I felt dreadful.[3]

In this section we present the reports of viva encounters selected from over 300 detailed questionnaires sent to us by the MRCP candidates over the last four years. We hope that going through these will give you a ringside view of the viva encounters, and prepare you for answering the initial, and responding to the supplementary, questions. We have made only minor alterations to the format in which they were written and thereby have preserved the atmosphere as perceived by the candidate. However, we have added footnotes whenever we felt that the scenario given by the examiner could have been treated in a specific way (e.g. *Ghost* or *Detective* Story, etc.), and wherever we thought that the account may lead the reader to the wrong conclusion. In the main, you are free to draw your own conclusions and prepare your own answers. The most important lesson to draw from these experiences is that you need to address the main concern of the examiner as suggested by the phrasing of his question.

As in Section 2, we have provided extra information in the footnotes whenever we felt that it would not be readily available in a textbook. Thus, we hope that this book will be helpful to you regarding the areas not well covered in standard textbooks or lecture notes.

To make the best use of this chapter, we suggest that you read each experience as if you are in the 'hot seat' answering the questions. Once you assemble all the information necessary to answer a question, you should practise narrating it to a friend, or to a dictaphone, and then assess the success of your performance. It may take several weeks to work through the entire book in this way, but it will leave you well equipped to cope with the viva in all of its diversities.

---

[2]   p. 141
[3]   p. 237

1

I was asked, firstly, about the **management of a 35-year-old man with mild hypertension** (BP 160/105). They seemed to be looking for how I would reassure the patient and his wife that no immediate treatment was necessary. They were happy that I would take a full history (they did not probe me on this), and I made sure to give an impression that I would look for all the secondary causes for a raised BP. They then coaxed me into defining how much endorgan damage there could be – retinopathy (and they asked me to describe the four grades[1]), nephropathy and cardiac effects (particularly **left ventricular hypertrophy**, which they asked for a definition of by **voltage criteria**[2] and LV 'strain'). They then asked me to describe briefly the measures to lower the BP before using drug therapy[3] – weight reduction, stopping smoking, etc. – which they seemed satisfied with.

I quoted the MRC trial on mild hypertension and they seemed happy with that.[4]

The second and final topic I was asked about was the **management of a patient** (a young woman in her early twenties) who presents with **rectal bleeding**. I started by saying the usual – full history and examination.

---

[1] **Grades of hypertensive retinopathy**
1. *Arteriolar narrowing* with undue *tortuosity* of the vessels, a *silver-wire appearance* of the arteries because of an increase in the central axial light reflex of the artery.
2. *Arteriolar-venous nipping* caused by the thickened arteriolar wall where it crosses the veins, resulting in venous dilatation distal to the crossing.
3. *Exudates and haemorrhages*: soft exudates (cotton-wool spots) suggest local ischaemia; haemorrhages and hard exudates (shiny spots with well-defined margins) reflect vascular leakage. Microaneurysms may occur which indicate irreversible changes in the capillaries.
4. *Papilloedema*.

[2] See p. 52

[3] **Nonpharmacological treatment of hypertension**
1. *Dietary salt*: several studies have shown that reducing salt intake reduces the blood pressure in hypertensive patients
2. *Obesity*: true hypertension, measured with an adequately sized cuff, will show a fall with weight reduction
3. *Alcohol* intake increases blood pressure and all hypertensive subjects should be questioned about this contributory factor
4. *Stress*: the effect of stress on blood pressure is difficult to quantitate. However, relaxation therapy has been shown to produce a fall in blood pressure (Br Med J 1985; 290: 1103)
5. *Smoking* is a risk factor for cardiovascular disease and it should be discouraged in hypertensive subjects. Antihypertensive drugs are less effective in smokers than in nonsmokers (Br Med J 1980; 3: 191; N Eng J Med 1984; 310: 951)
6. *Vegetarian diet* has an antihypertensive effect, and a return to a 'normal' diet raises the blood pressure again (Br Med J 1986; 293: 1468). Further, vegetarian meals are a cheaper way of reducing the intake of animal fat and thereby the serum cholesterol level. Hypertensive subjects should be encouraged to declare two or three days of the week as 'vegetarian days'.

[4] 1. Medical Research Council Working Party 1985. MRC trial of treatment of mild hypertension: principal results. British Medical Journal 291: 97–104
2. Medical Research Council Working Party 1988. Stroke and coronary heart disease in mild hypertension: risk factors and the value of treatment. British Medical Journal 296: 1565–1570.

Unfortunately, I got cornered by them on the infective causes of diarrhoea after talking about travel abroad. I quoted *Campylobacter*, *Yersinia*, and *Salmonella*, but they really had to encourage me to remember *Shigella* and amoebic dysentery – my mind went completely blank. They asked me what was the general name given to bloody diarrhoea of an infective origin, and I thought of everything except dysentery – so simple but under the stress of the viva I simply couldn't remember!

I then told them about the importance of sending a specimen of stool to exclude infection, but this girl obviously had **ulcerative colitis**. She had bloody diarrhoea and tenesmus. They asked me which type of inflammatory bowel disease it was likely to be. I said ulcerative colitis and they were happy with that. They then asked me about the treatment. I told them about local or systemic steroids, intravenous rehydration and transfusion if necessary, but they were more interested in the development of **toxic megacolon**. They asked me how I would check for this, and seemed to be satisfied with serial abdominal X-rays. They were quite complimentary to me when I talked about the dangers of sigmoidoscopy and rectal biopsy in this case. They were also happy with my decision to refer to a surgeon if medical management failed.

Impressions: I thought I had done badly on the short cases, having been taken to see two hearts, and also had not done particularly well on the long case (which I was not asked to examine with the examiners as it was a case of neurogenic diabetes insipidus).[5] After the viva, where I was asked on only two topics, I was convinced I had failed and was very depressed walking away from St Stephens.

The examiners in the viva were both very pleasant and not aggressive, and I thought gave me a lot of help with the questions – this again worried me as I thought they were probably feeling sorry for me. I was examined in a small room with a long rectangular table, the two examiners on one side and myself on the other. The time went incredibly quickly. There was a sympathetic registrar outside to keep one away from the wards and his parting words were 'Don't worry, I'm sure you have passed'.

(*Passed*)

---

[5]   This was a patient with post-traumatic diabetes insipidus, and the candidate had taken a rather inadequate history and had not asked about menstruation, galactorrhoea, etc.

2

The viva was the last part of the examination. There were three pairs of examiners and three of us. The examiners stuck well to their timetable so that at no point did any of us have to wait for more than a minute or so. The examiners I had for the viva had both come up from London, their names being familiar to me. They were both polite and introduced themselves; one was a little more brisk than the other but the terms *'hawk'* and *'dove'* would be too extreme to describe their behaviour. The viva took place in a side ward which had been set up for the occasion and the environment was as comfortable as it could be under the circumstances. I was not asked what job I was doing or had done, nor if there was anything I was particularly interested in.

The first examiner was basically asking about **acute tubular necrosis (ATN) and trauma**. He did this by way of a scenario: **'You are on ITU awaiting a 20-year-old man who is in theatre following a *road traffic accident* – what would you anticipate?'** It seemed to take me a long time to get towards the right answer (after a few offerings to **'any other abdominal organs that you would consider?'**), when I finally realised that he wanted to talk about the kidney. I then went straight into ATN without even considering other causes of oliguria such as perioperative ligation of ureters, etc. (I was not doing my current job then.) After this initial rough start, we maintained a reasonable dialogue covering the **course and management of ATN**, and especially the **management of hyperkalaemia**. The examiner was a renal physician and, perhaps because I knew this, I had subconsciously assumed that he would not be asking questions about his own topic. I had considered every organ bar the kidney! To be fair, beyond asking about the **indications for dialysis in hyperkalaemia**, the word dialysis did not come up, and it was very much a general physician's, rather than a nephrologist's, approach to ATN.

The second examiner, a rheumatologist, asked about acute **mono-arthropathy**, again via a scenario: **'The casualty officer refers . . . .'** I gave a differential diagnosis and a management plan. He had specifically been considering **gonococcal arthritis** and the closest I got to it was 'septic' and he seemed a little irritated, although not unduly so, by this. He really wanted to be reassured that I would ignore negative blood cultures if I believed the patient to be 'septic', and the overall key seemed to be ensuring that I was safe rather than omniscient. He then asked two questions relating to a **raised uric acid**, again in the form of a patient in the outpatient clinic. For the one with a very high level we discussed causes such as myeloproliferative diseases; for the other, a businessman with borderline levels, I said that I would repeat the test but did not mention that I would not perform it when the patient was fasted[1] – he had to tell me this. We also covered whether to commence allopurinol in a patient with a history of attacks of gout and he seemed not to agree with my answers.[2]

Finally, the viva covered how I would set up a **public health campaign aimed at hypertension** in a city such as Glasgow. I was entirely unprepared for this question and was a little unsure of epidemiological evidence to support my proposed manoeuvres.

Impressions: Generally, neither examiner could be described as being awkward or unfair. I felt that I had probably failed the viva (I still do) but this had been entirely due to a poor showing on my part. Both examiners, contrary to the generally understood policy, asked about subjects related to their own speciality although, in retrospect, the scenarios they devised were really within the realms of general medicine and did not require any specialist knowledge. I think it is important not to be put off by this. I think it is also important to admit that you don't know an answer or didn't know at first when they asked (as happened to me); similarly, my experience was that when I was on the wrong track they attempted to lead me back.

The scenario type question in its various forms seems very popular but they do usually seem to have an underlying topic at which they are aiming. As with all the other parts of the exam, it is important to put mistakes behind you and to take each question afresh.

(*Passed the exam*)

---

[1] Hyperuricaemia is a characteristic feature of starvation probably due to a decreased uric acid excretion caused by the associated dehydration and ketoacidosis. Uric acid is reabsorbed in the proximal tubule and then secreted in the distal tubule. Conditions in which there is increased proximal tubular sodium resorption are generally associated with a fall in uric acid clearance and a rise in plasma urate level. Among these are **dehydration**, **salt restriction**, **volume depletion** secondary to diuretics (frusemide), **hypertension** and inadequately treated **diabetes insipidus**. The anions of many organic acids (ketoacids, lactate) interfere with the distal tubular secretion of uric acid, thereby increasing the plasma urate concentration.

[2] Most physicians do not prescribe allopurinol unless a patient has had two or more acute attacks of gout, or has urate deposits. In the early stages, it is advisable to combine allopurinol with a regular daily dose of colchicine (e.g. 0.6–1.2 mg) to prevent the recurrence of acute attacks.

3

The whole examination was in the private wing, and the vivas were held in a private patient's room.

The entire viva rested on hypothetical situations.

'A 19-year-old girl was brought into casualty, moribund and cyanosed with a rash developing on her legs. No heralding illness.'
(It was obviously **meningococcal septicaemia**).

He was clearly impressed by my practical approach: 'After a cursory examination I would set up a drip, take cultures, check clotting, etc.'

'What IV fluid?'

'N/saline,' I answered. He said, **'I'm glad you're dealing with the true problem'**. He asked the dose of penicillin and the route. We discussed the blood pressure, the use of steroids, Waterhouse–Friderichsen syndrome,[1] etc. He asked the mortality, and a leader in the *BMJ* which I had read six months ago, helped to give the correct answer.

'How would you manage a surgical patient who you are called to see with postoperative oliguria?'

I planned the approach – history, examination and special investigations to differentiate the prerenal, renal and postrenal causes, emphasising the latter. He asked what could be done to decrease the period of oliguria, saying, **'think carefully before you answer'**. I said a loop diuretic, and he replied there was no evidence for this and prompted me to say mannitol.[2]

The other examiner then took over.

---

[1] Haemorrhagic infarction of the adrenals often occurs in fulminant meningococcaemia (Waterhouse–Friderichsen syndrome). It was first observed by Ernest Gordon Graham Little, a London physician, in 1901, but the credit goes to Rupert Waterhouse (b. 1873), a Bath physician who described the syndrome in 1911, and to Carl Friderichsen (b. 1886), a Danish paediatrician who described it in 1918.

[2] The use of mannitol also has its detractors and hazards (pulmonary oedema). The anticipated therapeutic effect is achievable if frusemide or mannitol is administered within two days of the onset of the oliguria. It has been proposed that the course of acute renal failure may be modified in one of three ways: (1) functional abnormalities may be reversed and the degree of organic damage reduced; (2) the length of the oliguric phase may be shortened; and (3) the diuretic phase may ensue and dialysis may not be required. However, there are no firm data to support these suppositions. Studies have demonstrated that the short-term use of frusemide does not improve the clinical picture of patients with *established* acute renal failure (Am J Med 1975; 58: 510; Nephron 1976; 17: 51). Nonetheless, it is justifiable to attempt to produce a diuresis with a single injection of mannitol 12.5 g or an infusion of frusemide 250 mg over an hour.

'A drunken alcoholic presents in casualty with a unilateral sixth nerve palsy'.

There followed a discussion of the relevant causes. I stressed that the clinical examination would determine the need for a CT scan (other signs, increased BP, fall in pulse rate, bruises, etc.). They asked what the pathology was in Wernicke's and which important vitamin was not present in *parentrovite*[3] – I didn't know.

'A young woman is *hyperthyroid three weeks after an IVP.'*

I was lost here, saying that iodine from the contrast could cause this,[4] and I asked whether she was clinically hyperthyroid – she was. I got stuck by not remembering how carbimazole worked.

'Does it block iodine trapping?' I asked. He said that this is a gland full of iodine. I said that this patient's thyroid gland was probably deficient in iodine. I then said she'd be better before most treatments had worked, but the whole question went badly.

Somewhere along the line, a question about **thromboses** in *dried-out* alcoholics arose. They coerced me into saying that there were antiplatelet antibodies in alcoholics[5] – in fact I thought it was not known – but I said it with confidence hoping it was right.

---

[3]   A bee-under-the-bonnet question. Parentrovite contains vitamins B and C but not all the members of the B group, e.g. pantothenic acid, biotin and vitamin B_{12} are absent. Although any one of the last-mentioned three vitamins may have been this examiner's 'bee', we suspect that he was a parenteral nutritionist and that he probably wished to discuss the suitability of a more comprehensive water-soluble vitamin preparation such as *Solivito N* for prolonged use. From an alcoholic's standpoint, the examiner's 'bee' may have been folic acid, which is missing both in *parentrovite* and in an alcoholic diet, since few heavy alcoholics are ever sober enough to consider, or can spare the time, to eat leafy vegetables.

[4]   The candidate was right in blaming the heavy dose of iodine which the patient received during the IVP. Expert thyroidologists tell us that this is possible even with modern contrast media, and that they have seen a wide variety of abnormalities in thyroid function tests after such radiographic procedures. Frank iodine-induced thyrotoxicosis (Jod-Basedow phenomenon) after the administration of contrast media is rare, but occurs in sensitive (i.e. iodine deficient) subjects or in those with goitres. In most such cases, the thyroid gland is free from TSH regulatory control.

[5]   This is one of those factual questions which sound straight forward enough but often carry a sting in the supplementary tail! (p.58). In this case, the candidate was apparently forced into saying that there are antiplatelet antibodies in alcoholics, for which there is no evidence. A galaxy of platelet abnormalities have been reported in alcoholics. Alcohol can cause thrombocytopaenia through a direct toxic effect which is not dependent on concomitant folate deficiency. Alcoholics not only have a reduced number of platelets, but impaired function and structural abnormalities (i.e. giant platelets with increased granularity) are also found in the circulating platelets. Alcohol seems to be working as a metabolic poison since there is a decreased intracellular adenosine 5'-diphosphate (ADP) and a reduced rate of its release following appropriate stimuli. A series of papers on the medical consequences of alcohol was published as a book by the New York Academy of Sciences in 1975 (Volume 252). The possibility that some of the effects may be due to an antiplatelet antibody was explored but no evidence was found.

Somehow, **milk-borne infections**[6] were asked about; he seemed to want to hear me say listeriosis – it was topical but I wasn't sure if it was milk-borne.

(*Passed*)

---

[6] **Milk-borne pathogenic micro-organisms**
1. *Tubercle bacillus* – seldom now in developed countries
2. *Brucella abortus* – usually from infected udders
3. *Streptococci* – may be excreted or from human carriers
4. *Staphylococcus aureus* – mastitis
5. *Corynebacterium diphtheriae* – from the throat or nasopharynx of human carriers
6. *Typhoid, paratyphoid*, dysentery bacteria – usually from human contact though *Salmonella*, particularly *typhimurium*, may be excreted in milk
7. Less commonly, *listeria monocytogenes, toxoplasma, rickettsia, campylobacter fetus*; polio and hepatitis viruses in developing countries.

4

The main problem was that the examiner always had one particular answer in mind and it became an exercise in mind-reading. Whatever else I said, however correct, didn't seem to count. It went something like this:

**Examiner 1
(a hawk):** 'We'll start with an easy question: What are the risk factors for ischaemic heart disease?'

'Smoking, high cholesterol, age, family history, hypertension, obesity.' [1]

**Examiner 1
(interruption):** 'What is much more important than any of those you mentioned?'

I couldn't think of anything. Long pauses! I went back over those I'd mentioned to make sure that they had heard them. They kept pushing this one question for what seemed like ages, then asked, '**Suppose you are a GP doing a routine medical, what would you check?**'

I said a few things and when I mentioned 'Check the urine,' they jumped on this and said, '**Wasn't diabetes a risk factor for ischaemic heart disease?**' I agreed that it was (I didn't think it was 'much more' important than everything else but I didn't argue).

Examiner 1: 'Do you know anything about sleep apnoea?'[2]

'Something', and then I proceeded to make a mess of telling them about it by only talking about the obstructive type and by not knowing the precise definition in terms of times per hour, which was what they had wanted.

---

[1]   Notwithstanding the bee under the examiner's bonnet (diabetes mellitus), this haphazard presentation would not distinguish the candidate from many a lay person's account, since many people have been made well aware of these by the media. Only a well-informed doctor such as a postgraduate physician would know that a bad family history of ischaemic heart disease is more important than the three factors – smoking, high cholesterol and age – mentioned *before* it. A methodical approach listing the risk factors in their order of importance, would have reduced the risk of interruption with a dangerous and unforeseen supplementary question.

[2]   A typical *Bedtime* Story question in which the candidate is invited to say as much as he knows. Apnoea (cessation of airflow for 10 s) occurs in normal people during rapid eye movement (REM) sleep, but the number of episodes seldom exceeds 30 during a normal 7–8 hour sleeping period. Prolonged and frequent episodes during *both* REM and nonREM sleep, associated with hypoxaemia occur in patients with massive obesity, maxillary bone hypoplasia, large tonsils, acromegaly, musculoskeletal deformities, myopathies, alcoholism and a wide variety of neurological disorders. Sleep apnoea is classified as *central* when there is a complete absence of thoracoabdominal movements, and *obstructive* when there are exaggerated and ineffectual thoracoabdominal movements (pharyngeal cavity narrows and the airflow ceases). *Mixed* episodes occur in most patients with the **sleep apnoea syndrome**. Excessive daytime somnolence, loud snoring associated with obstructive apnoea, early morning headaches, depression, chronic fatigue and impotence are the presenting features. Weight reduction in obese patients and abstinence from alcohol are effective in reducing the frequency of apnoeic episodes. Tracheostomy should be considered in cases with persistent obstructive apnoea.

Examiner 2:   'Tell me about *water conservation.*' I obviously looked slightly taken aback, because he added, '*in the body*'.

I thought they wanted to know how the kidney worked, and after a preamble about the importance of the skin in conserving water, which didn't seem to interest them, I embarked on a discussion about volume receptors and osmoreceptors and the loops of Henlé. It turned out that they were really wanting to talk about **inappropriate ADH**,[3] and there followed a question about the approach to a patient with a low Na^+, which was much more straightforward but I had already lost a lot of time.

Examiner 2:   'You are a GP and are called to see a patient whom you *diagnose as having a pneumonia*, what do you do?'[4]

There followed a relatively straightforward discussion on the criteria for admission, likely organisms and the first-line antibiotics based on the British Thoracic Society survey.[5]

I tripped over my chair on the way out, forcing the metal leg over the concrete floor with a noisy effect.

(Failed; obtained a score of 4/10 in the viva and also failed in short cases.)

---

3   p. 46
4   Numerous candidates reporting back to us have complained that it is unfair to be asked to pretend to be a general practitioner in a higher examination for hospital practice! In most cases, the examiners are asking for an initial clinical assessment which a hospital practitioner should be able to provide. It is also possible that a GP may ring you for advice and you would have to look at the problem from *his point of view*!
5   British Thoracic Society 1987 Q J Med 62: 195.

5

I greeted the two examiners and I had barely sat down when the first examiner asked:

Examiner 1: **'Tell me the indications for *oral hypoglycaemic drugs*.'**

I said failure of dietary control in a type II diabetic. The examiner, who was rather aggressive[1] pressed me to tell him how I would know if the diet had worked.[2] I said by asking the patient; I should have said by looking at the weight chart.

Examiner 1: **'What oral hypoglycaemic drug would you use?'**

I said, 'Glibenclamide.'[3]

Examiner 1: **'Why glibenclamide?'**

I said it is a once-a-day drug and works by increasing the release of insulin.

Examiner 1: **'What other drug would you use?'**

'Metformin, particularly if one wants them to lose weight.'

Examiner 1: **'What *side effects of metformin* do you know?'**

'Lactic acidosis.'[4]

Examiner 1: **'Have you seen a case of lactic acidosis?'**

'No'.

Examiner 1: **'What would you warn the patient about?'**

'Not to drink excessive amounts of alcohol.'

Examiner 1: **'Tell me the uses of *occupational therapy*.'**

I said that occupational therapy is used in helping a person who has suffered major trauma to learn to live as normal a life as possible. I gave an example of a patient with a stroke who can be helped by various home aids and can be re-educated to dress and feed himself. I forgot to mention home visits but mentioned alterations in the house such as installation of special kinds of doors.

---

[1] The candidate had not given a complete answer and it is not surprising that the examiner was getting a little agitated.

[2] Inadequacy of dietary measures for type II diabetes mellitus is indicated, in obese patients, by persistent hyperglycaemia in the face of weight loss (which suggests that the patient is adhering to a low calorie intake).

[3] Short and unsupported answers invite questions of the examiner's choosing, and the candidate then loses control over the ensuing discussion.

[4] The main side effects of metformin are gastrointestinal, especially diarrhoea which is sometimes transient. Lactic acidosis is very rare with metformin, occurring almost exclusively in patients with renal or hepatic impairment. See also p. 121

Examiner 2: The other examiner, who was more gentle, took over and asked me about **medical problems associated with flying**, in particular the cardio-respiratory ones. I mentioned hypoxia[5] which he was not pleased with and asked, **'What other problems?'** I said, 'Deep venous thrombosis.' He said, **'Good – why?'** I said, 'Venous stasis.' He added, **'Excess alcohol consumption in planes also contributes.'**[6]

He followed by asking about a man who went to East Africa and came back with a **headache (of sudden onset)**. I mentioned meningitis and subarachnoid haemorrhage. What he wanted was **cerebral malaria**.[7]

Finally, he asked about the **management of type II respiratory failure**. I gave a comprehensive account very quickly, as that was my easiest question.

(*Passed*)

---

[5] See p. 228

[6] The water content of the air in the cabins of aeroplanes is low because it is obtained from the outside, where the water content is negligible because of the high altitude and low temperature. Under these circumstances it is advisable to maintain a high fluid intake with low osmotic fluids, together with some degree of physical activity (e.g. regular walks up and down the aisle). Excessive alcohol consumption causes an osmotic diuresis and compounds the dehydration and venous stasis.

[7] Patients with malaria can get headaches without cerebral involvement.

6

Examiner 1: 'A 55-year-old female presents with *jaundice*. How would you investigate?'

Answer: 'A full history regarding previous jaundice, transfusions, intravenous drug abuse, tattoos, travel abroad, drug history, anaesthetics, alcohol, and a family history of Wilson's, Gilbert's, etc. I'd ask if she had any pain suggestive of gallstones or pancreatic carcinoma.'

Examiner 1: 'All negative!'

Answer: I'd examine her for jaundice, xanthelasma, Kayser–Fleischer rings, palmar erythema, Dupuytren's contracture, spiders, enlarged lymph nodes, palpable liver, spleen or gall bladder, tender right upper quadrant, etc.'

Examiner 1: 'Examination was normal.'

Answer: 'Investigations – FBC (note MCV, platelets, ESR); coagulation screen; U&E, LFT and gamma GT; hepatitis A, B; smooth muscle and antimitochondrial antibodies, ANF, Rh factor; urinalysis for urobilinogen and bilirubin.'

Examiner 1: 'Bilirubin 60; alkaline phosphatase 300; AST and ALT 50–60; others normal.'

Answer: 'Ultrasound?'

Examiner 1: 'Normal.'

Answer: 'Liver biopsy after a coagulation screen.'

Examiner 1: 'Evidence of extrahepatic obstruction.'

Answer: 'ERCP.'

Examiner 1: 'Why not question the ultrasound and biopsy results first?'

(*Diagnosis: sclerosing cholangitis.*)[1]

---

[1]   An interesting *what dunnit?* clinical story, excellently played by the examiner and the candidate. More than half the cases of **sclerosing cholangitis** are associated with **ulcerative colitis**, males predominate over females, and the peak incidence is in the third or fourth decade. Endoscopic retrograde cholangiopancreatography (ERCP) is of great help in showing the beaded, irregularly narrowed and somewhat attenuated *intrahepatic bile ducts*. However, the definitive diagnosis and the exclusion of a carcinoma can only be made at operation.

Examiner 1:   'A woman aged 39 presents to her GP with *acute breathlessness*. However, on arrival at the A&E, she was found to be quite all right. How would you investigate?'

My approach was to suggest asthma which was probably treated by the GP, foreign body, arrhythmia, LVF or pulmonary embolism.

(*Diagnosis:* **Phaeochromocytoma** – *acute hypertensive crisis with LVF.*)[2]

Examiner 2:   'Tell us about the *haemolytic uraemic syndrome* with reference to recent publications in the Lancet.'

Examiner 2:   'What are genetically engineered materials?'[3]

Examiner 2:   'What is retrovir and its place in AIDS?'[4]

I was a little lost in the second half.

(*Passed*)

---

[2]   The manner with which the first question was conducted should have alerted the candidate that this examiner enjoyed *Detective* and *Ghost* Stories. The scenario presented in the second question satisfies the criteria for a *Ghost* Story (p.74) with a number of possibilities (as were given by the candidate) and a *ghost-link* that the patient was normal when examined in the Emergency room. Of all the contenders mentioned by the candidate, an episode of left ventricular failure, precipitated by either an arrhythmia or a paroxysm of hypertension, is the only condition compatible with a normal clinical examination. Often, the crisis has passed off by the time the patient is seen. In some cases of phaeochromocytoma, hypertension is truly intermittent and can be lethal. The candidate could have looked for an additional *ghost-link*, by enquiring whether the general practitioner had found anything abnormal (e.g. signs of LVF, hypertension, etc.) and whether the patient had received any treatment before being sent to the hospital.

[3]   p. 30

[4]   Retrovir or azidothymidine (also known as zidovudine, AZT and Compound S) is identical to thymidine with the exception that an azido (N_3) group has been substituted for a hydroxyl group. It is monophosphorylated by cellular enzymes. The triphosphate form inhibits retroviral reverse triphosphatase. Clinical studies in humans have shown that AZT can ameliorate most of the clinical and immunological manifestations of HIV infection.

7

The viva was my last section of this examination. I thought I had probably done reasonably well in the short cases just prior to this, and I was a bit euphoric (on adrenaline)! It was desperately hot; the organising registrar had given me a glass of water and I stood waiting for about three minutes while I sipped this, feeling as though I could tackle most things (not typical of my usual self!). I was then called into a small office. I looked superficially relaxed and smiling which I think probably helped to give the impression that I was confident and not overawed.

The examiners were friendly; they stood up and shook hands, smiled and introduced themselves. We all sat down. The first question was, **'Can you tell me what the *chi-squared test* is?'** I replied that it is a statistical test which is used to compare and examine the significance of a difference between an observed and an expected event. The next question was about when it would be particularly helpful.[1] I wasn't sure and said so, although I think I did try to be positive by saying that I thought it might be helpful when examining observed and expected death rates in large populations. This wasn't the answer he wanted but he seemed extremely pleased that I was able to say anything at all about the chi-squared test! The following questions I can't remember in detail but were about the definitions of *standard deviation, normal distribution* and *parametric* and *non-parametric* tests.[2]

He then asked me what I would do if I were called to see a **post-op thyroidectomy patient who was unwell, breathless and had a tachycardia**.[3] I said I would be thinking of a **thyroid crisis** or infection[4] (it was obvious he wanted the former so I concentrated on it). I said I would give potassium iodide, carbimazole and treat any heart failure with O_2 and diuretics. I then said that the patient might have been given potassium iodide already preoperatively and I got side-tracked into a discussion about how and when to give it preop, and what were its dangers. I didn't know most of this and had to say so.

---

[1]   The *chi-squared* test is a measure of the extent to which the observed numbers in the cells of a contingency table deviate from the values that would be expected if they were all identical. The test is used where the data are grouped, particularly when comparisons have to be made between more than two groups.

[2]   Appendix 1 and p. 47

[3]   This is a good example of a *what dunnit? Detective* Story, and the examiner has a single diagnosis in mind. **Thyroid crisis** consists of hyperpyrexia and an exacerbation of the features of thyrotoxicosis; it usually occurs within 48 hours of operation and is probably due to a release of hormone from the thyroid at operation or soon thereafter. This complication is uncommon nowadays as a result of an improved preoperative preparation. This entails rendering the patient euthyroid by antithyroid drugs, and then treating with iodine (potassium iodide 5 mg three times a day) for two weeks before surgery. Thyroid crisis is a serious complication and should be treated vigorously with rehydration, antithyroid drugs and large doses of iodide by mouth (10 mg four-hourly for four doses followed by six-hourly). Sympathetic blocking drugs such as propranolol are helpful in reducing sympathetic overactivity, and the temperature should be reduced by fans and tepid-sponging in cases of hyperpyrexia.

[4]   The candidate should also have considered the possibility that the patient might have bled into the wound, causing asphyxia.

This must have taken 10 minutes because the other examiner then took over. He asked me what I would do if I were called to see a **patient in casualty who claimed to have vomited approximately 500 ml of bright red blood**. (He first asked me which firm I was on; I was working at the Chalfont Centre for Epilepsy at the time so I told him this as quickly as possible!) I said I would first quickly examine the patient to assess his circulatory status before taking a history. He pushed this aside amiably and asked what would I do if he was not shocked and was able to talk. I said I would take a history and ask especially about alcohol intake, because one of the commonest causes of haematemesis is oesophageal varices. He asked me what else I would ask about and I couldn't think, but eventually he prompted me along to say 'NSAIDs'. We then went on to the examination. I mentioned all the features of chronic alcoholic liver disease I would look for (or most of them!) and we then went on to the management. I said I would cross-match blood, arrange FBC, chemistry, clotting, CXR, etc., and admit the patient for observation. He then asked what would I do if he continued to vomit blood. I said I would resuscitate him as necessary and arrange for an urgent endoscopy and sclerotherapy. He asked what I would do if he continued to vomit blood after **'your friendly endoscopist has performed sclerotherapy'**. I said I might use vasopressin, and he agreed, **'that would be worthwhile'**. He pushed me further – patient still vomiting blood despite vasopressin – and I said I would put down a Sengstaken tube (I hedged answering this for nearly 60 seconds because I went blank and couldn't remember the name!). He asked if I had ever put one down, and I said no, and he said it could be very difficult. At this point the other examiner chipped in with, **'Do you know where they are kept on the ward?'**, and I said no. He said, **'In the fridge'**. I then said that if I couldn't get the tube down I might ask my friendly endoscopist to do it which went down well and made them both laugh! The last question was, **'Tell me about antituberculous treatment'** – so I talked about using three drugs instead of one and why. We got on to the history of antituberculous drugs, which I did know once (and now!) but couldn't remember then. He asked me about the length of treatment and I gave two examples of common regimes. It was spoilt by the fact that I just couldn't remember the name of pyrazinamide! However, the examiners were friendly and smiling throughout.

(*Passed*)

8

The interview was held in a side room of a large ward and I was asked to wait outside for a few minutes before being invited in. Both examiners were extremely polite and pleasant throughout. The first question was asked by the elder of the two, who had a trimmed grey beard and half-moon spectacles (very much fitting the image of a professor, which his name badge proclaimed). He asked me what would go through my mind if I was requested, as an admitting registrar, to see someone who had **just returned from a holiday in Bangladesh and was now complaining of fever and malaise**. I said the first thing to go through my mind would be malaria, and a brief discussion on prophylaxis ensued. He then told me that the patient said he had been taking chloroquine tablets for a week before his trip and daily thereafter. We talked about resistance and drug treatment (in very scanty detail) and he then asked me for any other illnesses which should be considered. I obviously appeared to stumble here and he said, '**Surely I haven't exhausted your knowledge of tropical diseases?**'

'No, no, no, no of course you haven't,' I replied – which at the time wasn't exactly true. Somehow I dredged up from the caverns of my mind a picture of *Salmonella typhi* and managed to blurt out '**typhoid**'. This brought a smile of relief to both our faces and I then managed to talk a bit about the signs and symptoms of this disease as well as a few complications.

His second question ran something along the lines of, '**A 42-year-old executive had a BUPA health check which revealed a *cholesterol of 7.1 mmol/l and a normal triglyceride level*. He has been referred to the medical outpatients for treatment where you are asked to see him. What treatment would you advise?**'

I said, 'That would depend on the cause of his hypercholesterolaemia; myxoedema and alcoholism would need to be excluded first. I would also like to assess his cardiovascular risk profile by weighing him, asking about his family and personal history of coronary artery disease, measuring his BP and assessing endorgan damage (if any) with fundoscopy, urine testing and ECG (although hopefully this would all have been done by BUPA).' Having stated all that, I said the first line of treatment would be a low-fat, high-fibre diet (assuming this was first degree hypercholesterolaemia). Only if this failed would I go on to the drug treatment.[1] He asked which drug I preferred in this instance and, like an idiot, I blurted out **simvastatin**[2] which one of my teachers had predicted as being topical and I should

---

[1] A sensible approach to this problem.

[2] Belongs to the statin class of compounds which are inhibitors of 3-hydroxy 3-methylglutaryl coenzyme A (HMG CoA) reductase, an early and rate limiting step in the biosynthetic pathway of cholesterol. Simvastatin reduces the production of cholesterol in the liver, and increases the number of LDL receptors in the cell, thereby increasing LDL clearance. This mechanism of action makes it suitable for use in heterozygous familial hypercholesterolaemia (a condition with reduced numbers of LDL receptors).

mention. The examiner wanted to know about **cholestyramine** which in my fluster I was unable to remember, nor its mechanism of action[3] which was his next question.

I was then referred to the second examiner. He asked me what I would do if requested to see a **25-year-old primigravida**, who was **36 weeks pregnant** and had been admitted to the antenatal ward with a history of nausea and malaise for a few days, and on the second day in hospital she was noted to be **slightly jaundiced**.[4]

I said I would ask about drugs, travel abroad, infectious contacts, urine/stool colour change and other symptoms, followed by a full examination. I would then carry out investigations with LFT, U&E, hep A and B serology, viral titres, FBC and liver ultrasound. He said all these were normal apart from mildly elevated transaminases, and that the next day her jaundice had deepened and she had become drowsy and a bit confused. What would I do next? I said I would transfer her to ITU, insert a CVP line, check blood gases and U&E and repeat LFTs and clotting. He then asked me the likely diagnosis which I said was **fulminant hepatic failure of pregnancy** and he agreed.

He then asked me an easy question about **TB meningitis** and one more which I have completely forgotten.

(*Passed*)

---

3   Cholestyramine is the chloride salt of a basic anion-exchange resin which, when administered orally, is not absorbed and binds bile salts in the intestine. The removal of bile acids increases the hepatic conversion of cholesterol to bile acids, thereby decreasing the concentration of cholesterol.

4   A very well presented *Detective* Story with the underlying diagnosis of **acute fatty liver of pregnancy** in the examiner's mind. This syndrome of acute hepatic dysfunction develops typically after the 30th week of gestation, and is manifested initially by constitutional symptoms (e.g. malaise, nausea, abdominal pain, etc.) followed in many cases by jaundice and encephalopathy, which occasionally progress to fulminant hepatic failure. The only known treatment is termination of the pregnancy. Milder cases without frank hepatic failure have a favourable prognosis.

9

The viva was the last part of my clinical examination; the long and short cases had gone fairly smoothly. While waiting to go in I was nervous not so much about what was on the other side of the doors, but whether I was going to be able to get to the station in time to catch the last train out of Edinburgh. It seems that British Rail cannot understand why anyone should want to travel south of the border after 5 o'clock, and my viva was due to start at ten past four. Nearly every candidate who was there at the same time as me had the same problem, which was something that could have been avoided if the College had arranged earlier vivas for the candidates having long distances to travel. I had to wait for four hours between the clinicals and the viva. Luckily for me the vivas were running exactly to time.

The examination took place in the large hall of the Royal College of Physicians of Edinburgh. At my examination table there were three examiners, the third being an 'observer' from the Sudan who did not take part in any way apart from wishing me luck. He did a very good job of melting into the background and didn't make me feel any more nervous than I would have expected.

Both examiners were very pleasant although one was rather deaf and kept asking me to speak up. The first examiner was completely poker-faced and kept saying things like **'Oh, really!'** and **'Are you quite sure?'** which was very off-putting. Even when I was very sure that what I'd said was correct I began to have doubts, but I'd decided before going in to the examination that whatever I said I would stick by it and at least appear confident even if I was wrong, and that if I really didn't know the answer, I would tell the examiner so. It was evidently a policy that worked because by the end of the first half I was ready to give up all hope!

The first examiner started by asking:

Examiner 1: **'What vitamin deficiencies would you expect to find in an alcoholic?'**

Having dragged me through folic acid and vitamin C, neither of which was the answer he was obviously looking for, I eventually came to the answer I should have come out with immediately, which was **thiamine deficiency**. There was an almost terminal air of tension which magically lifted with this answer, and there were smiles all round. This didn't last long!

Examiner 1: **'What are the *effects of thiamine deficiency?'***

After a lot of grubbing around we got through the various neurological sequelae.

Examiner 1: **'Why do patients with thiamine deficiency get oedema?'**

My mind was a blank. 'I don't know,' I said. But he wasn't having any of this nonsense and kept on like a dog with a bone and eventually had to tell me the answer – had I heard of **beri-beri**? 'Yes, I'm afraid so,' wringing my hands and wanting to curl up and die. There was a pause. Perhaps we were about to leave the dreaded vitamins and go on to something more hopeful, but no.

Examiner 1: 'What about the effect of *vitamin deficiencies on the eye?*'

We discussed vitamin A and night blindness, the biochemistry of visual purple and eventually came on to Bitot's spots and keratomalacia.

Examiner 1: 'Describe the histology of Bitot's spots.'[1]

This was one of the moments when I decided to be bold, as there was a little voice at the back of my mind telling me that I knew the answer if only I could dredge it up. At everything I said the examiner raised his eyebrows and asked me if I was quite sure and did I really mean that, all designed to put me off. I'm very glad that I stuck to my guns because I looked up the answer straight afterwards and found that I was correct in all that I had said.

Examiner 1: 'What other vitamin deficiencies affect the eye?'

'I don't know.'

Examiner 1: 'What about *pernicious anaemia* and the eye?'

'**Proliferative retinopathy** due to severe anaemia?'

Examiner 1: 'Yes, what else?'

'I don't know.' The answer he wanted was **retinal haemorrhage**.

Examiner 1: 'Other vitamins and the eye?'

'Pyridoxine causing optic neuritis.'

Examiner 1: 'Yes, any more?'

'Vitamin K causing bleeding.'

Examiner 1: 'Yes, any more?'[2]

I really had reached the end by now. He finally let it go. I had spent nearly the whole first half of the viva squirming in a most unsatisfactory manner and scoring only a few points despite a good deal of hard work. Just before the bell went he asked for the causes of **sudden onset of confusion in an elderly woman**. I was much happier with this and managed a respectable list.

The second examiner was much more pleasant and encouraging. He asked about the management of **acute colitis**, a subject I knew well, and later about the **extraintestinal manifestations of inflammatory bowel disease**. He wanted to know which skin lesion was associated with ulcerative colitis. I couldn't remember the name but was able to describe the appearance of **pyoderma gangrenosum** which seemed to do almost as well. I was also asked about the **seronegative arthritides** and we touched

---

[1] Bitot's spots (named after Pierre Bitot, a French physician) are small white foam-like plaques containing epithelial debris and masses of *xerosis* bacilli. These are found in xerosis conjunctivae associated with vitamin A deficiency, but are not specific to it since they can be found in healthy eyes.

[2] **Malnutrition amblyopia** (retinoneuropathy) develops in patients with an inadequate and unbalanced diet, in particular with deficiency of vitamin B. Patients with this condition are unable to read small print, especially in bright light. **Ariboflavinosis** causes angular conjunctivitis (and angular stomatitis) with burning and itching sensations in the eyes.

briefly on HLA groups. The examiner was very positive and sympathetic, and seemed to realise that I was still squirming at the memory of the first part of the viva. He gave me every opportunity to show what I knew and managed to look pleased whenever I said something right. Even so, I felt dissatisfied with my performance and worried that I might have blown the whole thing with my lack of knowledge of vitamins.

(*Passed*)

10

I was waiting for the examination with someone I knew, which helped, but I don't think I have ever been so scared in my life! The viva was in a Sister's office with lots of space. The examiners were cool and completely nonreacting throughout; they gave an air of being cold and calculating.

The first examiner asked only about **oral hypoglycaemic drugs**.

Examiner 1: 'What is the role of the oral hypoglycaemic drugs?'[1]

I said the main role was in those noninsulin-dependent diabetics who could not be controlled on diet alone, i.e. (i) obese and (ii) elderly patients. However, they also expected me to include very high blood sugars in the newly diagnosed elderly patients.

Examiner 1: 'What factors would suggest that they are inappropriate treatments?'

I replied: (1) young patients; (2) thin patients; (3) recent weight loss; (4) failure to control the blood sugars adequately; (5) previous ketoacidosis.

I was then asked about the complications of the different types of oral hypoglycaemics and the effect of the half-life of the drugs on the patients they were suitable for.[2]

Examiner 1: 'When should *biguanides* be used?'[3]

Examiner 1: 'Should old people be changed from chlorpropamide to a shorter acting drug routinely?'

Examiner 2 was the youngest and the most aggressive examiner that I have encountered. The first topic was on **stroke rehabilitation** (lasting four-fifths of the time).

Examiner 2: 'What factors may cause problems in stroke rehabilitation?'

I mentioned intercurrent disease, such as diabetes mellitus, ischaemic heart disease, chest disease, and poor vision. He got very irritated and said **'What else?'** I said social factors, age, motivation. Again he got irritated, **'What factors connected with the stroke?'** I said dominant/nondominant side, receptive/expressive dysphasia, hemianopia, sensory inattention/anaesthesia. I was trying to avoid mentioning dysphagia as I had forgotten

---

[1]   p. 110

[2]   This and the last question from this examiner reflect his concern about the occurrence of troublesome hypoglycaemia with chlorpropamide (biological half-life 35–40 hours) and glibenclamide (half-life 12 hours). These drugs should not be used in the elderly, in whom short-acting sulphonylureas such as tolbutamide or glipizide should be given. The long-acting sulphonylureas may cause neuroglycopaenia in elderly diabetic patients because of chronic or recurrent unsuspected hypoglycaemia.

[3]   Biguanides (phenformin and metformin) increase cellular uptake of glucose in the presence of insulin, reduce hepatic glucose synthesis, reduce the absorption of glucose from the gut, and decrease appetite. Phenformin is the more toxic of the two; it can cause lactic acidosis, toxic damage to the liver and kidney, and is not generally used in the UK. Neither drug is in use in the USA. Most physicians in the UK reserve metformin for the treatment of noninsulin-dependent diabetics who remain obese despite all attempts at dieting. The biguanides can be used with a sulphonylurea in resistant noninsulin-dependent diabetics, with insulin in older patients who require a large dose of insulin, and in patients on insulin who are overweight.

everything about a recent BMJ leader on dysphagia in stroke, but I did eventually mention it and then got involved in a hideous discussion on the pathways in the brain which were involved in swallowing. It rapidly became obvious that I knew no neuroanatomy and he seemed horrified that he had to tell me the names of the pathways between the cerebral cortex and the brain stem nuclei. He did not look at all impressed.

His next question lasted for the remainder of the time:

Examiner 2: **'What advice would you give to a patient on discharge from hospital following a myocardial infarction?'**

I came out with all the standard information, but he looked very dissatisfied and kept saying **'Yes, but isn't there anything else?'** I've no idea what he was getting at.

The final question was on the **management of ventricular tachycardia** as the bell went.

Impressions: I had been expecting to be asked about recent advances/topical issues and I had them all worked out. I was totally amazed to be asked such 'old-fashioned' medicine and I don't think my revision made any difference to my answers. Everything I said was from common sense and from what I have seen and done in the wards. Luckily, I had just finished four months of diabetes and stroke rehabilitation.

(Passed)

11

The viva was half an hour late. We were supposed to sit on numbered chairs corresponding to the numbered tables at which the examiners sat. I got up to chat to a colleague and the candidate who was due in the session after mine sat down in this chair. On release into a large and confusing examination hall, where the numbers were not very visible and people were moving in and out, we both arrived at the same table. The examiners seemed slightly irritated at the other candidate's mistake (although no attempt had been made by the ushers to stop him). I don't know how he fared. They both introduced themselves to me in a friendly way and shook hands.

The first examiner was extremely pleasant and reacted positively throughout. I was asked about the **biological markers of depression**[1] and talked about **alcoholism** and the dexamethasone suppression test. I was then asked about **investigating Cushing's syndrome.**[2]

The next question was:

Examiner 1: 'You are called to see a *young man in casualty with chest pain of sudden onset* – proceed.'

I suggested tension pneumothorax (which seemed to be the answer he wanted) and was then asked about the clinical signs. What would I do if he was extremely distressed and the X-ray department couldn't do a CXR for 20 minutes? What would I do if I put my needle in the wrong side? The examiner seemed to accept my answers and didn't challenge them.

The other examiner was much more reticent – no nonverbal feedback. He asked another clinical question:

Examiner 2: 'You are referred *a woman of 16 weeks' gestation who is having palpitations* – how will you manage her?'

After a lot of waffle about excluding mitral valve disease, I was prompted to the diagnosis of **Wolff-Parkinson-White syndrome**. I was then asked about the treatment and guessed a small dose of propranolol. The examiner seemed pleased and said that this was an actual patient he'd met in clinic that morning and that he had done exactly that. He then quickly asked me:

Examiner 2: 'How would you assess the *size of a myocardial infarction* and which parameter is the most accurate?'

Impressions: Neither examiner tried to hassle me or challenge my answers. At the end of the interview they both stood up and shook hands again. The overall impression was positive. I was quite surprised (having listened to the usual stories) to be treated so courteously.

(*Passed*)

---

[1]   p. 56
[2]   p. 63

12

Two unsmiling but fair examiners in a small side room off the medical ward.

The viva started with me being given **an ECG which showed atrial flutter, right axis deviation and right ventricular hypertrophy**. I described these and said it could be secondary to chronic lung disease and mentioned **cor pulmonale**. We then discussed the causes and treatment of cor pulmonale with a bit about the physiology of heart failure.

We next talked about thrombolysis[1] – the GISSI study[2] – and then the examiner asked me if I had ever used **streptokinase**. We talked about how to give it, the side effects, and follow-up including early stress testing. The examiner then said that this gentleman's brother now comes to you and asks should he be taking an aspirin every day, and we went on to discuss the British and American physicians' primary prevention studies. We also talked about **secondary prophylaxis** and the use of **beta blockers**.

Talking about other risk factors led on to the treatment of **mild hypertension** and I mentioned a few of the recent trials, including the MRC trial.[3]

I was asked the side effects of the antihypertensive drugs and asked which ones I would use in different situations, e.g. **in an asthmatic** or in somebody with a proven **supraventricular tachyarrthymia** (he wanted verapamil here).

The bell went and the registrar came in to say the time was up – this examiner had taken me for the whole 20 minutes and apologised to the other examiner for not giving him time to talk. He replied by saying that we had made a good duet!

(*Passed*)

---

[1]   p. 31

[2]   Gruppo Italiano per lo Studio della Streptochinasi nell Infarto Miocardico 1986 Effectiveness of intravenous thrombolytic treatment in acute myocardial infarction. Lancet 1: 397

[3]   Medical Research Council Working Party 1988 Stroke and coronary heart disease in mild hypertension: risk factors and the value of treatment. British Medical Journal 296; 1565 – 1570

13

Waiting for the viva was nerve-racking, especially as it took place nearly four hours after the clinical examination. I was probably hypoadrenal by then! The viva started about 10 minutes late and was conducted in a large hall with about seven pairs of examiners. The presence of other candidates being examined at the same time was not apparent to me, since my attention was intensely focused on other things! The examiners were very pleasant when I approached them and made strenuous efforts to put me at ease.

The first question centred on how a patient might present with **cirrhosis**; there then followed a listing of clinical signs in this condition. The examiner wanted as many as I could give and possible explanations for some of them, e.g. spider naevi and gynaecomastia (he gave a clue – **'what other conditions do these occur in?'** Answer: pregnancy). Then he asked about **ascites** (**'Imagine you are my registrar'**), wanting to know exactly how it would be managed – doses of drugs, volume of ascitic tap, transudates and exudates. He asked what side effect might occur with the treatment (interested in the electrolyte changes from diuretics); at this point there was a definite upgrading of the pace. Then a change of tack: **'How would you manage a *patient with an ESR of 100*?'** I managed to side-track the examiner into discussing myeloma. **'How does *myeloma* present? List 4 radiological appearances of myeloma.'** (I could only name three.)[1]

'What do *plasma cells* look like?' I answered, 'Blue cytoplasm and clockface nuclei' (I'm not sure if these were correct!).[2]

The next examiner then started on the applications of genetic engineering. I started with synthesis of hormones, viz. insulin. I was asked how to clone a gene, which I fortunately knew, and I used key words such as restriction enzymes and plasmids.[3] He said that growth hormone was also manufactured this way (unknown to me) and he asked me how growth hormone had been obtained in the past – I didn't know. He told me and then asked me about the likely problems. I answered by talking of the risk of HIV, hepatitis B and Jakob-Creutzfeld disease from using human brain tissue.[4] We then discussed **Duchenne muscular dystrophy** and the use of genetic engineering in the diagnosis of genetic disease. (Fortunately I knew this)

I was then asked about the management of a **patient in casualty with a serum sodium of 110 mmol/l**. I outlined the clinical presentation, e.g. dehydrated, oedematous, and mentioned the likely diagnosis in each case. I mentioned **pseudohyponatraemia** in passing, and discussed when and why it occurred.

---

[1] Punched out osteolytic areas in the skull and clavicles; diffuse demineralisation in the extremities, particularly in the early stages; spotty or diffuse osteosclerosis; localised osteoblastic activity may occur with intensive radiotherapy; and a solitary plasmacytoma may be seen as a cystic soap bubble.

[2] Unnecessary use of romantic terms (such as 'clockface') leads to uncertainty. A simple 'blue cytoplasm with an eccentric nucleus' would do.

[3] p. 170

[4] p. 263

I was then asked if I knew what 'beer drinker's potomania'[5] was. I didn't know the term but knew that alcoholics after a binge can induce hyponatraemia. I was asked how much fluid I could drink before it would affect my sodium. I answered by saying a very large amount, 24 litres in a day and my sodium would still be unaffected. Why do beer drinkers get hyponatraemia then? I was led to the answer – inability to excrete a solute load due to low urea in the urine.

I was unaware the bell had gone.

Impressions: I felt the viva was difficult and that I had not done particularly well at the start because I was not very lucid initially. They wished to increase the tempo but I was dragging my feet. Towards the end of the viva I was talking about subjects I knew, fortunately, and was more relaxed. It is obviously impossible to know all the answers. An impression of being at the sharp end managing real problems seems to be important. They were polite throughout. Incidentally, one of the examiners turned out to be the President of the College!

(*Passed*)

---

[5] **Acute hyponatraemia** occurs in some beer drinkers who manage to take 10–15 litres of beer without much food in a period of a few hours. The beer provides the necessary calories but virtually no protein and only a few electrolytes. As the urine volume is large and the solute intake low, the amount of *obligatory* solute excreted easily exceeds the quantity ingested, resulting thereby in a hypo-osmolality state.

14

I wasn't kept waiting for long. The examiners were in a small room behind a desk (the same room that this pair of examiners had used for the long case discussion). They were polite. Boredom had not quite set in as it was still the morning of the first day.

The first examiner asked me about the '**bends**'. At first I didn't think I knew anything about the topic but I answered the question, I think, relatively well. I said that the bends was the name given to a syndrome due to nitrogen coming out of solution in the blood during overrapid decompression in divers. The treatment was prevention, oxygen and recompression followed by gradual decompression. I then went on to list all the various presentations I could think of. I mentioned **adult respiratory distress syndrome** (I'm still not sure if this is right).[1] I was interrupted, predictably, to be asked about that. I gave a definition, a list of causes and a sketchy outline of the treatment without mentioning fluid restriction, PEEP or inotropes, but I was not interrupted very much at all. The bell went before the examiner really had time to probe deeper.

The second examiner gave me a harder time. His first question was about the **advice I would give to a businessman going on a trip to Bangkok**. I started my answer with a list of all the immunisations he would need (tetanus, typhoid, polio, yellow fever, hepatitis A – not all of them came to mind at once) and mentioned the need for malaria prophylaxis.

I said that I would telephone the Hospital for Tropical Diseases for advice about the drugs used for prophylaxis, as I was aware that there was a lot of resistance to various prophylactic drugs in Thailand, and he seemed to like this. However, he was scathing about my suggestions for avoiding mosquito bites and thought that a mosquito net would not be necessary in a Bangkok hotel. We then discussed **HIV risks**. I did not get a full and fluent answer out quickly, and as a result was badgered by the examiner.

I was then asked about **lead poisoning** and the signs and symptoms it might produce. I started talking about neuropathy (and for some reason gave a list of the differential diagnosis of a motor neuropathy, which wasn't at all called for and was not appreciated).[2] I mentioned encephalopathy and that a plain abdominal X-ray would occasionally show evidence of lead ingestion.[3] I also remembered that basophilic stippling on a blood film sometimes indicated lead poisoning. The examiner then said, '**Apart from neuropathy and haemopathy, what does lead poisoning cause?**' I mentioned

---

[1]   The term is applied to a state of acute respiratory distress from severe oxygen insufficiency in patients with previously normal lungs, and it is associated with an increasing number of unrelated conditions (hypovolaemic/septic shock, embolism, trauma, aspiration of gastric contents, disseminated intravascular coagulation, diabetic ketoacidosis, drugs, pancreatitis, etc.). On the other hand, decompression sickness presents with skin irritation, limb pains (bends), chest pains, and in many cases with CNS signs due to nitrogen bubbles in the cerebral or spinal circulation.

[2]   The peripheral nerve involvement is almost exclusively motor and involves muscle groups used extensively (e.g. wrist- and foot-drop).

[3]   The candidate was presumably thinking of lead-induced megacolon which has been reported in lead poisoning.

all the other things again. I couldn't think of any causes of lead poisoning other than paint ingestion.[4] I then suddenly remembered lead lines but I thought they were on the teeth rather than the gums.[5] The examiner asked me about this again and for some reason I still thought that lead lines were on the teeth! Then the bell went again and I was ushered out. I found that I answered questions much less easily when repeatedly interrupted by the second examiner; the first examiner let me get away with considerable omissions which the second would not have tolerated I'm sure.

(*Passed*)

---

[4]   Metal smelter workers or miners, storage battery workers, pottery makers, workers in car manufacturing plants, ship building and paint industries, house painters, demolition workers, petrol sniffers and environmental pollution from leaded petrol exhaust fumes.

[5]   A gingival blue, blue-black, or grey line is found in up to 20% of adult patients but is uncommon in children.

15

I had travelled the twenty or so miles from Falkirk to Edinburgh after the clinical, which I felt had gone very well. In no rush, I had an unhurried lunch and made my way to the College building. Ten of us sat in a semicircle in the new Library awaiting our turn to enter the examination hall. Some of us sat exchanging nervous pleasantries and discussing cases from our clinicals, while others maintained an edgy silence.

About five minutes late, we were asked to go into the hall where the pairs of examiners sat at tables dotted around the edges of the hall. I approached my two examiners who stood, confirmed who I was, and introduced themselves with hands offered to be shaken. Needless to say, if the clinical has gone well then one's confidence is running high at this point. The examiner on my left started with asking me what I knew about the **laboratory markers of alcohol abuse**. Remembering my first attempt at the MRCP, my initial thought was, 'You're not going to get me this time!' There followed a discussion on haematological markers – high MCV, low platelets[1] and why these occur, and then high gamma GT. My only mistake, which the examiner corrected, was to say that a single alcoholic binge could give a high gamma GT. The examiner seemed satisfied and moved on to ask me how I would go about **investigating a patient with anaemia and a high reticulocyte count**. After a few seconds' thought, I answered that this would indicate either blood loss or haemolysis and I would first take a history (the golden rule – start at the beginning). He seemed pleased by this. There followed a discussion on the questions I would ask about blood loss. These covered past episodes of anaemia, drugs, a family history of anaemia, and racial roots. We then side-tracked on to familial haemolytic anaemias and a more detailed discussion of hereditary spherocytosis followed. This took up the rest of the first half of the viva, and as far as I could see I was having no problems. 'Why couldn't it have gone like this the last time?' ran through my mind.

Examiner number two then said, '**Tell me about the *risk factors for ischaemic heart disease***'. Those few words rang through my head quickly followed by, 'PASS'! From recent editorials and personal interest I could murder this question. I spoke briefly and fairly uninterruptedly first on smoking, then hypertension and went on to hypercholesterolaemia and its various nuances associated with ischaemic heart disease. The examiner, sensing that I was going to talk myself out of time, interjected. '***How come Eskimos have high lipids and a low incidence of IHD?***'[2] This threw me slightly and I only told about half the story but it seemed enough, and I was then

---

[1]   p. 106

[2]   The low prevalence of coronary artery disease in Eskimos has been attributed to their high dietary intake of eicosapentaenoic acid (EPA) from excessive consumption of fish and marine mammals. However, even on a Western diet, Eskimos have plasma arachidonic acid (AA) levels far below those seen in Europeans, while dihomogammalinolenic acid (DGLA) levels are higher in Eskimos. These low AA and high DGLA levels seem to be due to a genetic abnormality, since they are found even when their EPA intakes are low. The genetic abnormality giving them high DGLA levels, their high dietary intake of EPA, their high physical activity and a lack of exposure to the stresses of a cash economy are all factors responsible for the low prevalence of ischaemic heart disease in Eskimos.

asked how I would **screen a population for cholesterol levels**. This did not proceed very well and I started to waffle about a GP-based service and struggled hard to define groups for testing. My confidence began to slip. The examiner had produced his desired effect (or so it seemed) and delivered the *coup de grace*, which unfortunately I didn't recognise as such. Our final subject of discussion was on the factors leading to a **decision to discharge the elderly from hospital**. I initially felt that this was a straightforward question,[3] and explained that it was a team effort enlisting the opinions of nursing staff, occupational therapists and physiotherapy services along with the social work department if necessary. Unfortunately, this did not suffice and he then asked how I would identify problems with mobility. Going for the obvious I said that I would ask to see the patient walk and enquire from nurses and physiotherapists how they found his/her mobility. Again, he didn't seem quite satisfied and asked what problems could affect mobility in the elderly. I dealt with medical problems, going through neurological, rheumatic and orthopaedic disabilities, and began to find myself lost for further thoughts. All the while he looked at me expectantly and when I finally dried up he asked, **'But what else causes problems with mobility?'**[4] At that the bell rang for time up and he said to me with a smile, **'Don't worry about it. It doesn't matter'**. I still don't know what he wanted. With this last exchange my thoughts of 'PASS' began to crumble, but on reflection, on my way from the exam hall, I couldn't see how I could have failed. I was also heartened by my boss's comment from a few days earlier, 'No-one fails on the viva alone.'[5]

(*Passed*)

---

[3]   Straightforward questions should be answered with due care, since an unstructured and haphazard presentation is likely to generate difficult supplementary questions.

[4]   The most important causes of immobility in the elderly are locomotor and neurological disorders. Locomotor problems include foot disorders (corns, bunions, trophic ulcers, onychogryphosis, etc.), bone disorders (fractures, osteoporosis, Paget's disease), any of the major arthropathies and diseases of the muscles (proximal myopathy, peripheral arterial disease, polymyalgia) and amputation of a limb. Neurological conditions are headed by stroke and Parkinson's disease and other disorders such as cervical myelopathy, multiple sclerosis, motor neurone disease, peripheral neuropathy, Charcot-Marie-Tooth, cerebellar disease, etc. Other conditions such as cardiorespiratory impairment, psychiatric disorders (e.g. depression, hysteria and dementia), repeated falls, pain, iatrogenic problems (sedatives, tranquillisers and hypotensive agents), prolonged bedrest, impaired vision and hearing and overprotection by carers can all contribute to cause immobility.

[5]   A dangerous piece of advice, see pp. 4, 5, 135, 203, 230.

16

The examiners were sitting in a side room and greeted me politely. The first one asked about the **risks of a myocardial infarction in diabetics compared to those in nondiabetics**. Did I know what the added **risk of smoking** was? I did. Then I was asked how I would bring home the risks to a patient in the clinic. I talked about making sure the patient was aware of the risks, knew about amputations and, if they were male, about impotence. I was asked the most common cause of **impotence in diabetics** (which I said was psychogenic) and **how to tell whether it was organic**.[1] Then I was asked what I would do if I found a diabetic with organic impotence. I said I'd probably get him to talk to a male doctor and to ask about his relationship with his wife, whether it was suffering, etc. Next, I was asked about **erectile aids**[2] so I talked about a couple.

Then the other examiner took over. I was handed some **liver function results** and told that they were from a nurse in a renal unit. They showed a hepatic picture so I talked about hep B and how it was more common in renal units (**'Oh, was it? Really?'**) and I mentioned AIDS. He liked that. Then I was asked about the **GMC recommendations on medical staff and AIDS**. I couldn't remember. Had I read the guidelines? I said no although I had and then had to try and redeem myself. He didn't seem at all interested when I finally told him the recommendations so I was convinced that they would fail me.

(*Passed*)

---

[1] The man with organic impotence (*erectile failure*) characteristically *never* has a normal erection, no matter what the circumstances, and yet has normal sexual drives and feelings. The psychogenic factors can complicate any impotence, and these can be revealed through a detailed enquiry into financial, psychological and physical circumstances. The majority of men in a hospital diabetic clinic complaining of, and of those on questioning admitting to having, impotence have a significant organic component, e.g. vascular factors (atherosclerosis) and/or autonomic neuropathy.

[2] Self-injected intracorporeal papaverine (some diabetologists use phentolamine and prostaglandin E_1) can be used to produce functional erection (Diabetic Medicine 1990; 7: 540). However, this therapy is relatively new, and long-term sequelae (e.g. fibrosis) may be seen in the future with frequent and prolonged use. There is also the danger of priapism, and this therapy should not be given unless there is a 24-hour service available (usually a designated urology unit) to deal with this complication. For this reason there is a case for offering **vacuum devices** (Br Med J 1988; 296: 161) as a first-line therapy. Further, this is the only nonsurgical option for those diabetic men who have a vascular component to their impotence, and who do not respond to intracorporeal papaverine. Patients with a psychogenic component should be referred to a Sexual Difficulties and Marital Clinic. **Surgical penile aids** are now rarely indicated.

17

The viva took place after the clinicals and I was in a state of profound shock thinking that I had failed![1]

The two examiners greeted me with smiles on their faces, shook my hand and sat down. The first examiner asked:

Examiner 1: 'You are in a busy medical outpatient clinic, the ophthalmologist from next door rushes around and asks you to see a young man with a *central retinal artery thrombosis* (CRAT). What would you look for on examining this young man?'

Answer: 'I would look for the stigmata of hyperlipidaemia and measure his BP.'

Examiner 1: 'Are these linked to central retinal artery thrombosis?'

Answer: 'No, but they would increase the risk of atheroma.'

Examiner 1: 'Is that relevant?'

I thought for a while, and then said: 'Usually CRAT are caused by emboli, so it would be important to look for an embolic cause, i.e. see if the patient is in atrial fibrillation, or if he has a dyskinetic apex (implying a ventricular aneurysm with a possible thrombus).

Examiner 1: 'I am glad you mentioned AF. What is so important about *AF in embolic disease?*' After several 'ums' and 'ers' I got to paroxysmal AF, which excited the examiner and he asked me, '**Why?**'. Eventually he gave me the answer.[2]

Examiner 1: '*What does CRAT look like?*'

I mentioned the pale retina with a cherry red macula.

Examiner 1 (excited): 'Why is the macula cherry red?'

Answer: 'It has its own blood supply.' This was wrong and he gave me the answer which I can't remember.[3] He then picked on the red pin on my suit.

Examiner 1: 'What do you use that for?'

Answer: 'Testing for central scotoma.'

Examiner 1: 'Do you use it for testing pain?'

Answer: 'No, I use an orange stick.'

---

[1]   We think that the candidate was dwelling more on his small mistakes than on his positive points: he had demonstrated his excellent examination technique in his long case (myocardial infarction and chronic active hepatitis) and in his eight short cases (including two with AIDS), as described by him in his communication to us. See Rule No. 1 in Section 1 of our *An Aid to MRCP Short Cases* (p.6).

[2]   The greatest danger of embolism is at the time when the rhythm changes from sinus to atrial fibrillation or vice versa.

[3]   At the fovea centralis, the retina is exceedingly thin and the underlying choroidal blood circulation shines through it, and looks like a cherry red spot against the pale retina after the occlusion of the central retinal artery. The fovea does not have any blood supply of its own and derives oxygen from the underlying choroidal circulation, which gives it its dark appearance as seen on fundoscopy of a normal retina.

Examiner 1: 'That's what I use! Why do you use an orange stick?'

Answer: 'It is less likely to spread hep B or HIV and less likely to draw blood.'

Examiner 1: 'Also if they are too sharp the patient won't feel anything! – Good.'

He then asked me about another ophthalmological referral. I got that right but can't remember what it was about.

Examiner 2: 'I am sure you have heard of that famous radio programme, "Just a Minute".' [4] (I shook my head.) 'You are going to talk for one minute about *Campylobacter pyloridis*.'

Answer: 'This organism has appeared frequently in the recent medical literature. It has been found to be associated with gastritis. People have found that treating the organism improves the gastritis. It can be treated with erythromycin. The organisms are sensitive to erythromycin but the indication for antibiotic treatment remains controversial. Although there is evidence that these organisms cause gastritis, a cause-and-effect relationship has not been firmly established, since they have been found in the gastric mucosa of normal subjects.'

Examiner 2: 'You've got 30 seconds left!'

Answer: 'I think it is better treated with bismuth. Bismuth-containing compounds are believed to eradicate gastric *Campylobacter*-like organisms from the gastric mucosa. For this reason some experts have advocated using bismuth-containing preparations to treat patients suspected of having *Campylobacter*-induced gastritis.'

Examiner 2: 'Never mind, you are a busy fellow and are called to casualty to see an *unconscious, pyrexial schoolgirl of 15*. How are you going to manage this?'

I mentioned the various causes to look for including overdose, meningitis, postviral, etc. He asked me what investigations I would perform. I mentioned FBC, U&Es, blood cultures, MSU and a lumbar puncture.

Examiner 2: 'Your clever SHO has done a drug screen and there is a high salicylate level in the blood. She also has a very high bilirubin and alanine transferase level. What are you thinking of?'

I mentioned **Reye's syndrome**. He then asked me about the metabolic complications of Reye's syndrome, which I answered perfectly.

Examiner 2: 'Now you are called to a surgical ward where a woman has collapsed in front of her relatives two days *after a cholecystectomy. She is hypotensive.* What do you do?'

Answer: 'I will examine her, take a history and look for signs of a pulmonary embolism or myocardial infarction.'

---

[4] An entertaining programme in which each contestant (usually a media celebrity) is invited to talk on a given subject for one minute without hesitation, deviation or repetition.

Examiner 2: 'She is hypotensive and looks very ill. What are you going to do?'

Answer: 'I will do a per rectum examination to see if she has had a GI haemorrhage.'

Examiner 2: 'There are no signs on physical examination and the patient is looking worse by the minute. The ECG and CXR are normal. The relatives are ringing their solicitors and the surgical team are flapping round like headless chickens. What are you going to do?'

Answer: 'I would now consider gram-negative septicaemia and put a central line in, take blood cultures, start broad-spectrum antibiotics and fill her up with plasma expanders.' Both examiners burst out laughing and I had to laugh.

Examiner 2: 'That is exactly what I would do! Tell me what antibiotics you would use.'

Answer: 'Cefuroxime and metronidazole.'

Examiner 2: 'Not bad but cefuroxime will not cover one organism, which one?'

I didn't know the answer was *Streptococcus faecalis*. The examiner said he would use ampicillin and metronidazole.

They both thanked me as the bell went and I was sent on my way.

Impressions: I found the examiners to be very friendly and I could establish a good rapport with them. I cannot remember all the details. The best way to prepare is to read the leading articles in the *BMJ*, *NEJM*, *Lancet* and *Hospital Update*. Secondly, one should do busy medical jobs. In the end, experience counts for more than knowledge.

(*Passed*)

18

We were in an outpatient room, just the two examiners and me. It was nice and quiet. I was asked difficult questions and this part was my downfall. Firstly, I was asked about a **young male accountant who wasn't coping at work**. What features in the history and examination would I look for? Eventually it turned out that they wanted a discussion on AIDS but it did seem a little remote to start with.[1] I was then asked about nonHIV retroviruses! They saw I was floundering but did not change tack, this lasted the whole of the first ten minutes.

The second examiner asked about **treating an old man with CCF in the community** and stressed he didn't want to know about drugs. It was a reasonable question and I relaxed a bit. He then asked about the **treatment of tuberculosis in pregnancy.**[2] I wasn't sure about rifampicin in pregnancy. The examiners were neither friendly nor aggressive; in fact they were totally neutral. There was no feedback at all. I had no idea of my result until it came.

(*Failed*)

---

[1] p. 18

[2] Ritampicin has been found to be teratogenic in animals but not in humans. Most experts treat pregnant subjects in the same way as they do nonpregnant patients with tuberculosis, i.e. two months of triple drug therapy (rifampicin, ethambutol, isoniazid) and two drugs (rifampicin and isoniazid) for the subsequent seven months. However, it must be done after a full discussion with the patient. Some experts omit rifampicin unless forced to give it by the severity of the disease.

19

My viva followed immediately after the short cases, in which I felt I had excelled; I was, therefore, very relaxed and felt that this would be a formality. I think that having a relaxed approach does help but this must be more difficult to achieve if things have gone badly so far. The viva took place in a side room off the main ward where we had seen the short cases. The examiners were courteous and friendly. The examination was definitely in two parts. The first examiner took me through the management of an outpatient with a common problem, **abdominal pain**. This was the part that I feel in retrospect I had to pass; if one can't deal logically and confidently with a routine problem then they will not be impressed. The second half of the examination went into some more obscure and theoretical aspects of **diabetes** and **renal disease**. The examiner was a professor of renal medicine. A lot of my answers were of the 'I don't know but perhaps . . .' variety, i.e. educated guesses, but the examiners accepted my ignorance. I think that at this point they were stretching me to see how far beyond the basics my knowledge extended, which really wasn't very far! I had been given a piece of sound advice by the senior physician for whom I had worked and who was an examiner, **'Know the basics well and forget about the small print, the examiners don't expect you to know it.'**

As I recall, the viva went like this (after all the bells, etc.).

Examiner 1: 'You see a new patient in the clinic with *pain in the right iliac fossa*. She's a woman of 23, what is your approach?'

Answer: 'Well, first of all take a good history.' (The examiner looks interested as I haven't suggested a diagnostic laparotomy as my first step!)

'Ask about . . . ' When I'd mentioned a variety of aspects of the history he stopped me.

Examiner 1: 'Good. Now which conditions are uppermost in your mind?'

Answer: 'Irritable bowel.' (My boss at that time was a GI specialist. Most new patients I saw had this condition or peptic ulcers.) 'Crohn's disease, renal disease, gynaecological problems.'

Examiner 1: 'Gynaecology! Good.' (I wondered if other candidates deny the existence of nonmedical possibilities when asked for a differential diagnosis.) 'So you examine the patient and find nothing untoward. Now what?'

Answer: 'I may think at this point that she has the irritable bowel syndrome, especially if I have elicited the following points from the history . . . If that were the case I would attempt to explain the nature of the condition to her as follows . . .' (My explanation goes along the lines of 100 people arranged in order of height from shortest to tallest, height not being a disease. Similarly arrange 100 people in order of sensations from their bowels from hardly ever to almost always, again bowel sensation not being a disease). 'I would advise on the following treatment . . . and then arrange to see her again in two months to see the effect of the treatment and also for any evidence of developing organic disease.'[1]

Examiner 1: 'Would you undertake sigmoidoscopy at the first visit? Why not? What investigations would you perform? Why? Tell me about the ESR in inflammatory bowel disease.'

I'm sure he must have asked me more than that but I can't remember what else. As I emphasised at the start, this is a fairly common clinical problem and he seemed genuinely interested to find out how I managed the case and whether, when our views differed, I could explain why I worked the way that I did. At this point he handed me over to Prof – who also started with a common problem.

Examiner 2: 'You are asked to go to casualty to see a *man of 45 who has been brought in after a fit, what do you do?*'

Answer: 'History again – including that from the ambulance man and relatives (to establish the nature of the seizure).'

Examiner 2: 'You establish that he had had a grand mal seizure, his first. What do you do, which is your investigation of choice?'

Answer: 'In someone of his age, having his first fit, I would suspect organic disease of the brain, particularly a tumour. I would therefore wish to have a CT scan of his brain. Our regional centre at Glasgow offers MRI scanning if need be.'

Examiner 2. 'This is normal. What other investigations would you arrange?'

Answer: 'Baseline haematological and biochemical tests.'

Examiner 2: 'They are all normal. Now what do you do?'

Answer: 'Explain to the patient and relatives what a fit is and that one fit doesn't make one an epileptic. Arrange to see him again in two months for review or sooner if further problems develop. Explain about driving. (throughout the viva the examiners seemed more impressed with my grasp of the practical than the elegant and obscure).

Examiner 2: 'Would you not start him on some treatment?'

Answer: 'No, he might never have another fit but could be unnecessarily on drugs for years. Drugs have side effects' (I listed a few) 'so I would prefer not to. I wouldn't if it were myself.'

Examiner 2: 'Tell me some of the *side effects of phenytoin and carbamazepine. Why do you think phenytoin interferes with vitamin D metabolism?*'[2]

My answers were good up to a point, then I got out of my depth so he changed the subject.

---

[1] This answer is a good illustration of how to take control and keep talking, thereby avoiding supplementary questions!

[2] Phenytoin and phenobarbitone induce drug-metabolising enzymes in the liver and accelerate the breakdown of calciferol. This effect may account for the lower circulating levels of 25-hydroxy cholecalciferol found in patients treated with anticonvulsants. Osteomalacia and hypocalcaemia do not usually occur unless there are other predisposing factors, such as poor nutrition or inadequate exposure to sunlight.

Examiner 2: 'Do you see many *diabetics* in the clinic? What do you examine them for?'

Answer: 'History of drugs, insulin use, other medical problems, any other related problems. Measure BP and look for peripheral pulses, reflexes, foot health, and urine for protein.'[3]

The last answer was the whole point of the question. He had now got me into his specialist territory from where I could not escape!

The remainder of the viva was about **renal pathology**, proteinuria and the measurement of renal function. I don't recall the details but felt that I was deliberately being stretched, but in a friendly way. By this time I felt that all three of us were sufficiently in tune, that they were able to accept my ignorance and guide my replies, rather as a tutor will listen to and encourage a slightly wayward but interested student.

Impressions: My advice about the viva must be to keep calm, tell them what you really think, rather than what you think they might want you to say, and don't be afraid to be amusing (as long as it's not too often!).

(Passed)

---

[3]   And annual fundoscopy through *dilated* pupils.

20

Both examiners greeted me in a friendly although slightly distant manner, and kicked off by asking me where I was currently working. The first examiner then started the ball rolling by describing a young lad recently referred to him with **polydipsia and polyuria**, and asked me in what way I would approach his management.[1]

As soon as I had mentioned the possibility of diabetes mellitus, the examiner interposed, **'Surprisingly, the blood sugar was normal.'** I then, in a very disjointed fashion, listed the causes of polydipsia/polyuria which provoked questions such as, **'What sort of *diabetes insipidus*? and 'How would you distinguish between them?'** The latter question caused me to get flummoxed and give a very jumbled although basically correct answer. The examiner then told me that this patient's Ca^{2+} was 3.2 mmol/l and he asked me how I would continue to investigate. I think I annoyed my examiner at this point by going all round the houses about the possible causes of hypercalcaemia, and by not putting **sarcoidosis** at the top of my list. He eventually dragged it out of me that this was the most likely diagnosis and asked me how I would investigate this. Again I annoyed him by going straight for the Kveim test (his comment being that I would have to wait several weeks for an answer) and the serum ACE level before mentioning a CXR and mediastinal lymph node biopsy. I also mentioned steroid responsiveness but this answer was ignored. We then got embroiled in a discussion of the main sites of lymph node enlargement on a CXR and the different sites usually affected by Hodgkin's disease and sarcoid which was eventually, with some prompting, prised out of me.

The bell rang as the first examiner was about to change the subject. The second examiner again introduced a clinical situation – **a lady who had been found by her GP to be hypothyroid** and was started on thyroxine,

---

[1] 1. *History* is by far the most important, particularly of associated features:
   a. Increased appetite and weight loss in diabetes mellitus
   b. Psychological disturbances in psychogenic polydipsia
   c. History of renal disease in nephrogenic diabetes insipidus
   d. Other clues suggestive of hypercalcaemia and hypokalaemia
   e. Drugs (lithium, demeclocycline, potent diuretics, etc.).
  2. Check blood sugar, serum electrolytes, urea and calcium.
  3. If the cause is still uncertain, determine the urine and serum osmolality:
   a. If the urine osmolality is greater than that of the serum, look for glycosuria and hyperglycaemia
   b. If the urine is iso-osmotic with respect to serum, check for evidence of renal disease and for evidence of diuretic abuse
   c. If the urine is hypotonic compared with serum, test the renal concentrating ability by restricting the fluid intake:
    i. If the urine becomes hypertonic – psychogenic or iatrogenic
    ii. If the urine remains dilute – nephrogenic or central diabetes insipidus. Check response to vasopressin. Urinary osmolality will increase in central diabetes insipidus.

with a worsening of her condition.[2] I was asked the likely cause and said she might be developing heart failure. This was not the answer he wanted and a long silence ensued after which I announced that I did not know. He then asked me about the tests of thyroid function. I got round to discussing primary and secondary hypothyroidism. I eventually realised that the lady may have secondary hypothyroidism and may have other **pituitary dysfunction**, e.g. **of ACTH**. I was then asked how I would **treat someone with hypopituitarism** and got this right, including the doses, except for forgetting to exclude a mineralocorticoid[3] and the subject was then changed to **the effects of alcohol**. Specifically, I was asked how alcohol kills people. I gave a reasonably structured answer and the examiner responded more warmly. In conclusion, I feel I annoyed my examiners by giving disjointed answers and by showing that I was unsure of several points, particularly by causing them to prise information out of me, even when I did know it. I did find it harder to know what they wanted from me than in my second viva (see viva experience 21).

(*Failed*)

---

[2]   The examiner introduced the *ghost-link* (see *Ghost* Stories, p. 74) leading the candidate to the diagnosis he had in mind. *Worsening of the condition* suggests that she already had symptoms which were worsened (i.e. thyroxine-aggravated adrenal insufficiency); the candidate missed this and introduced a new clinical setting, heart failure.

[3]   Supplemental mineralocorticoid therapy is unnecessary because of the partial preservation of aldosterone secretion.

21

My examiners both greeted me in a friendly manner although they kept me waiting whilst they discussed the previous candidate. The first examiner started by outlining the history of a drug addict coming in with a **cavitating lesion on his CXR.**[1] I jumped the gun somewhat by assuming that the patient was possibly HIV positive, and there ensued a discussion about lung disease in HIV. However, my examiner didn't appear too bothered and brought me back to the causes of cavitating lung disease and their investigation and treatment. The subject then changed to a discussion of the ethical implications of **testing for HIV**, and what I would do if the drug addict refused HIV testing[2] to which I was noncommittal, being unsure of the examiner's feelings in the matter. They didn't push me hard on that, though. The examiner then changed the subject to **diabetes** and asked me to pretend that he was the mother of a diabetic adolescent and to give her **advice on the management of her daughter**. I found it extremely difficult to treat him as anything other than an examiner and answer in the way he wanted; this was complicated by the fact that every so often he interposed as an examiner and asked a question such as whether fine control of diabetes influenced the outcome of long-term complications, the evidence for this, etc.

Fortunately, the bell went and the subject changed. The second examiner had a sense of humour and quickly put me at ease. He started by asking me what **advice** I would give **to a man going to Lagos** next week, excluding AIDS since we had already discussed this. I mentioned typhoid and cholera vaccines, hep A gamma globulin, and malarial prophylaxis (at which point he asked me about **chloroquine resistance**). I didn't know whether Lagos was such an area, but he seemed happy with that (I knew who to contact to find out). He then pushed me, much to my horror, on to **yellow fever** and quickly discovered that I didn't know the cause. He kindly didn't pursue the subject except to make an aside, that I probably wasn't old enough to remember when yellow fever stopped the building of the Panama Canal!

He then introduced the final topic of the viva, **cor pulmonale**, and pushed me on the physiology of this before discussing its treatment. I turned the subject to oxygen concentrators since I had done a respiratory job and also had read a recent paper on it. So we discussed the assessment

---

[1] This looks like a *Ghost* Story with a number of equally credible diagnostic possibilities, and we suspect that the examiner had a definite diagnosis in mind while he offered a *ghost-link* (viz., drug addict) to lead the candidate to it. The candidate's suggestion of AIDS was reasonable, but a more satisfactory way of dealing with such questions (see pp. 74–78) is to offer a number of possibilities and then, with the help of the examiner's response, narrow down to the *real* one. In this case, the candidate should have mentioned TB, *Staphylococcus*, AIDS, *Klebsiella* as the principal contenders, leaving a mycetoma, a cavitating rheumatoid nodule and a carcinoma as the outside possibilities. In clinical practice, HIV testing would not be the first investigation carried out on a patient (even a drug addict) with a cavitating lesion in the lung. The candidate should have tried a more plausible searching cue and suggested that he would examine the injection sites for evidence of any infection.

[2] p. 90

of a patient's suitability for an oxygen concentrator and, again, the physiology relating to why they were thought to be effective. The final bell interrupted this subject. I forgot to mention that having made a mess of discussing yellow fever, when we got on to cor pulmonale, I redeemed myself by knowing the commonest cause of this in Egypt – schistosomiasis!

(*Passed*)

22

The viva was held in the Hall of the Royal College of Physicians, Edinburgh. It began ten minutes late. The hall was unexpectedly noisy; I had expected to be alone with the examiners. There was an 'observer' from Iraq on my table who was introduced to me. However, I was too nervous to worry about his presence.

Examiner: 'Let me take you back into my past. I was asked by a colleague to see his 19-year-old son, who had been *acting strangely for the past two days* and on the preceding night had tried to strangle his mother. What would be your approach?'

The discussion centred around trying to differentiate between acute psychosis, the psychiatric manifestations of physical disease and substance abuse. When it was decided that the patient was a psychiatric case, I was asked what I'd do if the patient refused hospital admission. I was asked the dose of chlorpromazine I would give.

Examiner: 'Tell me about *type I* and *type II* respiratory failure.'[1]

Only after the examination did I realise I'd reversed the explanation for type II respiratory failure, saying that the normal person uses O_2 levels for driving respiration rather than CO_2. The examiner made no comment and I don't think he noticed!

I was asked **how to treat respiratory failure**, including when to ventilate and when to use positive pressure on the ventilator.

Examiner: 'A lady with a history of *breast carcinoma is admitted with a calcium of 4.0 mmol/l*. What would you do?'

I answered this well.

(*Passed*)

---

[1]   Some British workers divide respiratory failure into two types: *type I* in which there is hypoxaemia with a normal or low P_{CO_2} and *type II* in which hypoxaemia is associated with hypercapnia.

23

The first question was, **'What do you know about *simvastatin*?'**[1] I launched into a discussion of the development and uses of **somatostatin** before I was stopped and corrected.

The examiners then asked who and how I would **screen for hyperlipidaemia**.[2] They disagreed with, or appeared to dislike, my suggestion that I would check a full fasting lipid profile before commencing treatment.[3]

They then gave me an outpatient case of a **60-year-old man from Belfast** (where I worked) presenting with **shortness of breath** and asked what the **relevant points of the history** would be. I mentioned smoking, occupational history (e.g. asbestos exposure in the shipyards, byssinosis in the linen mills), and whether he had any hobbies such as keeping birds. They said I had missed a very important point and after some prompting I realised that they wanted me to mention TB (which is *not* as common as they suggested).

Finally they outlined a case of a 40-year-old man at outpatients with **severe occipital headache for three years**.[4] I said I'd take a further history regarding the site of the ache, associated factors, etc., but they got really impatient and said that it must be obvious what the diagnosis was. Eventually, after trying to defend my view that more information was necessary, I said that the most likely diagnosis was tension headache. The reply to this was, **'Is that your way of saying that the patient is a nutcase?'**

Before I could reply the bell went for the end of the viva and they dismissed me.

(Passed)

---

[1]   p. 116

[2]   p. 34

[3]   The candidate has not given the full details of the discussion. The examiners' disapproval of the suggestion about the treatment may have been because the question was about screening and not the treatment.

[4]   In a condition such as headache, where the list of causes is as long as a large textbook of medicine, the examiners often offer a *ghost-link* (e.g. occipital, pain over the temple/ mastoid/orbit, unilateral headache, etc.) to lead the candidate into some specific entities. The examiners' impatience was probably because the answer about history and associated symptoms was not specific to tension headache.

24

I was met by my superficially (and only initially) friendly examiners after a sweaty-palmed few minutes' wait standing outside a closed door. My clinical had not gone well,[1] which did nothing to quieten my nerves. After shaking hands with the examiners (a gesture initiated by me which seemed to surprise them), I was offered a chair and the first examiner set the scenario of a **15-year-old girl brought into casualty unconscious**. She had had a headache for a few days and had gradually become more and more drowsy and lapsed into unconsciousness. I had to take it from there. Remembering to start 'at the beginning', I wanted to take a history from any accompanying person and carry out a physical examination. Apart from an unconscious girl this was entirely fruitless and no other information was available.

'You can have three investigations', was the next comment. After a blood glucose and U&Es, I antagonised the examiner by asking for a CT scan (these two blood tests were normal). Having retracted this and asked for blood gases he said that she was acidotic. I then asked for a salicylate level – **'Undetectable'**. Then I was asked, **'Have you heard of a condition affecting young people who have a high AST and encephalopathy?'** After a few seconds' thought, **Reye's syndrome** was tentatively offered. I was met with a slightly more satisfied **'Yes'**, and this seemed to be the diagnosis I was expected to have sought from the beginning.[2]

---

[1] Managed to hurry through six short cases; missed gouty tophi on both pinnae of a patient when asked to look at his hands, did not notice an a-v fistula in a patient when asked to examine his abdomen, missed hepatomegaly by rushing the examination in a lady with hepatosplenomegaly and did not examine the pulse and precordium properly when asked to examine a patient's heart.

[2] Questions about an unconscious patient should always be treated as *Biblical* Stories, as apparently this candidate did. However, the discussion somehow degenerated into a guessing game (as in *Detective* Stories), probably because the candidate did not mention a lumbar puncture before asking for a CAT scan, since the possibility of meningitis and encephalitis should have been seriously considered. The examiner might have offered some encouragement had the candidate mentioned LFTs when he asked for urea, electrolytes and blood glucose levels. Incidentally, it is surprising that this severely ill patient with Reye's syndrome did not have hepatomegaly, hypoglycaemia or any electrolyte disturbances.

This was followed by a discussion of **ascites, its treatment** and the **mechanisms of its production**. We spoke briefly about the **pharmacology of spironolactone** and the viva seemed to be taking a turn for the better. However, little did I think that worse was yet to come. The second examiner opened with the question, **'What can you tell me about the process of care?'**[3] This is an exact quote, as the words are engraved on my memory. A blank stare and some fast thinking did not provide an acceptable answer, and I

---

[3]   The question has been phrased rather ambiguously, but the candidate should have sought clarification and asked about which particular care process the examiner wished to hear. We suspect that it was the modern nursing care process, whereby two nurses, a senior and a junior nurse, are given the task of *complete care* of a fixed number of patients, as opposed to the old *task process* in which each nurse was given a single task for the entire ward. However, a more comprehensive answer about the process of care would be something as follows:

Care systems

Care in hospital is given by many different people. The patients have the most direct contact with the doctors and the nurses, but one also has to remember the important roles not only of the administrative and clerical staff, but also of the domestic and portering personnel. All these people contribute to a patient's care within the hospital setting.

The multi-disciplinary approach to care is best demonstrated in the departments of medicine for the elderly. Here, a major input is made by the paramedical staff (physiotherapists, occupational therapists, etc.) and hospital social workers.

Care in the community is given informally by a vast army of relatives, friends and neighbours. These are supported where necessary by the district nursing services, social services (home carers, meals on wheels, day centres, luncheon clubs, etc.) and the voluntary organisations (Crossroads, Help the Aged, Age Concern, etc.).

For people with specific chronic disabilities, there are local branches of support groups such as the Parkinson's Disease Society, Multiple Sclerosis Society, Motor Neurone Disease Society, etc. The Disabled Living Foundation cares for certain patients by providing aids and adaptations for the home.

Some patients, particularly the very frail, elderly and disabled, require such an intensive degree of nursing care that it is necessary for them to be cared for in hospital continuing care wards or in private nursing homes. Terminally ill patients should be cared for in the most appropriate setting, whether this is at home with their family, supported by all the relevant services including the Macmillan nurses and any necessary respite care, or as an inpatient in hospital or in a hospice.

The changes soon to be introduced with the reorganisation of the National Health Service, and the implementation of the new community care bill (Griffiths), will inevitably alter the way that patients are cared for. The government hopes that there will be a greater emphasis on primary care and preventive medicine, and that care will be given in a much more individualised package. However, the problems of funding remain unsolved.

Everyone at some stage in their life will need 'care' from some agency or another. The essential features of 'caring' are that it should be adequate and be given with sensitivity and dignity.

could not get to grips with what he wanted. Some questions on statistics followed: **'Give an example of a *type 2 error'*.**[4] **'What is the power of a study?'** Only the last of these questions was met from me with anything approaching a decent stab at an answer.

His only question relevant to clinical medicine was about **weight loss in a middle-aged man**,[5] and as far as I could see my only slip was not mentioning thyrotoxicosis, which seemed the one diagnosis he wanted. The last question of the viva was again nonclinical. *'What is prescription event monitoring?'*[6] In retrospect I should have known this, but in the heat of the moment I again fluffed it.

I left the room and headed for the car convinced (and rightly so) that I had failed.

Impressions: My impression after this attempt was of being treated rather unfairly, an opinion shared by a number of people, including MRCP examiners, who I spoke to afterwards. One even offered to put in an objection to the College (an offer I refused). My months of reading, practice exams, etc., could not have prepared me for the content of this viva, and on a number of occasions I admit to considering not going for another attempt.

(*Failed*)

---

[4] Judging from the question that followed, the examiner did expect some understanding of statistical methods. In a statistical test which, for example, might be carried out on data comparing the efficacy of two different drugs, the result is usually stated to be significant at some level, e.g. $p < 0.05$, or not significant ($p > 0.05$). As it is not known in advance whether one drug is actually better than the other, either way the conclusion of the significance test may be in error. The situation is summarised in the table below.

Truth	Test result	
	Significant difference between drugs	No significant difference between drugs
Real difference between drugs	Correct	Type 2 or β error (the test fails to detect a real difference)
No difference between drugs	Type 1 or α error (the difference found is erroneous)	Correct

A *type 1 error* occurs when a significant difference is obtained by the test when, in reality, there is no actual difference between the two drugs. By analogy with a screening test, this may be viewed as a *false-positive* result. The probability of making a type 1 error, usually represented by the letter alpha (α), is the same as the p value; for example, an α of 0.05 indicates that the likelihood of erroneously finding a significant difference between the drugs is 0.05, or 1 in 20.

By contrast, a *type 2 error* arises when the significance test fails to detect a difference when in fact there is a real difference between the drugs. This would be a *false-negative* result in a screening protocol. The probability of a *type 2 error* is denoted by the letter beta (β). The concept of *statistical power* is more widely used than β. This is defined as the probability of obtaining a significant test result when a difference truly exists, and is calculated as $1 - \beta$ and it is analogous to the sensitivity of a screening test.

[5] Questions on weight loss are better tackled by relating it to appetite and food intake.

[6] In this study, being carried out in Southampton, events occurring against the prescription of a drug during a specified period are being monitored. However, its superiority over the yellow card system is rather doubtful.

25

One of the examiners came to get me and shook me warmly by the hand. He jokingly remarked that I had cold, sweaty palms and encouraged me to relax. He introduced himself and his colleague, who also offered his hand. The room was small but adequate. I sat at the opposite side of a standard table.

I can remember five questions (three from the first examiner and two from the second). They were relaxed and friendly, which helped me. Four of the questions were everyday clinical settings, and they stressed that I should pretend that I was in OPD or in an A&E room.

1. A classical clinical situation of **primary biliary cirrhosis** was given and I was asked to comment. I went straight for the diagnosis, which seemed to please them, and then described relevant history/examination/ investigation, etc. The role of, and findings at, liver biopsy were discussed. They then asked what I would tell the enquiring husband about the prognosis.

2. *'What can you tell me about trace elements?'*[1] This threw me a bit, and the other examiner made some remarks on it. I agreed which seemed to please them. I then waffled a bit from basic medical sciences and then remembered about zinc and parenteral nutrition. I said that there was a skin rash but I did not know what it was called. They told me, and they seemed happy.[2]

3. A clinical setting was given of a **young student with a headache**. It was compatible with a subarachnoid haemorrhage, and I gave a short dissertation and was questioned about LPs and the risk of rebleeding. We then went back to the original setting and I was pushed to making another diagnosis. I was then told that the answer was **migraine** and most students had them before exams, **'Hadn't I in the last week**?' Before I could stop myself I said 'No, but I'll have one afterwards,' which fortunately made them laugh.

4. A clinical setting was given of a case of **aortic dissection ripping off one of the spinal arteries**. I discussed the management but they did not

---

[1]   p. 54

[2]   *Acrodermatitis enteropathica* (eczematoid plaques around the mouth, on the face, hands and anterior surface of legs) is a rare autosomal recessive disorder characterised by an inability to absorb zinc. An acquired form also occurs in certain clinical circumstances (e.g. malabsorption syndromes, prolonged parenteral nutrition, dietary phytate, cirrhosis, postgastrectomy, alcoholism, renal tubular disorders, malignancy, etc.).

seem to agree about the possible role of surgery.[3] I had seen it used successfully but luckily I was not too dogmatic.

5. I was given a history of a patient with a tropical disease – during the course of the discussion I managed to 'admit a case of **lassa fever** to a DGH' for observation and was reprimanded jokingly.

(Passed)

---

[3] Surgery is usually indicated when the dissection involves the ascending aorta which poses a threat of retrograde dissection, rupture, acute aortic regurgitation, and life-threatening tamponade. Dissections involving the descending aorta are generally managed conservatively unless there is evidence of an increase in size, rupture or severe and uncontrollable pain.

26

It was a large hall with a series of viva tables around the edge. The viva came after an awful short case,[1] my nerves were a bit shattered and I was demoralised. I knew that a good oral was needed.

The first examiner, a pharmacologist, asked me about a long list of drugs some mad GP had prescribed – **their side effects, interactions, dosages** and **indications**. It went OK until my list of nausea-inducing drugs included chlorpromazine! He was just going to ask me about **anaemia in rheumatoid arthritis** (which I was looking forward to talking about) when the bell went, and I was handed over to the second examiner. He was less friendly and I never quite got on his wavelength! He asked me what I would say in a speech to GPs defending the need for **referral of all hypertensives** to hospital. I gave a muddled and unstructured answer. He asked me about **hypokalaemia** and **hypertension**. He persisted after I had exhausted my list and eventually said that I was **'clearly unaware that one-third of essential hypertensives had hyperreninaemia and hypokalaemia.'**[2]

I admitted my ignorance and we moved on to the niceties of the histological classification of **nonHodgkin's lymphoma** – a subject I had managed to carefully avoid up to now! I was OK when we got down to the clinical features and staging, but not when it came to the exact prognosis and management of each subgroup! He eventually asked me if treating NHL should be left to the experts. I breathed a sigh of relief and uttered a wholehearted, 'Yes'.

I have had no personal experience of treating such patients but should have known a bit more!

(*Failed; passed three months later*)

---

[1]   Diagnosed hepatosplenomegaly with ascites in a patient with polycystic kidneys.

[2]   Notwithstanding the methodological problems that are encountered in measuring renin, most studies suggest that about 60% of hypertensive subjects have normal and 30% have *low* values. Renin levels are low in blacks, females and older subjects. In essential hypertension, renin levels follow a continuous distribution curve with a predominance of lower values because of the larger proportion of blacks and older people in the hypertensive population (JAMA 1977; 238: 611).

27

The viva started approximately five minutes late but the examiners were very friendly and did all they could to put me at my ease, which was much appreciated as I was extremely nervous. The stem questions as I remember them were as follows.

Firstly, I was asked about **acholuric jaundice**, leading on to a discussion of bilirubin production and excretion, the causes of haemolytic anaemia and the treatment of hereditary spherocytosis.

The examiners then said: **'Imagine you're my registrar and I bring in a patient for investigation who is generally unwell with a markedly *elevated ESR*. How would you proceed?'**[1] After briefly discussing infectious causes, the discussion centred on (1) **multiple myeloma** – the diagnostic criteria, X-ray changes; and (2) **temporal arteritis** and **polymyalgia rheumatica** – their diagnosis and treatment.

The third question concerned the **effects of alcohol** on the body – cardio-myopathy, cirrhosis, peripheral neuropathy, Wernicke's encephalopathy. They asked me for another reason, apart from a low thiamine intake, why alcoholic patients should develop Wernicke's. I couldn't think what they were getting at but they wanted me to say 'vomiting'.[2]

'What do you understand by the term accelerated hypertension?' We firstly discussed the histopathological changes and where they were found, and then went on to the indications for the treatment of an elevated BP, how quickly it needed to be done, and what agents should be used. They then asked me the clinical and physiological aspects of **hypertensive encephalopathy**.

The viva concluded with a discussion on the merits of hypertensive control in reducing the risk of CVAs but not MIs, and why this should be so.

Impressions: Altogether, I felt that the viva had been fair. I was able to answer most of the questions asked me and they seemed generally satisfied with my responses. However, I failed the viva and I am sure this was because I was not sure enough of myself and my answers were often faltering and indecisive.

(Passed the exam)

---

[1] A typical *Ghost* Story with many diagnostic possibilities and the examiner having a probable one in mind. The candidate should have attempted to explore the *ghost-link* by asking the patient's age or/and the principal complaints on presentation, which would have narrowed down the possibilities. Alternatively, the possible diagnoses could be grouped under two headings: (1) where the raised ESR was the only haematological abnormality (collagen disease, subacute infections, malignancy, etc.); and (2) in which there were other abnormalities, e.g. anaemia, leucoerythroblastic anaemia, etc.

[2] Thiamin deficiency can be due to a lack of adequate nutrition (alcoholics depending entirely on alcohol for calories, prolonged and inadequate parenteral nutrition, systemic diseases such as hepatic failure and malignancy, and starvation) or due to nonretention of ingested nutrients (persistent vomiting – hyperemesis gravidarum, gastric malignancy, gastritis, haemodialysis, digitalis toxicity, etc.).

28

We started with the first examiner asking me to discuss the **medical consequences of pregnancy**.[1] I knew next to nothing about this but built a fairly coherent answer on a discussion of teratogenicity (e.g. warfarin), the use of alpha-methyl dopa in hypertension, and the effects of increased cardiac output in, for example, mitral stenosis. The examiner seemed quite happy with my answers though I made some quantitative errors. I was then asked to discuss the **management of asthma** which I did along fairly conventional lines.

The second examiner then asked me to discuss the investigation of **haematuria** and, after some general discussion, asked me if this could be related to a sore throat. I talked about poststreptococcal glomerulo-nephritis for a while, and he then asked me if I had any idea what might be wrong with a young man who developed haematuria whenever he suffered from an upper respiratory tract infection. This triggered a memory of a *BMJ* editorial and I offered **Berger's disease**[2] as the diagnosis. He seemed quite impressed with this and fortunately I was able to discuss the pathology and prognosis of this quite fully. He then asked me for examples of diseases caused in man by *Chlamydia*[3] and I was able to list trachoma, psittacosis, arthritis and Fitz–Hugh–Curtis syndrome[4] and to give brief details of each. By this time I was feeling very happy with my performance and felt quite disappointed when the bell went. Throughout the viva the examiners were pleasant and polite, never interrupted my answers and seemed quite interested in what I had to say.[5]

(*Passed*)

---

[1] The question as reported is rather vague; presumably the examiner wished to know the *consequences of various medical conditions* in pregnancy. This is an important area and one can either deal with it system by system, or pick a few principal examples (e.g. hypertension, diabetes mellitus, bronchial asthma, mitral stenosis, phlebothrombosis) to discuss.

[2] A focal glomerulonephritis with mesangial IgA deposits occurring in children and young adults, and characterised by *recurrent haematuria* that occurs with, or follows within 24–48 hours, a viral upper respiratory infection, a flu-like illness or a gastrointestinal syndrome. The eponym, Berger, is applied because in 1968 Jean Berger reviewed 55 kidney biopsies of children with so-called benign or idiopathic haematuria, and noted a high frequency of mesangial IgA deposits. Progression to renal failure occurs in about one-fifth of patients.

[3] The genus *Chlamydia* contains the species *C. psittaci* and *C. trachomatis*.

[4] This eponym is applied to a perihepatitis which typically occurs in women with concomitant or recent pelvic inflammatory disease. The hepatic capsule is principally involved, and 'violin-string' adhesions may develop between the anterior abdominal wall and the liver surface. There is usually a high titre against *Chlamydia* but it may occur with gonococcal infection as well. The condition is characterised by upper abdominal pain and fever. Laparoscopy is used as a therapeutic measure to rupture the adhesive 'violin-strings'.

[5] No doubt inspired by the candidate's sound knowledge and good presentation.

29

My first surprise was seeing the name of one of the examiners, which I recognised. I was a student on his firm in Oxford (I told the invigilator who said that he might not ask any questions – but he did, and took up much more than half the time).

The viva exam was in a side room on a disused ward; there were no problems with the venue. The examiners were a cardiologist (judging by his questions) and a haematologist, both straightforward and friendly. The Oxford consultant obviously recognised me; he handed me **an ECG** which showed anterior ST elevation but no q waves, saying *'You see a 45-year-old man with chest pain for three hours in casualty.* **What would you do?'** I said, 'Resuscitate, take a history, examine, arrange a chest X-ray and then transfer to CCU for thrombolysis'. He asked how long all that would take. I said 45 minutes where I last worked, and it would be safer to give the streptokinase on a CCU (he was obviously angling at saying to give it in casualty).[1] He asked what trials of **thrombolysis** I knew about and I mentioned a few. We talked about entry criteria and results. He asked what I would look for when examining a man with an acute MI.

Next, he asked about the management of a 25-year-old patient with a **single fit**. I said history, examination, baseline blood tests and no CT (pointing out that a structural abnormality would be very unlikely if there was no neurological deficit). He mentioned driving, and I said I would proceed no further pending another fit.[2]

Next, he asked about the management of a **subarachnoid haemorrhage**. He asked about the diagnosis, and what to do in Oxford where the CT scanner is miles from casualty. Next, he asked about vasospasm, which I said a few things about but a bit vaguely.

He tried to be aggressive at times but it didn't really seem to be in keeping with his character, so he quickly went back to being quite benign.

Next, the other examiner asked about **macrocytic anaemia** in the elderly when both the B_{12} and folate were normal. I said that the possibilities

---

[1]   It is equally possible that the examiner was exploring whether the candidate knew the pros and cons of giving streptokinase outside a CCU (e.g. inadequate monitoring and treatment of life-threatening arrhythmias).

[2]   The history should explore any familial link, a past occurrence and any precipitating causes (e.g. alcohol). The examination and investigations should exclude a primary cerebral cause (although at this age it is likely to be idiopathic) and the patient should be followed up. Driving a private vehicle is not allowed for a year; longer, if the fit occurred during driving. Driving of an HGV should be stopped indefinitely. It is advisable to record this advice in the patient's case notes.

included hypothyroidism, alcohol, liver disease, myelodysplasia and sideroblastic anaemia, and we talked a bit about these.

Next, I was asked about the causes of a **lymphocytosis**.[3] It took a bit to drag lymphoma out of me as well as infective causes, and then we briefly talked about **B** and **T cell** markers and the bell went.

Impressions: Obviously a bit stressful but nothing too bad.

(*Passed*)

---

[3] *High* ($\geqslant 15 \times 10^9/1$) – infectious mononucleosis (mostly T lymphocytes in the peripheral blood), pertussis, acute and chronic lymphocytic leukaemias

Moderate – viral infections (infectious mononucleosis, mumps, measles, hepatitis, coxsackie, varicella, etc.); toxoplasmosis, brucellosis, tuberculosis, typhoid fever; neoplastic disorders (Hodgkin's disease, lymphomas, chronic lymphocytic leukaemia).

30

I did the viva last and went from the short cases to the viva with less than five minutes between the two. We were in a small office with no other candidates; both examiners appeared friendly and relaxed and put me at ease. They did not ask where I worked or in which speciality.

The first examiner said, **'You are in casualty and have a patient in *acute pulmonary oedema*. What would you do?'**[1]

I thought it would be best to start with the basics and said that I would sit the patient up to make him more comfortable and give him 24% O_2.[2] If he was well enough I would try to obtain a history, e.g. of previous IHD or similar episodes of breathlessness or of acute chest pain preceding this attack. Then I would examine him to confirm my clinical suspicions and get a CXR and ECG. I then said that the mainstay of treatment for this condition was still intravenous frusemide. The examiner agreed and did not ask for the dose. He asked what I would do if the pulmonary oedema did not respond quickly. I said that I liked to use intravenous nitrates, providing that the systolic BP was $\geqslant 100$ mmHg, to offload the left ventricle. I then said that in the long term, the patient could be treated with oral diuretics, nitrates and captopril.

He seemed pleased with my answer and went on to ask about the **side effects of captopril**. I told him about first-dose hypotension, which is sometimes very severe, about loss of taste, skin rashes and renal failure. He asked me what else,[3] but I didn't know any others.

He then asked me about **drugs and the elderly** and how the **pharmacodynamics** were different. I talked about the smaller body mass and impaired renal and hepatic function. He then asked me specifically about the side effects of diuretics.[4] I listed postural hypotension causing falls, dizziness, dehydration, diabetes, urge incontinence, gout and renal failure.

He then asked me about other drugs, such as **anxiolytics**. I replied that they had a longer 'hangover' effect in the elderly, and in some cases had the reverse effect to that intended, e.g. temazepam causing agitation and confusion. He agreed with this and then passed me over to his colleague who had so far been silent.

The second examiner's first question concerned **vitamin B_{12} metabolism**. Again I thought it better to start at the beginning and began to list

---

[1] In such medical emergencies, it is always well to set out the immediate therapeutic goals: (1) *Reassure* the patient and sit him upright to ease his breathlessness and allay anxiety; (2) *Improve oxygenation* by giving 100% humidified oxygen; (3) *Reduce venous return* by giving 5 mg of diamorphine and 40 mg frusemide i.v.; (4) *Identify* and treat *underlying* and *precipitating* factors; (5) *Monitor* vital signs frequently. An intravenous cannula should be inserted to obtain i.v. access. Once a degree of stability is achieved, urea, electrolytes, arterial blood gas tension, ECG and a portable chest X-ray should be obtained. Further measures (i.v. nitrates, introduction of a Swan-Ganz catheter, correction of hypotension and arrhythmias, etc.) should be undertaken if necessary.

[2] Inadequate, unless the candidate was suspecting a coexisting chronic hypercapnoeic respiratory failure.

[3] Troublesome dry cough.

[4] Diuretics occupy the top of the list of drugs prescribed, and of those causing side effects in the elderly.

the sources of B_{12} – I said liver, red meat and vegetables. He said **'Are you sure about vegetables?'** I replied 'Yes'. **'So who gets B_{12} deficiency?'** At this point the penny dropped, 'Vegans – therefore there is no B_{12} in vegetables'. He then asked me to carry on, so I told him about intrinsic factor in the stomach and absorption at the distal small intestine. He asked how B_{12} was carried in the blood.[5] I didn't know. He then asked how it was stored. I said 'In the liver'. He then asked me what we need it for, so I started to tell him about cell metabolism and about megaloblastic anaemia, skin and gut mucosa changes. He just kept saying **'Mmm'** and I had no idea whether I was telling him what he wanted to know.

He then said, **'I had a *patient of 50 years of age with a serum calcium of 2.96 mmol/l,* what do you think of that?'**. I told him that it was high, but that it should be checked after a fast. He then asked me for the five main causes of hypercalcaemia. I could only remember four – malignancy, hyperparathyroidism, sarcoidosis and the milk-alkali syndrome. After a lot of prompting I finally got **myeloma**. He then asked for the **treatment** and I said intravenous fluids, steroids and possibly mithramycin or calcitonin. He just nodded and asked if I thought steroids were effective. I said I thought that they worked well in the short term. He nodded but was obviously not happy with this answer. He then asked how I would differentiate between **malignant and nonmalignant causes of hypercalcaemia.** I started listing tests such as serum angiotensin-l-converting enzyme activity levels, PTH, bone scan, etc. Again he was not satisfied and then asked what would happen if steroids were given to each type of patient.

I could see what he wanted me to say, so I said it – that is, that the patient with hyperparathyroidism would not be affected in terms of lowering the Ca^{2+} level (however, I am not sure if this is true).[6] He nodded and then asked me **the nerve supply to the hand**. I said ulnar, radial and median. He asked me the sensory areas supplied by each and I was able to tell him correctly.[7]

The viva then ended.

Impressions: I left feeling that if I had failed the clinical examination it would have been on the viva as in the last half (the second examiner) I was struggling somehow to get on the same wavelength as the examiner. I don't think I said anything particularly wrong, but I got no feedback and found this rather unnerving.

(Passed)

---

5   By B_{12}-binding proteins: transcobalamin, I, II and III

6   The corticosteroid suppression test is occasionally used to differentiate between the various causes of hypercalcaemia. It is based on the empirical observation that proliferative disorders and hypervitaminosis D respond to the administration of 60 mg of prednisolone given in daily divided doses for 10 days, whereas the same treatment only rarely results in a fall in serum calcium level in primary or ectopic hyperparathyroidism.

7   Asking a basic question like this at the end does tend to confirm the candidate's suspicion, that the examiner was not fully satisfied.

31

The Inverclyde Royal Hospital was not the easiest place to find (25 miles from Glasgow). No directions had been given on how to get there (I would advise people to look at a map well beforehand).

I felt fairly nervous but we were greeted very well and tea and biscuits were provided. My viva followed on my long and short cases directly, therefore I had time to warm up!!

I was called into a small room, 8'×10', and introduced to the examiners. From my long case I had found out that one examiner was a chest physician; I don't know what the other was, probably a gastroenterologist.

Examiner: 'Tell me what you know about the management of *oesophageal variceal bleeding*?'[1]

(I had already rehearsed this answer with my registrar.) I gave the details of resuscitation and the use of a Sengstaken tube including portal pressures (which impressed them!). Very easy supplementary questions if you have learnt the subject – it all took approximately ten minutes.

Examiner: 'You are called to A&E to see a 20-year-old man with left-sided *pleuritic chest pain* and shortness of breath of *sudden* onset. What is your first diagnosis? What would you do?'[2]

Answer: 'Pneumothorax – I would take a chest X-ray and then drain it appropriately or leave if the pneumothorax is small and the patient is stable.' There then followed a discussion about chest drains and pneumothorax. I had just finished six months of chest medicine so this was a good five minutes.

Examiner: 'A 60 -year-old man with a *lung carcinoma* develops polyuria and polydipsia. What is the diagnosis?'[3]

Answer: 'Hypercalcaemia.' There then followed a discussion on the treatment. I got into a mess with diphosphonates.

Examiner: 'How do they work?'[4]

Answer: 'I can't remember.' The examiners did not seem to mind too much and did not press the matter (five minutes).

---

[1] This question was phrased as a *Bedtime* Story and the candidate made the most of this opportunity by talking for ten minutes.

[2] A good example of a *Detective* Story.

[3] This was another good *Detective* Story from the same examiner. Some examiners are known to bring a collection of well-prepared *Detective* and *Ghost* Stories for the viva.

[4] Diphosphonates are stable analogues of pyrophosphate which may lower blood levels of calcium, probably by a direct effect on osteoclastic reabsorption of bone. Pyrophosphate modifies the crystal growth of calcium hydroxyapatite by adsorption onto the crystal surface, where it inhibits either crystal reabsorption or growth, thereby suppressing a rapid turnover of bone.

Examiner: 'You are called to see a 75-year-old woman on an orthopaedic ward who has had a *fit*. What are your thoughts?'[5]

Answer: 'Is she a fitter anyway?'

Examiner: 'No.'

Answer: 'Does she have any signs of a stroke or raised intracranial pressure – due to head injury?'

Examiner: 'No.'

Answer: 'This may well be due to a fat embolus.'

Examiner: 'What else would you look for and do?'

Answer: 'CXR.'

Examiner: 'Look for a petechial rash especially in the conjunctivae.'[6]

Bell went! I shook hands with the examiners, thanked them and left.

Impressions: I knew the viva had gone well as there was nothing very difficult and they did not seem to be 'gunning' for me. I'm sure that they could have been much more severe if they had wanted to be.

(Passed)

---

[5] Superficially sounds like a *Detective* Story (as were the two preceding questions), but this time the examiner provided the *ghost-link* by stating that the patient was on an orthopaedic ward, and there were other possibilities which should have been mentioned without asking questions. Fat embolism is a complication of injury and surgical trauma of limbs, and the symptoms usually develop within 2 – 3 days.

[6] A petechial rash appears over the upper half of the body (often precedes other symptoms), especially over the chest and conjunctivae (but not on the face or the back) in some patients with a fat embolism.

32

The viva started on time.

There was a large hall with at least ten tables with pairs of examiners, i.e. several candidates were being examined at one time. The examiners were courteous and introduced themselves.

Examiner: 'An unwell patient with *ulcerative colitis* presents to the A/E department.'

I discussed possible diagnoses and clinical signs, e.g. perforation, megacolon, haemorrhage, the presence or absence of bowel sounds, etc. Investigations – bloods and X-rays. Management – I discussed various aspects of conservative *vs* surgical treatment.

Examiner: 'A young footballer started *fitting* on a football field.'

I gave a differential – tumour, infection, idiopathic, metabolic. The examiner led me towards viral encephalitis and asked for the investigations. I said an EEG and a CT scan. Treatment–if herpes I would use acyclovir.

Examiner: 'A middle-aged lady *on warfarin* presents with a *GI haemorrhage*. Her primary diagnosis is mitral valve disease.'

I discussed causes of bleeding, the role of endoscopy, etc.

Examiner: 'What if her INR[1] was greater than 10?'

This led to a discussion on the treatment of overanticoagulation. The examiner felt that vitamin K should have been given and seemed annoyed at this.[2] I disagreed with the examiner by saying that I would give FFP but not vitamin K, since one would want to keep her anticoagulated in view of her valve disease. He also seemed annoyed when I said one would check the haemoglobin level. He asked me if I didn't think that one's clinical judgement was sufficient to diagnose anaemia. I said, 'No' (the other

---

[1] International Normalised Ratio $= \dfrac{\text{Patient's prothrombin time}^{\text{ISI}}}{\text{Control prothrombin time}}$

where ISI is the international sensitivity index provided by the manufacturer of rabbit thromboplastin used in the test. For adequate anticoagulant control, the INR should be maintained between 2.0 and 3.0, as recommended by the British Society for Haematology (J Clin Path 1990; 43: 177).

[2] Reversing the anticoagulant state with vitamin K_1 will render the patient refractory for about two weeks, and it will take longer to re-establish good anticoagulant control. However, strong disagreement with the examiner and annoying him was unnecessary, since a smaller dose of vitamin K_1 (5 mg) can be given to reduce the haemorrhagic tendency without cancelling the anticoagulation. In fact, many experts prefer this approach to FFP.

examiner seemed to agree with me on this one). **Drug interactions with warfarin** were then discussed.

The final question concerned the **differential diagnosis of collapse** in an old lady. The examiner led me towards the sick sinus syndrome and the role of pacemakers.

Impressions: Overall, one pleasant and affable examiner, the other one more taciturn and showed annoyance with my answers on two occasions. I was upset at having been in direct contradiction on two points; I felt that this was my weakest performance.

(Passed)

33

Both examiners were friendly and polite.

Examiner 1: **'We're going to talk about *diabetic ketoacidosis* — start by giving me some 'numbers' that we're dealing with!'**

I thought this was an odd request. This was not only a slightly peculiar question but he also proceeded to hinder my attempts at giving him a verbatim 'management of DKA' style answer by asking me further specific questions.

I gave him the standard 'numbers' he wanted.[1] He then asked me at what serum K^+ level would I start giving K^+ in the infusion.[2] I can't remember other specific questions but it was all reasonably straight-foward. Then he said:

Examiner 1: **'You're the medical registrar instructing the house physician. What instructions will you give him after about 18–24 hours, when the patient's glucose is back to normal but he still has ketones in the urine?'**

I said that he still needed insulin and I would give him alternate pints of normal saline and 5% dextrose. He wasn't happy with this and said that it should be 5% dextrose continuously. He concluded by saying, **'Never mind, you cured the patient and I suppose that's all that matters.'**

Examiner 2: **'What do you know about *acute phase reactants*?'**[3]

I mentioned C-reactive protein, other proteins, the role of interleukin-1 and the concomitant decrease in albumin and various hormone-binding globulins.

He then asked me if I knew the **mechanism of hypoalbuminaemia in inflammation**. I replied I didn't know and he said that I should 'hazard a guess' as I was doing OK so far. I surmised that the hepatic cells were using all available protein for acute phase reactant synthesis – he seemed to

---

[1]   On average, an adult loses about 6 litres of fluid, 500 mmol of sodium and 350 mmol of potassium. Nitrogen losses are also considerable, and important trace elements such as magnesium may be seriously depleted.

[2]   p. 41

[3]   Infections, trauma, inflammatory processes and some malignant diseases induce a number of host responses called acute phase changes. Although a variety of new proteins is synthesised in the liver, there are changes in many other organs (e.g. fever, leucocytosis, thyroid dysfunction, impaired glucose tolerance, anaemia, hypergammaglobulinaemia, etc.). There is a dramatic increase in the synthesis of several unique hepatic proteins that are not produced in health (e.g. C-reactive protein) and of many others that are normally present (e.g. fibrinogen, prothrombin, haptoglobin, ferritin, etc.). Of all the acute phase proteins, C-reactive protein and serum amyloid A protein are clinically important as these serve as indicators of disease. Interleukin-l, cachectin (tumour necrosis factor), and interferon are responsible for inducing acute phase changes.

think this was reasonable.[4] He then went on to ask me about the regulation of hormone-binding globulin levels normally and in inflammation. All I really knew about was the regulation of sex hormone-binding globulin, which I discussed until we ran out of time. I felt the viva had gone well.

P.S. The first examiner asked at the end, **'How many cases of DKA have you managed?'**

I thought, 'What's he getting at here? What's the perfect reply? If I say dozens he will think I ought to have known that one should keep them on 5% dextrose. If I say only one or two he will think I am too inexperienced.' So I said three (which was in fact the truth).

(Passed)

---

[4] Although the liver is producing increasing amounts of a number of proteins, hepatic albumin synthesis is decreased. This may be because amino acids are required for the synthesis of hepatic acute phase proteins, immunoglobulins, collagen, clonal expansion of lymphocytes and for the proliferation of fibroblasts.

34

I did my viva last with no gaps between any of the three parts. After the short cases had seemingly gone so badly, I was very distracted and demoralised when I went in to face my two examiners.[1] They were reassuringly friendly, however, and I decided immediately that I had to put the 'shorts' behind me and concentrate on the job in hand. The first examiner asked me, '**Tell me about the staging of *lymphomas* . . . why do we do it?**'

Elation! Having done a haematology job I knew my ground and I was away. He then asked, '**How would you treat these cases?**' I said it would depend on the nodal size, location, and if aggressive therapy was indicated. He said (with a twinkle in his eye), '**We're very aggressive in Scotland!**'

I launched into the CHOP/bleo[2] regimen, and when asked about the side effects I was able to give at least one characteristic effect of each drug. He seemed very satisfied and moved on.

He asked me, '**What *sugars* are we interested in measuring in the *blood*?**' This seemed tricky and I decided to give the obvious one (glucose), then skirted around to get on to the urine and Benedict's reaction, fructose and galactose (going back to erythrocyte galactose uridyl transferase). I was then asked the **basis of the 'BM' measurement**. I answered that well.

This first examiner appeared very happy and I was more confident now. I was directed to examiner number 2, a larger-than-life character who started with, '**I don't believe in beta blockers. I think they're awful drugs. Persuade me that they have a use in clinical medicine.**'[3]

He kept interrupting my answer with words of agreement and comment. He then moved on to **ARDS (adult respiratory distress syndrome) and the theories of its causation** (fortunately I'd done an ITU job which helped me to answer this question). Finally, he asked about **septicaemic shock and its treatment**.

By the time I'd had my 20 minutes I felt I had done myself justice, but the all prevailing feeling was that I'd 'blown' it on the short cases.

(*Passed*)

---

[1]   The short cases were: diabetic retinopathy (he was asked why it was not hypertensive, which sank his heart!); stasis ulcer on the leg (was told the patient had psoriasis, and he was doing a dermatology job at the time!); spastic paraparesis (the patient was wearing stockings and the time was short!), and primary biliary cirrhosis (he pointed to what he thought were xanthelasmata and which the examiners thought might have been impressions caused by the patient's spectacles!). The candidate passed the examination; presumably his own marking was more strict than that of the examiners! See also footnote on p. 132.

[2]   Cyclophosphamide, hydroxyldaunorubicin (adriamycin), oncovin (vincristine), prednisolone, bleomycin.

[3]   The phrasing of the question suggests that this was a bee under the examiner's bonnet, although he may have been simply exploring the foundations on which the candidate's practice of using beta blockers was built.

35

The first question was a clinical problem about an elderly man who had presented with a **unilateral headache**. He asked what I would be concerned about.

'**Temporal arteritis**', I said. He then asked about other clinical manifestations and the features of **polymyalgia rheumatica**. He asked about the investigations and I offered that I'd do an ESR and temporal artery biopsy, and then start steroids. The examiner got a little upset when I said we could get biopsies performed on the next available list with no delay.[1]

He then asked about the **histology of the biopsy** and how it differed from the histology of polyarteritis nodosa.[2] I had no idea and told him so. He then went on to ask how a diagnosis of polyarteritis could be made. We discussed cytoplasmic antibodies and renal arteriogram/biopsy. He seemed satisfied and then asked, 'Tell me about the **value of dieting**.' Fortunately by then it was halftime.

The other examiner said, '**I have discharged a 40-year-old man with an** *uncomplicated myocardial infarction*. **What would you offer him?**' We chatted about beta blockers and aspirin or anticoagulants. He asked what investigations I would do, and I said serum lipids and exercise ECG. '**Why would you do this?**' and I said to see if there is ST depression.[3]

He got a little unhappy at this and said, '**Surely the patient would complain of angina!**' I answered, 'He could have silent ischaemia.' I also said that I would perform angiography. He got really upset at this and wanted to know why. I said he was a young patient and we needed to know. He then said, '**The patient was an** *HGV driver*, **what would happen to his licence?**' I said he would lose it.

'**Is there any way he can get it back?**'

'Not that I know of.'

'**Who would you ask?**' The DVLC in Swansea was not the answer he wanted. He then told me that if there are no q waves and the angios are normal he can drive an HGV.[4]

'**How could he have a myocardial infarction with normal angios and no q waves?**' I mentioned, 'Subendocardial MI with an arterial spasm.' He then quickly went on to ask about the **rare causes of GI haemorrhages**.

(*Passed*)

---

[1]   A medical registrar should be capable of performing a temporal artery biopsy (a bedside, or as the Americans say an office, procedure) and not have to wait 24 hours and overburden the surgical list. Starting the treatment as soon as possible is important, particularly as the examiner had asked what the candidate would be concerned about (blindness).

[2]   Giant cells are the hallmark of giant cell (temporal) arteritis. Unfortunately, these are not unique to this condition and they do occur in some other forms of destructive arteritis (e.g. Buerger's disease). On the other hand, fibrinoid necrosis and fragmentation of the elastic lamina with microaneurysms occur in polyarteritis nodosa.

[3]   Exercise testing is now widely used to identify patients who might benefit from coronary bypass surgery. A poor prognosis is indicated by an exercise test that reveals ST segment depression on the electrocardiogram of more than 2 mm, angina, failure of the blood pressure to rise and ventricular extrasystoles. Patients who perform poorly on exercise testing may be recommended to have coronary angiography with a view to having bypass surgery.

[4]   Persistent ST-T changes, q waves, angina, or if the ST-T changes have returned to normal but reappear on exercise testing (ST depression of 2 mm or more) will ban an HGV driver from driving (Medical Aspects of Fitness to Drive, London 1985).

36

The viva and clinical exam were on separate days because the clinical was held some distance away from Edinburgh. This was therefore the first part of the exam I sat, and the worst! The oral was in a large hall where about eight other people were also having their vivas and this was distracting. I did not know either of the two examiners and they were very slow to introduce themselves. The questions were as follows:

1. **Cholesterol production and metabolism**. Mechanism of action of the lipid lowering agents and drug interactions.
2. **Anticoagulation during pregnancy**.
3. **Medical complications of a nuclear disaster**. Methods of minimising problems and avoiding excessive exposure. Despite the fact that I knew nothing about this subject, the examiner was very persistent and continued on it for most of his time.
4. **Treatment of hypothyroidism** in an elderly person with ischaemic heart disease.

I answered most of these questions very badly, and felt that I had probably failed this part of the exam. This was a very discouraging start to the rest of the clinical the next day.

I felt that my oral questions should have been more clinically orientated than they were.

(*Failed the viva; passed the exam*)

37

The viva was held in a comfortable room; the two examiners were a pleasant and very unaggressive duo. The viva was last and I was feeling slightly let down after the short cases.[1] I wanted to make up ground but I felt that they were bored of asking questions.

Examiner 1: 'A young man with *cardiomyopathy* is referred to your clinic. His GP has been increasing his *frumil*[2] but he is still in failure. What do you do?'

I asked for his BP and was given it (low) and then mentioned avoidable factors like alcohol. I said I would admit him, stop the amiloride, lower the dose of frusemide and give him captopril in a small dose, and watch his BP carefully. He eventually managed to get me talking about arrhythmias and the complications of these, viz. sudden death. I told him about amiodarone and talked of its negative inotropicity[3] and then talked about digoxin. The conversation spluttered out. Neither of us looked very satisfied. The examiner was obviously looking for a more comprehensive management of intractable heart failure.[4]

The other examiner asked me something about **respiratory physiology** although I can't remember exactly what it was. He received a preclinical textbook reply. He then asked me about the **nonanalgesic drugs** that relieve pain.[5]

I started on tricyclic antidepressants and psychic pain but this obviously wasn't what was wanted. I floundered for a while until *tegretol* came to mind. He then asked me what pain-relieving uses this might have, and I felt he probably didn't know about postherpetic neuralgia and carbamazepine and I couldn't think of any others. He mentioned what he was thinking of but I've forgotten – it wasn't as good as *tegretol*.

Impressions: I wasn't very impressed with my performance; while I hadn't said anything stupid I didn't feel I was winning any prizes. The examiners, while very pleasant, were obviously (and understandably!) bored out of their minds, and I felt that I had passed the viva by keeping it simple and by not irritating or stretching them.

(*Passed*)

---

[1] The candidate forgot to tell the examiners to move off the table while defibrillating *Annie*!

[2] A combination of frusemide and amiloride.

[3] Intravenously administered amiodarone causes only a slight and transient negative inotropic effect. Oral amiodarone may even enhance cardiac performance by decreasing systemic and coronary vascular resistance (Goodman and Gilman's 1990 The pharmacological basis of therapeutics, 6th edn. Pergamon Press, Oxford).

[4] pp. 31, 64

[5] **Nonanalgesic pain relievers:**
Anticonvulsants (phenytoin, carbamazepine) in trigeminal neuralgia
Antidepressants in postherpetic neuralgia
Amphetamines in postoperative pain
Tricyclic antidepressants in diabetic neuropathic pain
Antihistamines in somatic and visceral pain
Phenothiazines in somatic and visceral pain
Steroids in inflammatory pain
Behavioural therapy in psychic pain.

38

My viva was held in a well organised North Tees Hospital. Both examiners in the viva seemed fairly friendly. The first examiner's question was unexpected in its type:

'Imagine you have returned from a tropical country and find you have diarrhoea – what are your thoughts?'

Since this was directed to myself being the patient as well as the 'doctor', it seemed somewhat unconventional and initially 'threw me' in my answer.

I answered by talking about the possible causes and how I might decide clinically and from laboratory tests about the specific cause. Each answer led to the examiner either adding a bit more information or asking more questions.

He seemed content with my answers, although the vague type of questioning and the random path that the questions and answers took made me wonder how well I had done. There were very few straight questions and answers.[1]

The second examiner asked me direct questions. Firstly, about the diagnosis of **pulmonary embolism**. Most of this was straightforward although I made the mistake of saying that on a CXR one might see *small* pulmonary arteries at the hilum and I was corrected on this. I felt that this was a major error and wondered whether I had failed the viva on this account.

Secondly, I was asked if I had taken part in any **clinical trials**. I told him that only in the sense of completing questionnaire-type forms from major drug companies with national ongoing trials. I was then asked how I would set up a clinical trial, e.g. to test drug A *vs* drug B. This I felt was a somewhat unfair question. However, I answered by reciting all the usual phrases that I assumed the examiners wished to hear, e.g. double blind, randomised, prospective, etc. I was asked what **statistical tests** I would use, I said Student's *t*-tests.[2] I was then asked how I would compare '**unmatched**' **data**.[3] I had forgotten the exact test since doing Part I MRCP. I said I didn't know the name although I knew there was a particular test used.

Finally, with about two minutes to go I was asked to tell the examiners

---

[1]   The uneven path the questions and answers took was probably because the candidate did not pick up the two important cues (tropical and diarrhoea) to organise his answer. He should have first focused on *giardiasis* (by far the commonest cause) and then crystallised all the principal causes:

Bacterial – *Campylobacter, Salmonella, E. coli, Shigella*
Viral – enterovirus, hepatitis associated virus, orbivirus
Protozoal – *Giardia lamblia, Entamoeba histolytica*
Helminthic – *Ascaris, Ancylostoma, Trichuris, Strongyloides*
Dietary – irritating food, food allergy, nonspecific food intolerance
Toxins – food poisoning, drugs, alcohol, etc.

[2]   Since the two drugs (A *vs* B) are being tested on the same population a *paired t*-test can be used.

[3]   We presume the examiner meant that the data were obtained from *two* populations which were not matched for age, sex or any other factors relevant to the study. For such data an *unpaired t*-test can be used. However, if the study design is such that the populations can be grouped in 2 by 2 contingency tables (for example, males and females asked for a 'yes' or 'no' for smoking) then the *chi-square* test is appropriate.

about the **bad effects of smoking**! This seemed such a major subject in so short a time that I 'grouped' and subheaded my answer, e.g. physical – higher IHD, BP; social – unpleasant smell, antisocial; financial – cost, etc. I had a few seconds to tell them how I would convince a patient to stop smoking. I used a similar technique to answer this.

Impressions: Overall, I felt the viva was my worst performance and had I failed I would have blamed the viva, since I had answered quite a few questions wrongly or had said 'I don't know'.

(*Passed*)

39

The first question was an attempt at a 'local' topic: **'What are the specific illnesses among Glasgow shipbuilders?'** The mention of asbestosis led to a discussion of the **epidemiology of lung cancer**. When smoking and asbestos had been covered, one examiner asked, **'What do I tell my patients who have never smoked?'** He liked my answer indicating that the disease could be regarded simply as 'bad luck'; though it became clear that he had really wanted other risk factors, e.g. radium and uranium mines.

He then changed the subject and asked, **'What is *pharmacokinetics* and what is *pharmacodynamics*?'**[1] The depth of knowledge required was really very limited. He asked about **first pass metabolism**[2] and I was about to give examples when he tried to help by asking me to name an **'ITU drug beginning with "L"'**. I was not able to come up with the required 'lignocaine'. Further questions on the pharmacodynamics of digoxin were fairly trivial. He asked me for the correct length of time after a dose that one would take a blood sample for an aminophylline level. I did not know this answer but I believe that I concealed my ignorance by pointing out that there were numerous different preparations of aminophylline/theophylline.

The second examiner, who had been silent, quizzed me on **polycystic kidneys** by asking, **'How would you advise an adult patient with polycystic kidneys?'**[3]

He tolerated me briefly confusing the mode of inheritance with the infantile form. It was not clear as to what extent he wanted an account of the disease, and to what extent he was assessing my ability to counsel patients. He liked my reluctance to advise patients against having children,

---

[1]   p. 54

[2]   p. 57

[3]   *General guidelines*:

1. Be sure of the diagnosis
2. Develop a good rapport
3. Provide accurate facts about the diagnosis, prognosis, risk of transmission to offspring and the options available (e.g. treatment, contraception, prenatal diagnosis, etc.). Do not press for any of these. Encourage questions.
4. Assure of continuing support.

Specific guidelines:

Adult polycystic kidney disease is heritable, and manifests itself (pain, haematuria, hypertension, proteinuria) between 30 and 40 years of age, progressing to end-stage renal failure by the fifth decade. Some patients live a normal life. Modern treatment with the successful use of haemodialysis and renal transplantation can provide many years of active life. The mode of inheritance is autosomal dominant with a high degree of penetrance but with variable expressivity. The problems for the counsellor are that the patients have entered, sometimes passed, the procreative years before the condition becomes recognisable. However, the carriers of the affected gene can be recognised by DNA testing and the help of a genetics centre should be enlisted. Most genetics departments maintain a register, and the patient may be known to the nearest centre.

and then broadened the discussion to **Huntington's chorea**, and to the implications of a gene probe to indicate affected subjects prior to the onset of the disease. To the question, '**What is a *gene probe*?**'[4] I quickly answered: 'A biochemical group that is attached to the chromosome and is subsequently associated with the gene in question by genetic linkage.' I have no idea whether there was any truth in this answer. I am sure that had he probed the discussion, my ignorance would have been exposed.

As I left the viva the first examiner said, '**Well done, keep it up**'.

(*Passed*)

---

[4]   The two strands of DNA have a mutual attraction because of their complementary base pairs, and can be dissociated and reassociated *in vitro* by heating and cooling. In this way it is also possible to form double-stranded DNA – RNA molecules. The reannealing reaction is highly specific and, under suitable conditions, occurs only between DNA or RNA strands which have complementary base sequences. This specificity allows researchers to look for a particular gene buried in a large amount of DNA. Thus, we might use a length of DNA with a complementary sequence which will anneal to a particular gene but not to the rest of the DNA. This is the principle behind using **gene probes** to screen for the genes we are interested in. Using an enzyme called reverse transcriptase, a complementary DNA copy of any messenger RNA can be isolated from mammalian cells. A second DNA strand can then be copied on to the newly synthesised cDNA using a bacterial DNA polymerase. In this way, cDNA duplexes are made which can be incorporated into plasmids and then grown in bacterial cells. Thus, it is possible to clone fragments of genomic DNA into plasmids or bacteriophage and to amplify individual genes in bacteria to make **gene probes**. When used as probes, radioactive bases are added onto the synthesised cDNA and, when made single-stranded, these will bind to complementary sequences in genomic DNA; this hybridisation will be revealed by autoradiography by virtue of the radioactive bases incorporated in the probe.

40

My viva was probably the worst part of the whole examination. It was held in the College. It started late and was very awesome! I had to wait for about 15 minutes (which seemed like hours) outside the exam room. I could see all these poker-faced examiners looking at us as if we were going to the electric chair! My examiners, however, were very nice. They shook hands, introduced themselves and even tried to crack a joke to relax me.

Examiner 1:   *'What do you know about counselling?'*[1]

There were questions about HIV infection – mostly about ethics, should partners, GPs, etc., be told.[2]

Examiner 1:   *'What would you do as a doctor, if you were found to be HIV positive?*[3] **Would you still work? Would you tell your patients?'**

It was difficult to answer really, I gave my personal views. They seemed surprised that I'd tell my boyfriend first! This made them laugh a bit though!

Change of tack. Examiner number 1, who was very nice (the *dove*), said:

Examiner 1:   **'I'm 45, overweight, a nonsmoker, I drink 10 pints per week, I see you and** *ask to go on aspirin to prevent a heart attack.* **How would you advise me?'**

This led to a discussion regarding the recent trials of aspirin and MIs/CVAs, risks/benefits, etc. This led to other risk factors – we talked about a Western diet, cholesterol and obesity. We then talked about alcohol and current drinking advice.

Change of tack again.

**Examiner 2
(the hawk):**   *'Whilst you mentioned aspirin, tell me about Reye's syndrome.'*[4]

Again, a recent *BMJ* leader, which I'd read the day before, came to my rescue! This led to a discussion about acute liver failure – causes, treatment, management, etc. This then led on to a discussion about the indications for **liver transplantation** in children (I thought very unfair in an MRCP general exam) and in adults.

We then talked about **primary biliary cirrhosis** and its treatment. Once again, that had been the subject of a leader in the *BMJ*.

---

[1]   p. 83
[2]   pp. 22, 33
[3]   p. 36
[4]   p. 28

We talked about the **ethics of organ transplantation**[5] and the role of the medical registrar in this – seeing relatives and gaining consent. We also talked about lung transplantation.

Then the *hawk* asked me about **immunosuppression and its complications**, about the drugs used, and in particular cyclosporin and its side effects.

Then the bell went. Thank goodness!!

Impressions: I had prepared for this viva by reading the *BMJ, Lancet* and *NEJM* and had picked out the major leading articles that I thought may come up. I was lucky – I had picked well. All the topics I was questioned on I had prepared quite well. The *dove* seemed very benign but the *hawk* was probing deeply into my knowledge.

I surprised myself by being quite relaxed once I had started. However, I'd had plenty of practice with SR's and consultants.

The examiners seemed interested and said that I'd done well at the end.

(*Passed*)

---

[5]   pp. 35, 91

41

The examiners were very pleasant throughout! I was asked to sit down and the first examiner said to me, **'I would like to indulge in a little role playing. Imagine I am an 18-year-old boy who has had two fits in the last week. Ask me some questions.'** I asked about the fits, whether they were witnessed, had he been drinking, and was cut short. He told me that the fits were typical grand mal convulsions. He then asked me what investigations I would like to do. I mentioned routine blood tests, a skull X-ray and, provided that there were no abnormal CNS signs, an EEG.

'**Would you?'** asked the examiner, **'Why?'**[1]

I was taken aback but decided to stick to my guns and explained that a normal EEG would not help, but an epileptiform focus would confirm the diagnosis. He seemed satisfied, and then asked what I would like to tell him. I explained that he was, by definition, an epileptic and would therefore need treatment. This would hold implications for his social and working life, emphasising the problems with driving. He then asked, **'What sort of *treatment* would you recommend?'** and there ensued a discussion on the relative merits and disadvantages of anticonvulsants, particularly aspects of toxicity and pharmacokinetics. This seemed to go quite well, although I was a bit shaky on the monitoring of drug levels.

We then moved to the second examiner, whose first question was, **'Imagine I am a dentist and I have in my surgery a patient with a heart murmur. What advice are you going to give me?'** I'd mugged up all the antibiotic recommendations for valve lesions so this went quite well. The next question concerned **dentists and HIV infection**. I'm not sure what the examiner was after here, and I felt sure that there must have been something recently in the literature about this subject. I said that the risks were low compared to hepatitis B, and talked about common-sense precautions, but I still felt I was missing something.

The last question was the one I had dreaded, as I had been meaning to look it up and had never got round to it! **Diabetic microalbuminuria**. Luckily the bell went shortly after we'd started on this topic, so I didn't quite unveil the depth of my ignorance of this subject!

(*Passed*)

---

[1]   Physicians in general, and examiners in particular, tend to vary in the way they respond to a suggestion about the use of an EEG in the investigation of epilepsy. It is often forgotten that an EEG, unlike an ECG, does not provide specific diagnostic information, and in many cases is only as good as the person requesting it. The timing of recording an EEG is important (not useful soon after a fit), and its limitations must be borne in mind. The diagnosis of epilepsy can often be established on history alone, but in cases of difficulty an EEG may sometimes help to confirm it; postictal tracings often show an excess of slow waves, and there may be brief interictal spurts between the seizures. Ambulatory recorders can be used whenever nocturnal attacks are suspected. In some centres full video and eight-channel recorder equipped sleeping laboratories are available for nocturnal studies. An EEG can be helpful in resolving the important question of whether the fits are secondary to a cerebral pathology, although CT and MRI scans can give more precise information about a space-occupying lesion. Discordant records from the two hemispheres (spikes on one side and normal alpha rhythm on the other) suggest a local pathology, such as mesial temporal sclerosis which is potentially remediable.

42

I was pretty certain that I had failed the long case and therefore I felt relaxed and warmed up for the viva.[1] I was surprised at the clinical orientation of all the questions. All were of the form **'you are in casualty and . . .'** These seemed much more relevant to clinical practice.

I had one female and one male examiner. Both started pleasantly and then developed fairly aggressive questioning. The male examiner visibly relaxed towards the end.

Examiner 1: **' A confused, aggressive 45-year-old patient presents in casualty.'**

They looked for (1) that I would not leave him with the police and (2) that I would consider the underlying illness. They asked about sedation – chlorpromazine.

'What dose?' (Not allowed to do this, I thought.)

'What others?' (No answer given.)

Every answer I gave was met by a further complication in the patient! The eventual aim was to consider a **cerebral abscess** which I eventually got to.

I then got the medical student lecture on, **'Everybody forgets the cerebral abscess – look in the ears.'**

Examiner 2: **'A 42-year-old man with an anterior myocardial infarction is brought to casualty.'**

Routine reply – ECG, venflon, get to CCU as soon as possible.

Examiner 2: **'What is the cause of the cardiac pain?'**

I gave a stumbling reply and was told, **'No, shall we move on'**?
The eventual point after much probing was **streptokinase**.
'Yes, I was involved in the APSAC trial.'[2]
The examiner said that no-one in general hospitals knows that all anterior MIs get streptokinase.

Examiner 2: **'A phobic patient presents, discuss her management in the OPD.'**

I discussed flooding and desensitisation, then drugs – diazepam and beta blockers.

Examiner 2: **'What is the other drug that reacts with Marmite?'** he asked with a smile.

Mental blank.

---

[1]   The candidate missed the diagnosis of an anterior myocardial infarction on the ECG which the examiners politely pointed out. However, he had presented the history and demonstrated the physical signs competently.

[2]   Anisoylated Plasminogen Streptokinase Activator Complex (APSAC) Intervention Mortality Study (AIMS) Group Lancet 1988; 1: 545

Examiner 2: 'Well, we will let you think about that,' he said as the bell went.

I learnt that you can pass provided you keep your cool and talk sense and admit to what you don't know. Also, 'aggression' in the examiner does not reflect a fail or a pass.

(*Passed*)

43

The viva carried on straight from the short cases with barely a pause. I prefer that to a long wait. It was the third part of my clinical examination and after my experiences in the short cases,[1] I really thought I had already failed, so I suppose I was more relaxed. It took place in a room of ample size off the main ward with two examiners. One was Dr P so I expected, and subsequently got, some questions on infections. I don't remember the other examiner's name but he started off by asking me questions about statistics which threw me, as I wasn't expecting them. He asked me for my definition of **standard deviation**[2] which I bumbled through. He then asked me if I knew of any other way of describing the same sort of idea. He was after '**confidence intervals**'[2] but I didn't really know what he was driving at, and began to feel that the whole thing was futile! He eventually prompted me, and when it was obvious that I was floundering he moved on to my great relief.

He then asked me what I'd do if someone came into my outpatient clinic complaining of **diarrhoea**.

I replied that my course of action would depend on the age of the patient, so he asked me to describe what I'd do with a patient of about 30 with a one-year history of diarrhoea. I explained that I'd start with history and examination as with any patient, and mentioned the usual investigations such as stool culture, sigmoidoscopy, blood count, plasma viscosity, electrolytes and barium enema, if necessary. I also mentioned dietary assessment, in which he seemed uninterested and asked me what I felt that might contribute. I mentioned excess bran and fibre intake in obsessive individuals, laxative abuse and alcohol; for some reason he seemed quite impressed with the latter. He asked me for a differential diagnosis and wanted to know some of the differences between **Crohn's disease** and **ulcerative colitis,** and also touched on the **irritable bowel syndrome**.

We then moved on to the story of an **elderly patient with diarrhoea** and I talked firstly about neoplastic disease. I think we also talked about malabsorption, but I don't remember much about that.

Then the second examiner took over. His questions flitted from one subject to another, so I apologise if the account is a little disjointed. He asked me what I'd do if, when I left the room after the viva, I came across one of the patients who'd **just collapsed**. I mentioned immediate observations such as colour, state of consciousness, and then went on to say that I would assess the airway, breathing and circulation. He asked me what I'd do if I found no major pulse. I said that there was some controversy about delivering a precordial thump to such a patient.[3] He asked me for the advantages and disadvantages and then asked me to demonstrate the

---

[1]   The candidate had four *long* short cases (hepatosplenomegaly, mixed mitral valve disease and aortic incompetence, tuberose sclerosis and malignant pleural effusion) and a fifth case as the bell went. As she had no feedback she was not sure whether she had got them all right.

[2]   See Appendix I

[3]   p. 35

precordial thump itself! I said the blow had to be very firm if it was to be effective. I don't know if I just had a lot of adrenaline flowing or whether there was just more echo in the room than I had anticipated, but my blow to the desk top sounded very loud indeed! I was then asked to state whether I would use this manoeuvre or not and I said I would. We then got on to cardiac massage, mouth-to-mouth breathing and bagging and finally to establishing the rhythm by an ECG monitor (I had forgotten to say I'd call for the crash team!). I was then asked for my treatment of ventricular fibrillation (shock) and asystole (initially atropine, later followed by adrenaline). I was specifically asked if I would shock someone in asystole. I said, 'No.'

We then got on to the subject of a **pericardial effusion**, its diagnosis and the emergency treatment of **tamponade**. I was asked to describe the different routes for aspiration of the effusion, which one was the safest and what structure may be punctured using the subxiphisternal approach (the coronary arteries).

We then moved on to the **treatment of malaria**. My memory of this is a little confused, but it was basically a question of what would I do if my houseman rang me, to say that a patient who had just returned from Nigeria had malarial parasites on his blood film. I said that I couldn't remember the prevalence of chloroquine-resistant *falciparum* malaria in Nigeria, but said I would like to know the percentage of RBC infected. I would then go and see the patient and give quinine, if in any doubt. He said that this situation had actually happened to him when he was away from the hospital when on call, and that he hadn't needed to see the patient. He agreed with the suggested treatment, i.e. quinine. I countered by saying that I felt I would need to see the patient to assess the supportive treatment that would be needed as well as the antimalarials. He seemed satisfied with this, but I sensed a note of discord. I felt the comment about not seeing the patient was unfair,[4] as I felt it necessary to gain a true picture of the overall condition of a patient with a potentially fatal disease.

I was finally asked about **malaria prophylaxis** in chloroquine-resistant areas. I suggested *fansidar*[5] but he said that it was currently out of favour with him (even though a GP friend told me that it was recommended to him the previous day by the London School of Tropical Medicine!), and so ended my viva.

(*Passed*)

---

[4]   From the examiner's point of view, details about the patient's general state could have been obtained from the house physician who had examined the patient and made the call.

[5]   After the report in 1982 on the resistance of *falciparum* malaria to sulfadiazine-pyrimethamine (*fansidar*), the recommendations for malaria chemoprophylaxis were changed to chloroquine 300 mg base weekly and sulfadiazine-pyrimethamine one tablet weekly (Lancet 1982; 1: 1118). A subsequent study compared the prophylactic efficacy and side effects of chloroquine phosphate 500 mg weekly with proguanil hydrochloride 200 mg daily against chloroquine and sulfadiazine-pyrimethamine. The combination of chloroquine with proguanil was recommended because it resulted in fewer side effects (Brit Med J 1988; 296: 820).

44

My viva was the final part of the examination and followed about ten minutes after the completion of the short cases. I was led into a small room, usually a consultant physician's office. There were two examiners, one 60 plus years and the other 40–45. The latter, a courteous gentleman, asked what cases I had seen so far. The older man, who appeared the more distant (but polite), looked over his half glasses and asked, **'How would you recognise a *deep venous thrombosis*?'**

We passed from the clinical recognition to the differential diagnosis, treatment and management, the long-term advice and the possible factors leading to the development of the condition. Finally, he went on to the associated complications, in particular pulmonary embolism.

Examiner 1: **'What would be the *indications for thoracotomy and embolectomy*?'** **'Have you ever seen these done?'** (No.)

Examiner 1: **'What sort of patient might you consider for one of these procedures?'** **'Do you feel they are worthwhile?'** (Sometimes.)

Having passed through this without any particular problem and with a number of reassuring nods, the bell went and the second examiner, who had been noting my answers during the first part, took over the questioning whilst passing a pink sheet across the desk to the older gentleman.

Examiner 2: *'How would you treat a patient recently admitted to the coronary care unit?'*

I started with the usual gambit about taking a proper history and performing a relevant examination. As I proceeded, it became clear that he wanted me to talk about the role of the **thrombolytic agents** and **beta blockers** in **acute myocardial infarction**.[1]

He asked how I would administer streptokinase and what would be the contraindications to this treatment?

Examiner 2: **'Have you ever used this treatment?'** (Yes.)

'Have you ever seen a definite benefit?' (Yes.)

'How would you know that it was effective?'

Suddenly he changed topic, saying, **'I know that a general physician is not meant to be an expert in this field but what do you know about the *treatment of psoriasis*?'**

Working at present in dermatology I gave several graded options and he nodded.

---

[1] p. 31

Examiner 2: 'What else can happen to a patient with psoriasis?'

After mentioning several dermatological complications, I mentioned psoriatic arthropathy, when he asked, 'How would you recognise *psoriatic arthropathy* clinically?' Then 'How would you treat a patient with this condition?'

I mentioned several methods of treatment, both medical[2] and surgical, including synovectomy, but he persisted.

Examiner 2: 'Anything else?' I admitted I could not think of what he meant. 'Joint replacement, of course.'

Another change of subject:

Examiner 2: 'A man 40 years old returns home from a holiday abroad and later that day turns up at your clinic complaining of a *change in stool habit and weight loss*. What would you think may be the cause?'

I mentioned several infective and tropical causes, then added, 'At his age I would not be happy unless I excluded an underlying sinister cause'. At this stage the bell sounded and without any further questions they gave me my leave quite cheerfully.

I knew that if the result depended on the viva I would be hopeful of passing.

(*Passed*)

---

[2]   p. 56

45

The viva was held in a medium-sized hall in which there were about eight pairs of examiners around the edge. My viva started about five minutes late. I was rather anxious and depleted of confidence.

Examiner 1: '**What do you see as the *major problems facing medicine in the 1990s?***'[1]

Answer: 'The ageing population.'

The examiner wanted me to be more specific:

Examiner 1: '**What problems?**'

Answer: 'Multisystem failure.'

Examiner 1: '**Which systems?**'

I listed various problems and then discussed iatrogenic causes of illness in the elderly. We discussed the problems of diuretics, but I failed to mention hyponatraemia, which I had extracted from me. Next came questions on **osteoporosis and osteomalacia** together with a discussion about **fractured femurs**. Then I described the biochemical changes and probably answered wrongly about the Ca^{2+}, phosphate and alkaline phosphatase. I also said that the dietary intake of vitamin D was more important than sunlight.

Examiner 2: '**How would you manage a four-months pregnant lady with a history suggestive of a *pulmonary embolism*?**'

I initially evaded the issue by describing the investigation and treatment in the nonpregnant state, and waffled regarding the pros and cons of the treatment, whilst desperately trying to remember the effects of warfarin on the fetus and the risks to pregnancy. The examiner saw this and offered that I should look it up, as he had needed to do when the situation had presented itself to him! I agreed.

I then had questions regarding the management of **acute renal failure**; finally he asked me about **renal transplantation** and its indications, and then regarding transplantation in **diabetics**. I suggested it was a grey area and the bell rang.

(*Passed*)

---

[1] A typical 'bee-under-the-bonnet' question in which the examiner's own answer is unknown, but the situation can be tackled by offering two or three credible examples (see p. 94). The candidate started off well by suggesting the 'ageing population' but did not manage a soft landing. He could have directed the examiners' attention to the decreasing tax-paying population, with the inevitable contraction of resources in the face of an increasingly dependent population and expanding medical technology.

46

The viva was held late. Although nervous I was somewhat calmer than I had been at my first attempt. This had a lot to do with my impression that my clinical section, particularly the short cases, had passed reasonably well.

The first question was: **'What can you tell me about *nosocomial* infections?'** I was unfamiliar with this term so the examiners asked me about 'hospital-acquired' infections.

I began by talking about infections in immunocompromised patients, but they duly stopped me and informed me that they wanted to discuss infections in general medical patients, not those on steroids, chemotherapy or with immunosuppressive disease status. At this stage, as you can imagine, the viva wasn't proceeding the way I would have wished it to. However, the examiners appeared pleased, if not relieved, when I suggested that the type of patients they wished to discuss were diabetics. Despite this I could not explain in the depth they wanted the reasons why diabetics were more prone to the 'normal infections', such as urinary tract infections and pneumonias.[1]

The next topic they picked was the use of **ACE inhibitors in congestive cardiac failure**.[2] This subject had also been chosen in the viva of my first attempt. I was now well read on it and there was a favourable response

---

[1] The normal host defence mechanism is impaired at several stages in diabetic patients:
   1. *Skin*. There is a higher rate of nasal carriers of bacteria (*Staphylococcus, Candida* and *Streptococcus*) among diabetics than nondiabetics. Because of impaired sight and sensations together with decreased moisture, skin breakdown is more frequent among diabetic subjects, particularly in the feet.
   2. *Blood vessels*. The high prevalence of atherosclerosis leads to ischaemia in diabetic patients. There is an increased permeability causing tissue oedema; autonomic neuropathy in the feet may cause arteriovenous shunting of blood away from nutrient capillaries to the tissues, such factors are conducive to bacterial proliferation.
   3. *Humoral immunity*. Serum complement is normal or increased. There are conflicting reports about the impaired killing power of polymorphs on various bacteria in diabetics.
   4. *Phagocytic function*. There is decreased chemotactic activity (i.e. the ability of polymorphonuclear cells and macrophages to get to the site of infection), impaired engulfment and intracellular killing.
   5. *Lymphocytes*. Cell-mediated immunity tends to be impaired in diabetics who are in poor metabolic control.
      There is universal agreement on the fact that hospital-acquired infections are commoner among diabetics than in nondiabetic subjects, and that they also develop more serious complications.
[2] pp. 31 and 64

from the examiners as I quoted papers such as the CONSENSUS Study.[3] I therefore managed to keep on the topic for some time, discussing some of the other effects of ACE inhibitors, such as the reduction of proteinuria in normotensive diabetics.

The third topic discussed was that of the care needed for the **terminally ill patient**. I volunteered that the wishes of the patient should be taken into consideration and that there should be a discussion with the family. Although I mentioned social support services at home, they also wanted me to mention the work of the **Macmillan Nurses**.[4]

(*Passed*)

---

[3]   The CONSENSUS Trial Study Group 1987: Effects of enalapril on mortality in severe congestive heart failure: results of the cooperative North Scandinavian enalapril survival study (CONSENSUS). New England Journal of Medicine 316: 1429. This was a controlled trial in 253 patients with severe congestive cardiac failure. A significant reduction in the mortality rate of 40% was observed at the six months follow-up, and 31% at one year. The improvement was entirely due to a reduction in deaths from progressive failure, with no change in the incidence of sudden death.

[4]   A charity organisation which supplies nurses for home care to terminally ill patients.

47

The first question was about the **mortality from an acute myocardial infarction** and I said 15%. He then asked me about the causes of the initial mortality, and I listed them: arrhythmias, cardiogenic shock and sudden death.[1]

I was then asked to take any of these and to discuss its management.

I talked briefly about **cardiogenic shock**, and mentioned diuretics, intravenous inotropes and ITU monitoring.

The next question was: **'A perfectly fit patient has a *left-sided pleural effusion* found at a routine medical examination. *What might be the cause of the effusion?*'**[2]

I discussed routine FBC, U&E, LFT, ESR, CXR, pleural tap for cytology, histology and a pleural biopsy.

I was asked about the difference between a **transudate** and an **exudate**.

This was followed by a question-and-answer session which I have summarised as follows:

Examiner 1: **'Take any type of *drug interaction* and give an example.'**

Answer: 'An example is synergy between trimethoprim and sulphamethoxazole.'

Examiner 1: **'Recent data suggest that this is not so. Now give another example.'**

Answer: 'Liver enzyme induction – barbiturates and warfarin.'

Examiner 1: **'Now give another example.'**

Answer: 'Aspirin and warfarin (protein binding).'

Bell

Examiner 2: **'What is the overall most important therapeutic measure in treating *diabetes mellitus*?'**

Answer: 'Diet.'

Examiner 2: **'Yes, leaving aside diet tell me about the *oral hypoglycaemics*.'**

A confused discussion followed regarding how the various kinds of oral hypoglycaemics work, and the pros and cons of each one.

Examiner 2: **'How could a patient with a *subarachnoid haemorrhage* present?'**

Answer: 'If conscious, with photophobia, headache and neck stiffness.'

---

[1] Sudden death would be covered under arrhythmias. The candidate should have related the mortality to various times after infarction, e.g. first hour, first month, first year, etc. The stated figure of 15% does not include the first-hour mortality, which can be as much as 50%.

[2] This is a *what dunnit?* scenario (see *Detective* Stories, p. 68), and the examiner's patient, being *perfectly* fit ('apparently' fit would have been preferable!), narrows down the possibilities to tuberculous, neoplastic (lymphoma, mesothelioma if over 45 years of age), postpneumonia, pulmonary infarction (haemorrhagic fluid) and possibly Meigs' syndrome (if female). The ensuing discussion about history, examination and investigations should concentrate on these conditions in an attempt to pursue the examiner's diagnosis.

Examiner 2: 'How would you investigate?'

Answer: 'The investigation of an unconscious patient includes a routine history from the relatives, physical examination, routine investigations, e.g. CXR, CT scan if available, and if not a lumbar puncture (as long as there are no signs of increased intracranial pressure!).'

Examiner 2: 'What would a subarachnoid haemorrhage look like on the CT scan?'

Answer: 'White!'[3]

Bell

(*Failed*)

---

[3]   An increased density of the subarachnoid spaces on the CT scan is the hallmark of a subarachnoid haemorrhage. A haemorrhage producing a haematocrit of more than a few percent in the cerebrospinal fluid would be detected in 95% of the cases by a CT scan, particularly within the first week of the haemorrhage.

48

We all shook hands. I was first asked:

Examiner 1: **'A 23-year-old man, who feels well, attends your clinic as a referral from his GP with a *Hb of 13.5 g/dl and an MCV of 105*. What are your initial thoughts?'**

I stated that I would ask about his general health and that I would take a full history, specifically about his alcohol consumption (they were nonplussed).[1] I also talked about any drugs he might be taking which may interfere with folate metabolism. I then mentioned that I would ask about any features of pernicious anaemia (PA) at which point he jumped down my throat stating that with a Hb of 13.5 g he could not have PA.[2] After that, I struggled through the causes of a high MCV, such as hypothyroidism. He went back to my statement about drugs and folate so I said folate malabsorption, which was what they had wanted. Unfortunately, his disagreeing so heatedly with my pernicious anaemia had put me off **malabsorption of B$_{12}$ and folate**. They seemed satisfied at this point, as they did not actually have to state the answer themselves, and I had by then explained why I had been reluctant to say malabsorption.

Next, I was quizzed about the **irritable bowel syndrome (IBS)** its symptoms, signs, causes and its relative frequency, and I was asked if I knew of any other systems involved.[3] I stated that women generally had worse period pains, but they said, **'That may be in the character of the person with IBS'**, to which my reply was, 'No'.

It was then over to the next examiner, who started by saying:

Examiner 2: **'A 50-year-old is admitted with a *left hemiparesis* but with nothing else to find. You are called to the ward two hours later when he has suddenly become**

---

[1]   The candidate missed a very important *ghost-link*; namely, the GP had already obtained a full blood count of the patient which makes it unlikely that the patient had presented to his GP with symptoms related to alcoholism. The most probable clinical scenario confronting the GP must have been a young man presenting with vague ill-health, multiple nonspecific complaints (tiredness, malaise, headaches, etc.), and possibly loss of weight – features that could not be tied into any referral, and the GP was obliged to look a little further and arrange a full blood count. Dwelling for a while on the reasons that took the patient to his GP would have led the candidate to **malabsorption and coeliac disease**, which was probably the *ghost* over the discussion.

[2]   Pernicious anaemia is extremely rare at the age of 23 (this patient's age). **Neurological symptoms** (symmetrical paraesthesiae, irritability, somnolence, perversion of taste and smell and visual disturbances) *can precede* the anaemia. In its early stages, the neurological syndrome can be reversed by vitamin B$_{12}$ therapy and therefore its recognition is very important. In untreated cases, the chronic and irreversible syndrome of **subacute combined degeneration** of the spinal cord, sometimes associated with **optic atrophy**, becomes established.

[3]   The examiner was probably thinking of the *associated* psychosomatic features, such as emotional lability, lethargy, headaches, chest pains and palpitations.

dyspnoeic and cyanosed. **On examination, he has bilateral crackles in the lungs to the midzones. What are your immediate thoughts?'**[4]

Answer: 'I would listen to his precordium for a systolic murmur – a myocardial infarction with embolism and a low BP could have caused the CVA, and he may have ruptured his septum or mitral valve secondary to ischaemic damage!'

Examiner 2: **'Common things occur commonly – no?'**

Answer: 'Although the findings are not classical of **aspiration pneumonia** that would need to be thought of.'

Examiner 2: **'Yes** (sarcastically), **I have just described a classical case of** *aspiration*–**have you ever seen one?'**

Answer: 'Yes, but normally the signs tend to be asymmetrical, as aspiration occurs usually down the right main bronchus.'

We then discussed the management, and she was not at all impressed by my idea of sucking out any vomitus that remained in the back of the throat!

(*Failed*)

---

[4] This is another example of a good *Ghost* Story, with four major possibilities for abrupt respiratory deterioration (acute pulmonary oedema, pulmonary embolism, pneumothorax and aspiration pneumonia), and one *real* one among the four in the examiner's mind. Listening carefully to the examiner's detailed scenario (and looking for the *ghost-link*), it is clear that she is discouraging the candidate from considering pulmonary embolism and pneumothorax, by stating that the patient had crackles up to the midzones on both sides. This, together with the neurological condition of the patient, should increase the index of suspicion for **aspiration pneumonia**.

49

The viva was held in a large hall and there were approximately 20 tables with two examiners and one candidate at each. It was, therefore, noisy and difficult to hear the questions asked.

Examiner: 'An 80-year-old lady is admitted to hospital after having *several falls*. How would you go about investigating the cause?'

Answer: 'I would take a full history and examine the patient, paying particular attention to any drugs she may be taking. The examination should look for any cardiovascular abnormality, e.g. arrhythmias (bradycardia, SVT, atrial fibrillation, etc.) and postural hypotension. I would carry out a full CNS examination.'

Examiner: 'What causes are there for *postural hypotension* in the elderly?'

Answer: 'Most commonly it is drug-induced, e.g. diuretics and beta blockers. Another possibility is autonomic neuropathy[1] due to diabetes mellitus.'

Examiner: 'You are the medical registrar on call, and the casualty officer phones you to say that a 23-year-old man has been brought into casualty after *collapsing* with *central chest pain* whilst playing squash. What is your differential diagnosis on your way to casualty?'

I asked more about the history and whether or not the patient was breathless, but the examiner insisted that I should not need to know any more details.[2]

Answer: 'The differential diagnosis would be: myocardial infarction – possible but unlikely; pneumothorax, dyspepsia, dissecting aortic aneurysm.'

Examiner: 'Tell me how you would manage the patient if he had had a *pneumothorax*?'

Answer: I discussed the different types of pneumothoraces and their management, and the insertion of intercostal tubes.

Examiner: 'How would you manage *atrial flutter* in the context of an *acute myocardial infarction*?'

Answer: 'I would deliver a synchronised DC shock of 40J.' I then discussed the treatment of atrial fibrillation with digoxin, if a DC shock fails.

Examiner: 'What do you think about *digoxin as an inotrope*?'

Answer: 'I believe it is a positive inotrope in the presence of atrial fibrillation. Some people also believe it to be a positive inotrope even in the face of sinus rhythm.'

(*Passed*)

---

[1] pp. 18, 66
[2] This is a *Biblical* referral story – an opportunity for giving a competent performance and not one for asking a lot of supplementary questions (see p. 59).

50

The first examiner was smiling and welcoming.

Examiner 1: 'A 50-year-old lorry driver is referred to you with a six-week history of *central chest pain that sounds cardiac in origin*. In outpatients, how would you go about investigating him?'

Answer: 'I would take a full history, paying attention to a family history of ischaemic heart disease as well as to how much and for how long the patient had smoked. I would carry out a full examination including a check on the patient's weight.' I was interrupted here by the examiner, who said that there was nothing to find on examination except for xanthelasmata on the eyelids. I proceeded to say that I would do a CXR to assess the cardiac size, a resting 12-lead ECG and a FBC to exclude anaemia and polycythaemia, both of which may cause angina. I would also request urea and electrolytes, fasting serum lipids and fasting blood sugar. If the ECG was normal then I would arrange an exercise ECG.

The examiner said that I had missed out an important routine blood test. I couldn't think what he meant. He said thyroid function tests. I just agreed, but I don't think I would do this routinely in this context unless there were clinical features of thyroid disease.[1]

He then said that if the exercise ECG was done and the patient attained a pulse of 120 with a BP of 90/60 and that he had started with a pulse of 80 and a BP of 140/80, what would I do? I said I would stop the test, as the fall in BP was an indication of poor cardiac function and to carry on could precipitate an infarct.

Examiner 1: 'What would you do about the treatment and about this man and his family?'

Answer: I discussed the **treatments for angina**. I said I would use beta blockers as a first choice providing that there were no contraindications (I stated them). The family would have to be screened for hyperlipidaemia. I then discussed the treatment of hyperlipidaemia.

The second examiner did not smile. He seemed cold and inflicted fear on me!

Examiner 2: 'Pretend that you are a GP. A patient of yours is living near a *nuclear power station*. She has heard that there is an increased *incidence of leukaemia* if you live near one for several years. She has come for advice about what to do as she has a 5-year-old son.[2]

Answer: 'It is true that there is an increased incidence of leukaemia if one lives near a nuclear power station.'

---

[1]   This candidate had already mentioned some 'routine' investigations (e.g. FBC, U&E and CXR) which many medical auditors would take issue with. Anaemia, polycythaemia and, of course, thyrotoxicosis (presumably) are all clinically recognisable conditions, and the investigations can only be justified if the clinical suspicion is high. However, *mild hypothyroidism* may be clinically unrecognisable, and should be looked for, along with a screen for hyperlipidaemia.

[2]   The candidate has been asked to pretend to be a general practitioner, but any hospital practitioner could be confronted with the same problem. As the ensuing discussion reveals, the question is highly relevant to hospital practice.

Examiner 2:   'Is that so? Some studies say not! How would you go about proving it?'

Answer: 'I would take a population living within a certain radius of a nuclear power station and compare the prevalence of leukaemia with another population.'

Examiner 2:   'What would you measure? Doesn't leukaemia occur in some areas more than others?'

I carried on saying what I thought were sensible things, and then I was interrupted by the examiner, '**Haven't you heard about longitudinal and lateral studies in statistics?**'[3] I said nothing! '**Let's ask you something else then.**'

Examiner 2:   'A woman, eight weeks *pregnant*, has been exposed to *rubella* and she comes to you for advice. What would you do?'

Answer: 'I would tell her that she must not panic because although she had been exposed to rubella, she may be immune and there may be nothing to worry about. I would measure the antibodies then and repeat two weeks later. If there were a rise then she will have been exposed and was probably nonimmune in the first instance. As she is only eight weeks pregnant there is a risk of teratogenicity (I stated the effects here). I would therefore advise abortion.'

Examiner 2:   'What if it is against her principles. What would you do?'

Answer: 'I would tell her of the risks she is taking, but would have to respect her decision and support her as best I could through her pregnancy.'

Examiner 2:   'Would you do anything else?'

Answer: 'No.'

(*Passed*)

---

[3]   *Longitudinal* studies explore the occurrence, or increase, of any phenomenon in a given population over a period of time, viz. leukaemia in Hiroshima and Nagasaki after the atomic explosion (Am J Epidemiology 1981; 14: 761). Other methods of establishing a *cause* and *effect* between infection or radiation and a disease are by maintaining a register for a certain disease (e.g. Cancer Register) and by studying *time-space clusters* over a given time period (Applied Statistics 1964; 13: 25). The examiner probably used the word *lateral* interchangeably with the longitudinal studies.

51

The viva began on time and was held in a large hall with pairs of examiners at each table. I admit that I was feeling reasonably confident as my turn approached, but this was soon dispelled by the attitude of the examiners, who behaved completely 'dead-pan' and remained expressionless throughout the viva. There was absolutely no feedback when I answered a question, just more questions!

Things began awkwardly when I was asked to give *my* **criteria for prescribing domiciliary oxygen**. I tried to give a general answer, discussing the types of patient that would benefit, as I didn't know the exact PO_2s, FVCs, etc. which was what they wanted.[1]

Next, I was asked what I consider was an unfair question: How I would justify my **expenditure in a coronary care unit** to the area health board? This was nuts! Junior SHOs have absolutely no say in where the 'readies' are spent.[2] I waffled a bit about the benefits of monitoring young patients with myocardial infarctions.

The next question concerned the **management** of a person found to have had a **myocardial infarction at home**, but it was now three days after the event and he was quite stable. He wanted one answer, that much I could gather, i.e. *not* to admit. They now seemed a trifle agitated that things were not running smoothly as regards my answers.

I was then asked about the **management of status epilepticus**. I trundled that answer out without difficulty but I got no hint as to whether or not they were happy with my answer.

Next, I was asked about the **investigation of ascites**, and I was telling them why I would perform a diagnostic tap when the bell went.

(*Passed*)

---

[1]   p. 215
[2]   They do have enough experience of coronary care units to justify the expenditure.

52

The viva was held directly after I had finished my major and minors. It was in a ward cubicle. I admit to having felt a bit tired after all that had gone before, and I thought that I had messed up at least one minor case.

The first question was about the **management of a 35-year-old man** who was found to be **hypertensive**. I told them how I would fully examine him and perform simple baseline investigations (U&E, CXR, ECG, urinalysis and MSU, 24-hr urinary catecholamines, IVP).[1] Once an IVP was mentioned they asked me about **renal artery stenosis** – how to definitively investigate it and whether to operate (doing selective renal vein catheterisation first and measuring renin levels).[2]

The next question concerned the **management** of a known **alcoholic** brought in with a **massive haematemesis**. I told them about putting in an intravenous line, giving blood and plasma, passing down a Sengstaken tube and giving ADH. They asked me what else I'd do and I wasn't sure – they suggested 'informing your surgical colleagues' and I agreed.

Then I was asked what would I think was the problem with an **elderly chronic bronchitic** admitted with an exacerbation that didn't clear up. The answer they wanted was **'lung cancer'** and it only clicked when they told me that the patient was a heavy smoker. This was after I had ventured a few other ideas like atypical pneumonia and pulmonary embolus. When I mentioned pulmonary embolism, they asked me what investigations I would perform to diagnose it. I went through ECG, CXR and then mentioned V/P scan. I was asked what percentage of the scans was positive in pulmonary embolism.[3]

(*Passed*)

---

[1] The last-mentioned two tests are not carried out as baseline investigations in straightforward essential hypertension.

[2] Renal arterial angiography is the definitive investigation but should be carried out by someone skilled in angioplasty techniques, so that an opportunistic therapeutic intervention may be undertaken at diagnosis.

[3] The predictability of a ventilation/perfusion scan depends on the size of the lesion: multiple segmental and lobar mismatches are diagnostic in 95% of cases compared with pulmonary angiography. V/P mismatches have a poor predictive value in segmental embolism. In other words, an abnormal V/P scan is almost always helpful, whereas a normal one leaves room for doubt, and one must consider it in conjunction with the clinical picture.

53

I felt very nervous as I thought the other two parts had gone all right and I didn't want to muck it up here! It was a small room with no windows. There were two serious and impassive examiners, who were not giving much away.

The first question was, 'What *advantages* are there of *being an Eskimo*!'[1] He asked about the **risk factors for ischaemic heart disease** and then about which ones were reversible. He seemed unimpressed even with the correct answers. I talked about the **results of the major hypertension trials** and the **lipid modification trials**.

He asked how I would **treat hypertension**. I went for the conservative answer, i.e. beta blockers, and was then asked about the newer agents, their indications and problems and 'Why wouldn't you use *captopril as the first-line treatment*?'[2] I trotted out some of the side effects. The examiner trotted out some side effects of beta blockers. He then let me off with a casual, 'It's a controversial area'.

I was then asked about the **causes of hypocalcaemia**, calcium metabolism, protein binding and then about the **mechanism of paraesthesiae in the hyperventilation** syndrome and in hypoparathyroidism.

He then changed to **hypercalcaemia** and there was a discussion of the mechanisms and the different types. 'What disease state causes *hypervitaminosis D*?' I didn't know and was told 'Sarcoidosis'.

The examiners then dismissed me, still not giving anything away.

Incidentally, I forgot the opening gambit: 'You are the last candidate of the afternoon, what effect do you think that has?'

I gave a noncommittal reply.

'Probably favourable', they said, then a rather threatening, 'Not promising anything!'

(*Passed*)

---

[1]   p. 129

[2]   At the time of this examination (1989), the recommendation of the Committee on Safety of Medicines was that ACE inhibitors should be used only when the first-line drugs are either ineffective or contraindicated. The manufacturer's 1991 data sheets advocate the use of captopril and enalapril as first-line drugs in suitable hypertensive patients; presumably the Committee on Safety of Medicines has relaxed its stricture. Candidates should consult the British National Formulary before the examination, and quote it as their source in controversial therapeutic areas.

54

I had the viva after my long and short cases. They all followed on immediately from each other and so there was no time to worry! The examiners were extremely friendly, and one of them started off by asking me, '**What would cross your mind if someone came into casualty with a *fever* and *headaches* shortly after *returning from Mombasa***' (they each asked me if I knew where it was!). I said that I would think of **malaria**. We discussed the investigations, treatment, clinical findings and prophylaxis. They asked if I knew whether Mombasa was a chloroquine-resistant area![1] I said I didn't know and would have to check with the School of Tropical Medicine

(I didn't feel very happy about that part).

Then they asked about the **yellow card system of reporting drug reactions.**[2] Next they asked what **Reye's syndrome** was.[3] I said an encephalitis associated with aspirin in children; they corrected me by telling me that it was hepatic encephalopathy. They then asked what was recommended instead of aspirin and I said paracetamol. They asked me if I thought aspirin and paracetamol were safe drugs. I said 'Yes' (considering the number that are consumed without adverse effects). He agreed and we went on.

They asked me about **sudden onset of blindness in one eye**.[4] I wasn't very fluent here and needed quite a bit of prompting. I can't remember the exact questions and answers but I tried working from the eye inside out.

I was then asked about the investigations that should be done on a 50-year-old man with a **single TIA**, including what I'd look for while examining him. They asked first what I'd do if a 40% stenosis of his carotid artery was found, and then about a 70% stenosis. For the 40%, I said I'd put him on aspirin and *persantin*. He asked, '**Both?**' I said it was controversial and some think that the *persantin* is a waste of time. He asked '**What dose of aspirin?**' I said that was also controversial but I'd give 300 mg on alternate days. For the 70%, I said I'd have to discuss the pros and cons of surgery with the patient. He asked, '**What would you say if it were your own father?**' I said I'd tell him to leave well alone–he agreed.

Impressions: During the viva they were much more responsive to my answers, telling me if I was correct or if they agreed or not, unlike the short cases.[5]

(*Failed the viva; passed the exam*)

---

[1]   Chloroquine-resistant *P. falciparum* has been reported in many parts of Asia, East (including Mombasa) and Central Africa, Central and South America. *Fansidar*-resistant organisms have been reported in Brazil, Indonesia, Kenya, Tanzania, New Guinea and Thailand.

[2]   p. 54

[3]   p. 28

[4]   *Thromboembolism* (from plaques in the proximal major vessels, valvular disease, mural thrombi, atrial fibrillation, recent myocardial infarction, blood dyscrasias – polycythaemia, macroglobulinaemia, etc.)
Vasospasm (migraine)
Vasculitis (temporal arteritis)
Haemorrhage in a tumour compressing the optic nerve
Retinal tear and detachment

[5]   Had seven short cases with many supplementary questions!

55

The viva was conducted in a room with two examiners, one male and one female. I was asked to sit down. The woman stared at me. The male examiner started with:

Examiner 1: '**I'll ask you a simple physiological question: explain to me *why asthmatics are hypoxic on air.*'**

I did not start off very well on this, but eventually got on to ventilation/ perfusion mismatch. However, this did not seem to satisfy him and the question was put at least twice more, despite my saying I could not answer him any further.[1]

The examiner then said,

Examiner 1: '**Now a clinical case: *what would you do about an eight-month pregnant woman who arrives in casualty fitting and has haemorrhages throughout her fundi?*'**

I said her fits need urgent control with diazepam and her blood glucose needs to be measured. The case then centred on the management of preeclamptic toxaemia![2]

The next question was:

Examiner 1: '***Describe to me the conducting system of the heart in detail and name the structures.*'**

I did not do this well. I could not remember the name 'Purkinje' and he asked me three times about this. I was then asked why left bundle branch block was pathological but right bundle branch block was not.[3]

---

[1] V/P imbalance *is* the principal reason for hypoxaemia in asthma, since bronchodilators may relieve airways obstruction without affecting Po_2 and aminophylline (which has a vasodilatory effect on pulmonary vessels) may aggravate it. An increase in the work of breathing caused by an increased airflow resistance and respiratory drive probably also contribute to the hypoxaemia.

[2] This was a cleverly delivered *Ghost* Story with the *haemorrhages* being the *ghost-link*. The examiner deliberately did not specify the retinal findings to suit either diabetes mellitus or hypertension. The candidate missed this subtlety and responded quickly with a diagnosis of diabetes mellitus (hypoglycaemic fits) rather than hypertension as the primary problem in this patient.

[3] They are both pathological, though right bundle branch block occasionally occurs in the absence of any other indication of heart disease. The left bundle branch cascades down as a broad sheet of fibres to the left side of the muscular interventricular septum. Because of its wide distribution, the interruption of the left bundle branch has been thought to be more serious than that of the right bundle branch, which is slender and courses down the right side of the septum without branching. However, an acute appearance of right bundle branch block with a pulmonary embolism or in an acute myocardial infarction is an ominous sign.

I could not give a straightforward answer and said that I honestly did not know. Despite this he asked me again. At this point the female examiner gave a huge sigh and turned her back on me. I thought, and still think, that this was rude and unhelpful. The conversation then went on to the **management of an 80-year-old man with a pulse of 30**. We discussed the management of complete heart block.

The next examiner started with the subject of **the law and epilepsy,**[4] describing hypothetical cases and asking for the legal aspects of whether such patients should possess a driving licence. I tried to sound convincing. I think I answered correctly in each case, although I was unsure at the time.

Examiner 2: **'Name common side effects of commonly used drugs.'**

I started with digoxin and was allowed to talk freely and then I went on to theophylline.

Examiner 2: **'What kind of arrhythmias? Why does it cause hypokalaemia? Why does salbutamol cause hypokalaemia?'**[5]

I had no idea.

Examiner 2: **'What about NSAIDs? Why do they have the side effect of water retention?**[6] **Come on, there must be many drugs used on the wards with common side effects.'**

She was very aggressive and determined to unsettle me.

Examiner 2: **'Tell me about the management of patients after coronary artery bypass surgery. What about their lipid levels and how do lipid levels affect their grafts?'**

I could answer the first part satisfactorily but said that lipids should have been investigated prior to surgery and should be under control by the time of surgery.[7] These comments seemed unacceptable. The bell went – I was glad. It had been very aggressive and uneasy. I was sure I had failed the viva (which I had) although the lady did manage to give me a weak smile on the way out.

(*Failed*)

---

4   p. 19
5   A bee-under-the-bonnet question! **Hypokalaemia** could hardly be considered a *common* side effect in association with the routine use of salbutamol; it occurs in sensitive patients when salbutamol is given intravenously, especially with hydrocortisone, probably due to an intracellular shift of potassium and its loss in the urine. Xanthine derivatives potentiate the effects of catecholamines and cause accumulation of cyclic AMP, thereby activating the sodium pump with an influx of potassium. These drugs also have a modest diuretic effect but do not inhibit potassium secretion in the renal tubule.
6   These drugs cause significant retention of sodium and chloride with an associated reduction in the urinary output.
7   Unfortunately, serum lipids are not checked before surgery in some centres. At some places, hypercholesterolaemia is not sought and treated even after bypass surgery. However, the message is gradually getting through!

56

My viva began pleasantly enough with Dr S, whom I remembered from my final examinations as being pleasant and friendly. However, now she was very stern and I found her manner abrupt, very definite and a little awkward to respond to.[1] The viva started 'averagely' and then plummeted to a struggle!

Her first question was about my last short case – the **resuscitation Annie**. **'Do you think that it was significant that the doll was wearing a tracksuit?'**[2]

I mentioned sudden death among athletes and was then asked about the other **diseases of joggers**.[3] After what seemed like ten minutes silence I said the only thing I could think of–the danger of being hit by a car! Then I blurted out about march fractures and 'march haematuria'. This latter name was corrected to march haemoglobinuria by my examiner. I was then asked to talk about the **causes and treatment of myoglobinuria**.

'Where is myoglobin deposited?'

'The glomerulus', I said. Again, I was corrected with **'Oh, I thought it was the tubules'**. Further questioning revealed more imprecise knowledge on my part, but then the subject was changed to **acute pneumonia**. Unfortunately, I had not read the very recent review on the subject in the *Drug and Therapeutics Bulletin*, but I had done an infectious diseases job, and I think my redemption was the fact that I could talk as though I'd had experience and had developed my own clinical impressions.

The next examiner asked me to tell him all I knew about **AIDS**.[4] A sigh of relief and I was off. Our only discussion was about the extent of the heterosexual epidemic, and it was apparent that he held strong views on this.

Impressions: The exam was on time, the conditions reasonable and at the end, and indeed throughout, the examiners were pleasant.

(*Passed*)

---

[1]   A classic example of the difference in the same examiner's attitude between Finals and MRCP!

[2]   A bee under the examiner's bonnet!

[3]   p. 28

[4]   A *Bedtime* Story question which the candidate apparently treated as such!

57

Examiner 1:   'How would you manage an aspirin overdosage?'[1]

I gave my reply and they seemed particularly interested in the order of management. It ended with a discussion of **other common overdoses**.

Examiner 1:   'Give me some examples of the nonmetastatic manifestations of malignancy.'

They seemed happy with the original subgrouping into endocrine and neuromuscular.

Examiner 1:   'Give some examples of cancer markers.'[2]

I gave some examples of CEA and α-FP. The discussion ended with whether breast cancer has markers.

Examiner 1:   'What is an oncogene?'[3]

They seemed happy with my reply and the examples I gave (luckily I had recently read a review article).

Examiner 2:   'A nurse shows you a patient with a foot ulcer – tell her what to do.'[4]

I got bogged down with the mode of action of various cleansing materials, but they changed the subject as soon as I started talking about pressure sites.

---

[1] p. 44

[2] **Cancer markers**

Experience with cancer markers has been disappointing: none of the ones tried has shown sufficient specificity and sensitivity to become a reliable diagnostic tool. With this reservation in the background, the following markers can be used as adjuncts to clinical assessment:

Acid phosphatase – carcinoma of the prostate but now replaced by the much more sensitive prostate-specific antigen

Alkaline phosphatase – bone and liver malignancies

Amylase – carcinoma of the pancreas

Alpha-fetoprotein – primary hepatoma, teratoma, gastric carcinoma, etc.

Carcinoembryonic antigen (CEA) – colonic carcinoma, neuroblastoma, urological malignancies, adenocarcinoma of the bronchus, breast and ovary

3,4-dihydroxyphenylalanine – mesothelioma.

[3] An oncogene encodes a protein that controls the malignant transformation of the cell. Oncogenes are genes present in normal cells but which have become altered in structure after infection by an oncogenic virus. The virus converts the RNA genome of the cell into DNA which becomes integrated into the host's chromosomal DNA, subsequently producing copies of the virus protein. Similar genes have now been found in normal cells and it is thought that these may have some protective value.

[4] p. 53

Examiner 2: 'What investigations would you do in a 16-year-old girl with primary amenorrhoea?'

They got annoyed when I suggested that this was still in the normal age range,[5] but I then proceeded with my answer and they seemed happy.

Impressions: I thought that the viva was fine. It consisted of about six pairs of examiners around a large room but it seemed 'private' at the time. Initially, I was quite perturbed by some previous candidates coming out to collect their baggage and telling their answers which were obviously ridiculous. This was morale boosting! Unfortunately, the candidates just before me came out looking either shell-shocked or close to tears! Altogether, the examiners seemed agreeable and it was quite interesting taking them down a line.

(*Passed*)

---

[5]   The age of menarche has steadily fallen in the Western hemisphere to around 12 years. Since the examiner had specifically asked for *investigations*, the candidate should have at least mentioned *karyotype* and basal *gonadotrophins*. If the question had been phrased as, 'How would you proceed?' or 'What would you do?', then it would have been pertinent to establish whether the girl's mother had been a late starter. The age of 16 years could be considered within the normal range if there was a family history of late menarche.

58

I was initially questioned on the **management of a male patient aged about 40 years presenting with dyspnoea**. My attempts at giving answers about cardiovascular or respiratory disease were rebuffed, and so I moved on to haematological causes. They were trying to get at hereditary spherocytosis as a cause! However, I did badly on describing the urinary findings in haemolytic anaemia.[1]

They then moved on to the **management of a lady who was gravida 1 and 33 weeks pregnant and who presented with an eclamptic fit**. For my part, I said I would control the fit as rapidly as possible, using the nearest drug to hand. They then tried to question me on my use of thiopentone and what I knew about it. Unfortunately, when it became clear that an anaesthetist[2] knows a lot about it they rapidly moved on to the **management of the hypertension**! I quoted hydralazine as being the drug I might use, although I admitted I didn't know the right answer.[3] They then became quite facetious and told me that I should not need to look it up, especially as my consultant might have gone home (!) and that I should be able to quote the right drug. They never said what that was.

The final session involved talking about the **renal problems of myeloma**, in which I quickly got bogged down. I was unable to give a lengthy description of amyloid kidney and that didn't seem to impress them. Fortunately, the bell went at this point. I felt I had failed the viva as they both had a very 'hawkish' attitude: against that, I did talk about the emergency case well enough.

(*Passed*)

---

[1]   In haemolytic anaemia, bile is characteristically absent from the urine as the predominant form of bilirubin in the plasma is unconjugated and is bound to albumin. Consequently, products of bilirubin degradation called *dipyrroles* appear in the urine and give it a dark colour resembling Coke or Chinese tea. The history of passing such urine, and not just the concentrated urine of water-deprivation, should be carefully sought from the patient. Haemoglobin released from the haemolysed red blood cells binds with plasma haptoglobin and, once these are saturated, haemoglobin appears in the urine and gives it a faint pink discolouration. Haemosiderinuria is reliable evidence of chronic haemolysis. In normal subjects, the iron concentration in the urine seldom exceeds 0.1 mg/day. In addition to haemosiderinuria, an absent or decreased plasma concentration of haptoglobins, unconjugated bilirubinaemia, anaemia, aggressive reticulocytosis and poikilocytosis are the important indicators of haemolysis. Urobilinogen is present in excess in the urine of patients with haemolysis: although it is colourless its presence can be detected by commercial dip-stix.

[2]   The candidate was a registrar in anaesthetics!

[3]   The suggestion is reasonable but the examiners were probably unconvinced because the candidate did not give the dose or the route of administration and admitted that he was guessing. An intravenous infusion of labetolol is preferable because the fall in BP can be controlled with ease.

59

Myself and two other candidates waited in a large hall outside three doors behind which sat our examiners. We had just finished our short cases and were led away from this venue by our designated medical students (who were very considerate). I was feeling pretty shattered by this stage and was left waiting for at least five minutes. My medical student finally asked the examiners if I could come in. They were obviously discussing one of the other candidates as I walked in. Both examiners were very polite and introduced themselves. The younger one of the two kicked off by asking me if I'd enjoyed the afternoon so far! I answered that I'd spent better afternoons! That actually put me at ease.

He then questioned me about **drug interactions**[1] and I had to name examples as I went along. I started with ones in the gut, e.g. tetracycline and milk; liver enzyme-inducers, e.g. phenytoin, and inhibitors, e.g. cimetidine; kidneys, e.g. probenecid and penicillin; protein binding, etc. He seemed happy with my answers.

We then moved on to **IgA nephropathy**[2] **and its natural history**. I wasn't too sure about this and waffled. I said that it was closely linked to Henoch-Schönlein disease and started talking about this when I was stopped.

He asked about **reversible factors in chronic renal failure** and wanted me to say hypertension and infection, which I hadn't done. He then decided to leave this subject (by saying that I didn't seem to like it) and asked his colleague to continue.

I was then asked to **define an isotope**![3] I was dumb-struck and mumbled something about electrons and protons. The next question was on the **uses of isotopes in the treatment of medical conditions**. I rattled on about ^{131}I and thyrotoxicosis and the pros and cons. Unfortunately, I mentioned that it was the treatment of choice in elderly thyrotoxics, to which he asked if I considered him elderly![4] I couldn't think of any other examples but eventually he managed to jolt my memory about ^{32}P. We talked about polycythaemia and its natural history and the side effects of ^{32}P. Finally, I was asked about the **treatment of thyrotoxicosis in pregnancy**. I was ecstatic since I'd just read about this in the car on the way to the exam!

I left the room feeling I hadn't done well enough but glad that it was over.

(Passed)

---

[1]   p. 53

[2]   p. 152

[3]   Isotopes are the atoms of the same elements with different mass numbers (e.g. ^{22}Na and ^{24}Na). As they emit radiation they can be used for diagnosis (detected by gamma/beta counters) and for the treatment of numerous disorders.

[4]   It is advisable not to sound dismissive about the elderly since most examiners are in that age group! It is particularly important not to offer 'elderly' age as the main reason for suspecting a carcinoma.

60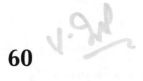

There was a little while to discuss the short cases with the other two candidates. This did my morale some good, but then it was utterly destroyed by the acid smiles of the two examiners in the viva. It was a small poky room with me sitting in the centre of a straight line joining the examiners.

I was shown a **CXR of a pneumothorax with old TB and emphysema**, and was asked:

Examiner 1: '**How would you treat this patient?**'

There was a discussion on when to insert the intercostal drains and, probably an important question, where I put mine. Also we discussed the possible complications.

I was shown the **U&Es from a fitting patient in a coma**.

Examiner 1: '**What would you do next?**'

I said a CXR to look for a tumour as it was probably SIADH. They seemed happy with that, but there then followed an awful discussion on the chemical pathology of the condition. It became quite clear that I didn't know how one got central pontine myelinosis.[1]

Examiner 2: '**How would you classify cryoglobulinaemias?**'

It became obvious that I knew virtually nothing about cryoglobulinaemias so they laboured the point.

Examiner 2: '**What serology would you perform on patients with vasculitides?**'[2]

---

[1]   p. 28

[2]   Superficially, the question appears like a *Bedtime* Story but the underlying objective of the examiner is to assess whether the candidate has a good grasp of the subject and whether, upon discovering a vasculitic lesion in a patient, he can think of the possible causes and arrange a battery of relevant investigations. Thus, the candidate can enumerate the tests and mention the relevant conditions as he goes on: ESR and C-reactive protein (mandatory in all vasculitides); ANF (connective tissue diseases); rheumatoid factor (rheumatoid arthritis, cryoglobulinaemia, Wegener's granulomatosis); immune complexes (necrotising lesions – connective tissue diseases, cryoglobulinaemia, neoplasms, etc.) complement (hypocomplementaemic vasculitis); cryoglobulins and hep B antigen (cryoglobulin-aemia); and antineutrophil-cytoplasmic antibody (Wegener's granulomatosis). Although only serology has been asked for, blood cultures must be mentioned (infective endocarditis, meningococcaemia). Alternatively, the candidate can present a loose classification of vasculitides, and mention the relevant tests as he enumerates the conditions.

Causes of vasculitides
Hypersensitivity angiitis – Henoch-Schönlein purpura, cryoglobulinaemia, hypocom-plementaemic vasculitis
Allergic vasculitis – drug reactions
Underlying infections – infective endocarditis, meningococcaemia
Underlying neoplastic disease – carcinoma, lymphoma, leukaemia
Connective tissue diseases – systemic lupus erythematosus, rheumatoid arthritis, poly-arteritis nodosa
Granulomatous vasculitis – Wegener's, Churg-Strauss disease
Giant cell arteritis – temporal arteritis, polymyalgia rheumatica, Takayasu's disease

I gave a rather stilted answer but I think it was probably alright.

Examiner 2: **'What patients would you not allow to drive?'**

They did not seem at all happy with anything I was saying and the discussion persisted for some time after the bell.

I got the impression that 90% of what I said was total rubbish, but as I stood up the first examiner said that I had been right to say that there is a cryoagglutinin[3] in syphilis. They then argued the point in front of me so I left.

Impressions: They were generally very impassive and with the total absence of feedback I felt I was floundering rather.

(Passed)

---

[3]   The candidate and the examiner seem to have christened cold agglutinin as *cryoagglutinin*, which is not the same as cryoglobulin. Simultaneous occurrence of cryoglobulin and cold agglutinin has been reported in chronic cold agglutinin disease, chronic lymphatic leukaemia and primary macroglobulinaemia (N Eng J Med 1977; 297: 538). About 5% of Waldenström macroglobulins are cold agglutinins. Cryoglobulin has been associated with a variety of conditions, including syphilis, Lyme disease and infective endocarditis.

61

The viva was the best bit!! It was after the clinical and I thought I hadn't done well enough in the short cases (I only had four short cases).[1] On the whole it had been a good performance, but it was bedeviled by self-doubt so I decided that I would have to give the viva everything I had. Although I had trained in Edinburgh and was HP to Professor M, a famous personality – not a disadvantage perhaps! – I had gone to London for my SHO jobs. One of the examiners was a renal physician in Edinburgh, who I knew by sight, and she first asked me about what I'd done since leaving Edinburgh – a good start!

Since I was about to do a renal job in London she asked me about the **K+ changes in metabolic alkalosis**, and we got into quite a technical discussion about distal tubular K^+/H^+ fluxes. That went well, and then she asked me what I wanted to do in medicine. I said cardiology so she asked me about **thrombolysis** which was easy to talk about since I'd just finished a cardiac job. I was asked if I'd done any Third World medicine and I said 'No' promptly to avoid any tropical medicine questions.

The other examiner then asked about **screening**. I quoted the Edinburgh breast screening trial results, so that went well. Then we discussed **hypertension**, and I'd read up the EWPHE[2] and other trials so I could quote papers directly as evidence for beneficial treatment. He then asked a much more basic question about **anaemia in an elderly woman**. He wanted a straight answer so I side stepped and classified anaemias first to prove that I wouldn't just say iron deficiency and leave it at that. This annoyed him a bit but the other examiner was nodding vigorously so I'm sure I scored points by being measured in my approach. Then the bell went.

Impressions: I felt the viva went well because I managed to steer the conversation on to my home topics of cardiology and renal medicine. I had a large amount of luck but quoting papers, I felt, gave me a huge boost and enabled me to talk about screening for hyperlipidaemia and hypertension which made me feel very comfortable. After poor short cases I felt that I had to score a high mark in the viva so I tried not to let the examiners do any talking, since that wouldn't have got *me* any marks! I started talking as soon as they had put a question using phrases like, 'Yes, well that is a crucial/key/important area' while I was thinking of the best reply. I think that practice in public speaking is important as well.

(*Passed*)

---

[1] Hepatosplenomegaly in a patient with polycythaemia rubra vera; retinal artery branch occlusion with lower quadrantanopia which the candidate had to demonstrate; subacute combined degeneration with some discussion about the extensor plantars; and a mixed mitral valve disease with tricuspid incompetence. The candidate missed the latter when asked to auscultate only, but picked it up later from a prominent *v* wave when the discussion concentrated on heart failure.

[2] European Working Party on High Blood Pressure in the Elderly Trial. Lancet 1985; 1: 1349.

62

The viva was conducted in a big hall at the Royal College in Glasgow with eight or ten tables placed round the edge. The viva was delayed by 20 minutes – I don't know why. We were taken up to wait outside in batches of eight candidates. The examiners were initially polite and pleasant.

The first question was, *'A young man of 26 years comes to the general medical OP with a history of a fit. He is an HGV driver. How would you investigate?'*

I told them I would take a history to establish the nature of the fit and then perform an examination. I was told the examination was normal. We then discussed the investigations and this led to a discussion on the usefulness of an EEG[1] as it may be normal in an epileptic. I was then asked about the treatment of a first fit. I said, 'Observe and inform the patient that he must tell the DVLC and surrender his driving licence.' The examiner said he would lose his job and times are hard. I agreed but said that unfortunately it is a legal requirement as fits are a proscribed illness in the driving regulations. He seemed satisfied.

The next question was on the **management of a 35-year-old woman with thyrotoxicosis**. I said drug treatment and was asked for how long. Then I was asked about other modes of treatment. I said surgery and was told that the patient had refused to have an operation. Then I said radioiodine. I was told the patient had not yet completed her family. This led into a discussion on the use of radioisotopes for the treatment of thyroid disease. I put differing views and commented that it is used quite readily in North America. Then I was asked to discuss the effects of carbimazole on the fetus.

Fifteen minutes were up so I was handed to the second examiner, who butted in quite abruptly and said he thought it was his turn to ask some questions!

He had a sheet in front of him which he said was a memorandum from the Royal College directing him to find the candidates' **views on talking to relatives**. Did I think this was important? I expressed the view that talking to relatives was *very* important because a patient is not ill in isolation but forms an important part of a family.

'Yes, yes', the examiner said, **'we know that.'** I then went on to say that I felt it most important to ask the patients' permission first before discussing their case with their relatives.

'So you feel that the information regarding patients' illness is their property?'

'Yes, very strongly,' I replied. There was some further discussion on how I would actually tell a patient that he had a malignancy.

Then the examiner asked me what I understood by **'informed consent'**. I gave him my definition. He then said a patient came to the hospital with a GI haemorrhage and the next day he said to the patient, 'You can have a gastroscopy if you want.' **'What do you think of that?'** he asked me. I felt a bit edgy here, as I was unsure of the point he was trying to make. He said

---

[1]   p. 173

that that was informed consent, **'Was it not?'** I said perhaps it needed to be qualified with a little more explanation. Then the examiner said loudly, **'Don't you think it was rather crass of me to say that to a patient?'** ('me' being the examiner himself). I felt very wary, not wishing to offend. I again repeated that I would try to explain in a lay person's terms what a gastroscopy entailed.

He then asked me if **gastroscoping a patient shortly after a GI haemorrhage** influenced the prognosis. I said I supposed it depended on whether there were facilities for the diathermy of any visible bleeding site. The examiner commented that obviously I had not been reading the same paper as him recently. I said I hadn't come across anything recently on this issue. (I had read all of the last 6 months of the *Lancet*, *New England Journal* and as many *BMJs* as I had time for).[2] He said, **'No, it did not affect the outcome, but I suppose it helped the surgeons if the patient bled again.'**

End of viva! It felt more like a job interview with so many ethical questions raised!

(*Passed*)

---

[2]   This was a hot topic in the late 1970s (before this candidate had entered a medical school!), when an editorial in Gastroenterology (1977; 72: 762) raised the issue about the usefulness of endoscopy in upper gastrointestinal haemorrhage. A British prospective study (Lancet 1977; 1: 1167) comparing emergency endoscopy and radiology concluded that there was no difference between the two as regards the management and outcome. However, endoscopy has a better diagnostic yield in **oesophageal varices** which is sometimes a surprise finding in a patient suspected of having peptic ulcer disease. Further, endoscopy offers a therapeutic opportunity for *electrocoagulation* and *sclerosis* of bleeding vessels both in variceal bleeding and in peptic ulcers (Gastroenterology 1990; 99: 1303, 1991; 100: 33). Surgeons favour endoscopy because it shows them the source of bleeding, which may be in the chest, and thus makes their task easy.

63

The viva followed straight on from the long and short cases. It was conducted separately, in a large room in the postgraduate centre. The examiners were Professor A (I think) and Professor B.

Prof A started with describing **a woman in her 60s who wakes up in the night suddenly blind.**[1] **'What are the causes?'** I got off on the wrong foot as I gave him a list of the causes of blindness in one eye. He interrupted crossly that he had said *completely* blind. I struggled a bit and finally said that a CVA might be the cause. He asked, **'Where?'** I struggled again but eventually said the basilar artery.

Then he described the case of **a woman in her 20s who had had a partial pneumonectomy in the past and was flying home from the USA when she developed severe polyuria and polydipsia.**[2] I started out saying that I would dip-stick the urine to test for glucose.[3] I was told that this was negative. He then orally gave me a list of her plasma electrolyte values. I need to see that sort of thing written down. I began to get mixed up with inappropriate ADH secretion and diabetes insipidus. Somehow, because he mentioned lung disease, I had it fixed in my mind that she had inappropriate ADH.[4] I got deeper and deeper trying to explain how to investigate this. The other examiner kept fiddling with his watch and looking up at the ceiling. He interrupted and said that there was no point pursuing this line. There had been numerous long pauses and now I just wanted to crawl away and die!

Prof B took over and asked me the **causes of Addison's disease**. I started off with a list of the causes of adrenal insufficiency. He pointed out that adrenal insufficiency is not the same as Addison's disease. I said the cause was autoimmune adrenalitis. He asked if autoantibodies to the adrenals could be measured. I said I supposed they could (but I did not recall ever testing for them). He asked what other organ may be attacked? I think I managed to produce the 'ovaries' eventually.

Then he gave me the case of a woman on steroid replacement for Addison's, and gave me another list of electrolyte values to hold in my head

---

[1]   This is a *what dunnit?* story, and the examiner has a single diagnosis (cortical blindness) but he is willing to hear about a few other possibilities. A sudden onset suggests a vascular cause (thromboembolism or spasm in the basilar artery – both cerebral arteries supplying the visual cortex originate from it), or a haemorrhage in a tumour compressing the chiasm, though hysteria must be considered as a possibility. A neurological examination looking for the associated signs should establish the precise diagnosis. In cortical blindness, the pupillary reflexes will be intact, and in a chiasmal lesion the loss of vision is unlikely to be complete.

[2]   This is another *Detective* Story. Unfortunately, the candidate has not provided the details of the plasma electrolytes (probably didn't remember) without which it is difficult to pick the examiner's diagnosis with certainty. We assume that the candidate was given a picture of a dilutional hyponatraemia (with a lowish osmolality) resulting from the patient's polydipsia. It would seem that this lady with a partial pneumonectomy panicked and developed psychogenic polydipsia. The possible reasons for her pneumonectomy are carcinoid, pulmonary tuberculosis, lung abscess, carcinoma or localised bronchiectasis.

[3]   This was a good beginning and turned this *Detective* Story into a *Ghost* Story with the examiner providing the *ghost-link* in the form of the plasma electrolytes.

[4]   This must have created a very bad impression, since polydipsia, far from being a feature, is dangerous in the syndrome of inappropriate ADH secretion.

and decide on the problem.[5] I worked out that she was not taking fludrocortisone – this at last was correct! Then he went on to talk about the **side effects of oestrogen and progesterone**. I gave a list of a few. Then he asked about **hormone replacement therapy in postmenopausal women**[6] and the risks. I said endometrial carcinoma and that in the USA a hysterectomy may be recommended. Then he asked about the benefits. I wanted to launch into a discussion of decreasing the incidence of osteoporosis and the risk of hip fracture but this was not the desired answer. He changed tack and asked what was the commonest medical emergency I had admitted (I was an SHO in haematology!). I was unsure about exactly what he wanted me to say so I said CVA. This was not taken well and eventually I suggested myocardial infarction. This was the link with oestrogen. At that time, papers had just been published regarding the beneficial effects of hormone replacement therapy on the coronary arteries of postmenopausal women. Needless to say, I did not come across this until I read an article in the *New Scientist* – by chance a week later.

Then he asked me what I did, I said SHO in haematology (or perhaps he asked this when I seemed unsure about the medical emergency bit). Then he said he had an **elderly woman who complained of stiffness when kneeling at the prayer rail at communion and who had an ESR of 100**. What was the diagnosis?[7] I said polymyalgia rheumatica. The viva then terminated. I heard one examiner say to the other as I left the room, **'I wasn't very happy with that, were you?'** Imagine how I felt!

(*Failed*)

---

5   We contacted Prof B who said that he would have suggested something like this: Na$^+$ 125, K$^+$ 5.0 and urea 12 mmol/l. Hyponatraemia and a high blood urea level suggested that the patient was salt deficient and needed fludrocortisone.

6   p. 27

7   A good *Detective* Story!

64

My viva came at the end of the exam so I didn't have much time to worry about it in particular! The examiners were polite and friendly. I think the room had a sea view but I wasn't really in the mood to appreciate it!

My first questions were on **microbiology** and my heart sank. '**What do you know about Strep bovis?**' I didn't know anything so the question changed to, '**An old man has Strep. bovis in his blood and a heart murmur — what are you going to do?**' Other questions were, '**What do you know about Strep. milleri?**' and '**What do you know about Listeria monocytogenes?**' In each case my one sentence answers were quickly followed by being *given* information. This examiner had recently seen a case of a hepatic abscess caused by *Strep. milleri*; *Strep. bovis* was a common bowel organism in the elderly, and *L. monocytogenes* was first isolated in the faeces of pythons (I found this genuinely funny!). Although I did my best to say what I could, I was a bit alarmed by the fact that the examiner did a lot of the talking. Afterwards, people said that a viva should be an exchange of information and I certainly felt that I had been educated!

His last question was about **H₂ blockers** – should they be sold over the counter? I said, 'No, because of the importance of excluding a malignant gastric ulcer before treatment.' He then asked for two absolute indications for their use. I said a proven duodenal ulcer and the Zollinger-Ellison syndrome. He accepted the first but was looking for hepatic encephalopathy as the second.[1]

The second half was less alarming. The examiner set the **scenario of a 20-year-old girl with her second grand mal fit**. He asked (accepting my answers each time):

Examiner 2: '**What is the management of a fitting patient in the street?**'

Answer: 'Maintain the airway.'

Examiner 2: '**What about the management of a fitting patient in casualty?**'

Answer: 'Oxygen, diazepam given intravenously or rectally.'

Examiner 2: '**What investigations would you undertake in this girl?**'

Answer: 'Plasma glucose, serum calcium, urea and electrolytes, EEG and possibly a CT scan.'

Examiner 2: '**What is the diagnosis?**'

Answer: 'By exclusion, the likely diagnosis is idiopathic epilepsy.'

---

[1] The candidate had given a textbook answer to this question, and the two conditions mentioned by him were regarded as being the absolute indications for the use of H₂ blockers, by every gastroenterologist we spoke to. H₂ blockers are also given for postoperative recurrent ulcers. In **fulminant hepatic failure**, H₂ blockers are given prophylactically to prevent **stress gastric ulcers** and complicating haemorrhage. This consideration also applies to other *critically* ill patients who are at risk from developing stress ulcers. They should be given to pregnant women undergoing anaesthesia to prevent the possible occurrence of **chemical pneumonitis** due to the acute aspiration of gastric contents into the lungs – **the Mendelson syndrome**. H₂ blockers are not of any benefit in hepatic encephalopathy due to chronic liver disease.

Examiner 2: **'What's the treatment?'**

I suggested carbamazepine (I said carbimazole in the heat of the moment which brought a look of surprise – he accepted my correction easily).

Examiner 2: **'What are the side effects?'**

Answer: 'Drowsiness, skin rash and interaction with the oral contraceptive pill.'
He mentioned neutropaenia which I had not said.

Examiner 2: **'What are the implications?'**

I mentioned the regulations on driving which I knew well. He asked about occupation and I first said there were no hard and fast rules except for HGV drivers. He corrected me, mentioning pilots, and also suggested that looking after young children and other sorts of occupations were potentially inadvisable. He also asked about the advice I should give the girl if she was taking the oral contraceptive pill. I said to use barrier methods in addition for three or four cycles, and if breakthrough bleeding occurs to increase the dose of oestrogen in the pill. He asked what the high-dose pills contained. I said '50' easily, but struggled with the units – finally settling on mcgs! (I felt this was more the women's magazine-acquired knowledge than the stuff I'd revised for the MRCP!!)

Overall this half went well. At one point I was keen to butt in with more information (not usually my style but I was getting caught up in the heat of the occasion). I was aware that we were both talking at the same time and he wasn't backing down, so I did as soon as I realised that I must be sounding out of turn.

I was comforted by my fellow sufferers being horrified by the microbiology questions afterwards.[2] Their indignation did something to allay my shock!

(*Passed*)

---

[2] An examiner with a lot of bees-under-the-bonnet!

65

The first question was: **'What is your view on routinely screening hospital patients for HIV?'** I talked about the need to have the patients' consent, and the implications for them of a positive result. I also talked about the dangers of its false-positive rate.

I was then given a **scenario of a patient being treated on the ITU for severe diabetic ketoacidosis who then passes red urine**.[1] I talked about the possibilities of drugs, haematuria or myoglobinuria. What he wanted to talk about was **rhabdomyolysis** in a severely ill patient. Then I went on to talk about the management of acute renal failure and the associated hyperkalaemia. The examiner was very keen on the basic practical day-to-day management, e.g. exactly how many times a day I would check the serum K^+, etc., and at what level I would consider dialysis or haemofiltration.

The second examiner then took over. He asked me to talk in general about **screening for disease**. I talked about the requirements, i.e. the need for a highly sensitive and specific test for a disease that is treatable and must be treated early, e.g. neonatal hypothyroidism and phenylketonuria. Then I talked about screening in general practice – urine testing for diabetes, BP checks, etc.

Following on from that, he asked me about the possible **causes of an unexpected high calcium on a routine biochemical profile**. I mainly talked about hyperparathyroidism, but managed to go a bit blank on its clinical manifestations; I completely forgot renal stones and nephrocalcinosis, and I couldn't think which 'bone problems' they had. They were very sympathetic and tried prompting me.

Impressions: The whole atmosphere was very friendly and not at all intimidating. They gave me lots of nonverbal cues indicating that I was on the right track most of the time.

(*Passed*)

---

[1] This question fulfils all the three criteria for a *Wild* Story (p. 85). **Atraumatic rhabdomyolysis** is a very rare complication of diabetic coma though myoglobulinuria is probably more common (Arch Intern Med 1963; 111: 76) than the frank manifestations of muscle lysis (e.g. muscular tenderness and weakness, heavy myoglobinuria, raised serum creatine phosphokinase level and oliguric renal failure). The mechanism is not well understood, but serum hyperosmolality (several cases have been reported in association with nonketotic hyperosmolar coma) and energy deprivation, due to nonutilisation of glucose, probably cause muscle dissolution. The condition should be suspected if the urine assumes a *deep brown* mahogany colour, and is confirmed by detecting heavy myoglobinuria and rising levels of serum creatine phosphokinase.

66

The viva started promptly in a small room with friendly examiners (perhaps partly because my name begins with Z!). There was some alarm on my part as I had discovered just before the exam that my viva examiner was an expert on the endocrinology of sex change! Happily, the subject did not come up. Instead I was asked about the **recent advances in the management of acute myocardial infarctions** and we discussed streptokinase. This led to questions about the indications for, and best timing of, angiography after the infarction.

The second examiner then asked me what I knew about the use of tumour markers[1] – I discussed α-fetoprotein, CEA and acid phosphatase. I was not pressed too hard, and was then asked for the **definitions of '*p* value' and '*regression coefficient*'.**[2] I was vague about the latter!

Finally, my examiner asked me **what I would tell a woman in her forties with disseminated cancer about her disease** in various circumstances: with a son of 15, married, single and so on. By this time he had clearly left the realm of scientific medicine well behind. It was by and large a genial viva.

(*Passed*)

---

[1]   p. 197
[2]   Appendix I

67

The first examiner wanted to know about the difficulties **prescribing in the elderly.**[1] My answer was rather vague initially, until he made it clear that he was wanting specific examples, some of which I managed to recall. He was very friendly and gave considerable prompting as to which direction he wanted the discussion to take (which was just as well since his questions were pretty nebulous).

The second examiner wanted me to go through the **steps required to diagnose diabetes**[2] in a young man with glycosuria. Whilst I was anxious to get through the relatively straightforward part of excluding false-positive urine tests and low renal thresholds, and to talk about anti-islet cell antibodies, he seemed to shy away from all this fancy stuff, and wanted to get back to being rather aggressive about my vagueness on the subject of the lag storage curve! I thought I might have failed the viva on this point, but the first examiner seemed quite sympathetic – perhaps he put in a good word.

(Passed)

---

[1]   Drug and Therapeutics Bulletin 1990; 28(20): 77
[2]   The World Health Organisation criteria for the diagnosis of diabetes mellitus (WHO Technical Report Series 1985; 720) have different thresholds depending on whether glucose is measured in blood or plasma, and whether the sample is venous or capillary:
  A. *Diabetes mellitus likely if random*:
      venous plasma glucose $\geqslant$ 11.1 mmol/l
      capillary plasma glucose $\geqslant$ 12.2 mmol/l
      venous whole blood glucose $\geqslant$ 10.0 mmol/l
      capillary whole blood glucose $\geqslant$ 11.1 mmol/l
  B. *Diabetes mellitus unlikely if random*:
      venous plasma glucose $\leqslant$ 5.5 mmol/l
      capillary plasma glucose $\leqslant$ 5.5 mmol/l
      venous whole blood glucose $\leqslant$ 4.4 mmol/l
      capillary whole blood glucose $\leqslant$ 4.4 mmol/l
  C. If the random glucose level lies between A and B, a formal 75 g oral glucose tolerance test is required:
      The diagnosis is likely if fasting:
      venous plasma glucose $\geqslant$ 7.8 mmol/l
      capillary plasma glucose $\geqslant$ 7.8 mmol/l
      venous whole blood glucose $\geqslant$ 6.7 mmol/l
      capillary whole blood glucose $\geqslant$ 6.7 mmol/l
  D. If the fasting value is less than C, then 75 g of glucose is administered orally:
      The diagnosis is established if two-hour levels are:
      venous plasma glucose $\geqslant$ 11.1 mmol/l
      capillary plasma glucose $\geqslant$ 12.2 mmol/l
      venous whole blood glucose $\geqslant$ 10.0 mmol/l
      capillary whole blood glucose $\geqslant$ 11.1 mmol/l
  E. *Impaired glucose tolerance (IGT) is diagnosed when the fasting value is less than C but the two-hour glucose levels are*:
      venous plasma between   7.8 and 11.1 mmol/l
      capillary plasma between   8.9 and 12.2 mmol/l
      venous whole blood between   6.7 and 10.0 mmol/l
      capillary whole blood between 7.8 and 11.1 mmol/l
  It is prudent to repeat the test annually in patients with IGT: some go on to develop diabetes mellitus; in some the status of carbohydrate intolerance does not change; in some it returns to normal.

68

I was feeling angry when I went for the clinical. Already I expected to fail. I was fed up spending time, money and energy attempting to please the College. I saw other people sailing through with less experience and knowledge than myself. White, male, public school types seemed to do best. My previous boss voiced his opinion (but not to me) that I would never pass because I was too easily intimidated. On the morning of the examination, however, I felt calm and determined. I wore a yellow suit (it reminds me of Van Gogh's 'Sunflowers') and carried a black handbag. When I entered Glasgow's College, the looks on the other candidates' faces were gratifying. One look at my outfit and they expected me to fail. Everyone else was in sober navy, black or brown (basically I didn't feel like spending another hundred pounds or so on a suit I would never wear again).

My viva was with two men in their fifties. The first asked me about **chemotherapy**. He wanted to know general principles only. This was straightforward. Once I started to become enthusiastic about various regimens he changed the subject. He gave me a clinical scenario: '**You're in casualty. You see a patient with *a stroke* and notice *a spleen*. What do you think?**' I immediately said **polycythaemia rubra vera**. He was pleased that I hadn't just said polycythaemia. I outlined the investigation, prognosis and management. I found this question quite easy as I had done a haematology SHO job at a busy teaching hospital.

He then asked me about the **management and investigation of unconscious patients in casualty**. This led into the management of **subarachnoid haemorrhages**, when and when not to lumbar puncture, and the place for CT scanning. This too was straightforward as I have had a lot of contact with the local neurological unit.

The second examiner was slightly more aggressive but I think that he was a little deaf and found my nervous shallow voice difficult until I 'piped up'. He wanted to discuss the **management of biliary disease** – surgery, endoscopy, ultrasound and drugs. I had read some relevant articles in the *BMJ* so I muddled through to his apparent satisfaction. I think that as long as I backed what appeared to be his opinions, he was happy.

Impressions: Both examiners were polite and pleasant. They gave the impression that they were prepared to give me a fair hearing. I suspect that they were both *hawks* who had been fed earlier that morning!

As I left the large hall in which the vivas were being held I met the eye of a female examiner. She looked me up and down and then gave me a rather ferocious frown!

(*Passed*)

69

This was my first viva examination and it was a disaster. Myself and nine others were conducted to a hall where we sat for ten minutes, when we were called out by number into the library/sitting room of the Royal College of Glasgow. It seemed so crowded!

My examiner presented me with an old piece of equipment saying,

Examiner 1: **'I got this from the museum. Have you any idea what it is, as it is pertinent to our discussion?'**

I confessed I did not recognise it.

Examiner 1: **'It's a set of *Southey's tubes*[1] used before we had powerful diuretics. Tell me how frusemide works.'**

I was unnerved and hesitant. I detailed its effect of promoting a sodium diuresis by acting on the ascending loop of Henle. There was a pregnant pause as he nodded at me (probably wanting its other mechanisms and actions of vasodilatation, which I did not mention).[2]

Examiner 1: **'What are its side-effects?'** These I detailed.

Examiner 1: **'What would you use for a pure water diuresis and which is used commonly in clinical practice?'**[3]

I mentioned mannitol and mercurials, neither of which was what they wanted. I then said that thiazides and acetazolamide would not act (silly thing to say), before admitting that I did not know.

Examiner 1: **'What about an intravenous infusion of alcohol?'**[4]

The other examiner nodded and said,

Examiner 2: **'Yes, used in neurosurgery.'** (My morale was now falling rapidly.) **'How would you treat congestive cardiac failure?'**[5]

This I detailed (but forgot to mention ACE inhibitors).

---

[1] Southey, a London physician (b. 1835), used a thin rubber tube threaded along a cannula into the subcutaneous tissue to relieve tense oedema. These tubes retained their use in severe cases of heart failure until the powerful diuretics, such as frusemide, became available.

[2] Even leaving the other actions aside, the answer was inadequate on the basics, since the candidate did not mention chloride. Frusemide inhibits the reabsorption of both sodium and chloride in the ascending limb of Henle and increases the excretion not only of the solute but also of water, by removing the gradient for passive water movement from the descending limb and the medullary collecting duct into the renal blood. Frusemide reduces vascular resistance, but as it also stimulates renal renin release some of its vasodilatory effect may be compromised by the activation of the renin-angiotensin system.

[3] Water itself is a diuretic when ingested in large quantities. Demeclocycline (*ledermycin*), a broad-spectrum antibiotic, is said to cause free water diuresis, and can be used in the treatment of the syndrome of inappropriate secretion of ADH.

[4] Alcohol causes diuresis by inhibiting the secretion of the antidiuretic hormone in the posterior pituitary gland.

[5] p. 31, 64

Examiner 2: 'What would be the *effect of standing too close to the Chernobyl reactor?*'

I detailed immediate, short-term and long-term complications.

Examiner 2: 'What has recently been in the news – in fact two nights ago – on *Alzheimer's disease?*'

I said I had not seen the news in a week!

Examiner 2: 'Well, what are the causes of Alzheimer's disease?'

I replied there was no known cause but there were a number of causes of senile and presenile dementia – which I listed (badly).

Examiner 2: 'What about trauma?'

I mentioned the punch-drunk syndrome, and then mentioned chronic subdural haematoma. **'Yes, that should have been top of the list'**, she said, looking irritated.

Examiner 2: 'What are the indications for domiciliary oxygen?'[6]

I was floored by this time and floundered through the question. In retrospect I should have listed them and then said no more but in desperation I resorted to bullshit! I buried myself by losing my nerve.

(Failed)

---

[6] Two multicentre studies (a British one and a larger American one) have shown that the continuous administration of oxygen via nasal tubes for 15 out of 24 hours a day can prolong life. The outlook was better in those who had hypercapnia as well. Before deciding to prescribe domiciliary oxygen (which incurs effort and expenditure), it is important to ensure that the patient has *given up smoking* (carboxyhaemoglobin of less than 3%) and that he *can tolerate oxygen* for long periods every day. The patients likely to benefit are those with:
1. Chronic hypercapnoeic respiratory failure (PCO_2 greater than or equal to 45 mmHg and PO_2 less than 70 mmHg).
2. Chronic bronchitis and emphysema (FEV_1 of less than 1.2 1, PO_2 less than 70 mmHg).

70

The viva followed the short cases which I felt I'd totally messed up. Therefore, I entered the room (reasonable size but spartan) feeling rather dejected. One examiner welcomed me into the room (he was a nice, fairly friendly chap) and the other (behind the desk) held out his hand – I assumed he wanted to shake mine and I held it out only to have him pluck my examination form out of the other hand. I was anticipating that I should fare reasonably well in the viva, since I could usually talk to anyone about anything and keep them moderately entertained but . . .

The first question was, **'We hear about *screening in the general public*. What are your opinions on screening?'** I thought, 'Oh God, what a tedious question.' I said, 'Well, it depends on one's definition, etc.' I was trying desperately to point out that I didn't really want to talk about this, and was hoping they'd ask about the management of diabetic ketoacidosis instead! The examiner continued, **'If you were a GP, what sort of screen would you wish to perform?'** I thought, 'Here am I, three years postqualification pursuing a career in hospital medicine and being asked, in a higher examination in hospital medicine, what I'd do if I were a GP!' I was not impressed!

There then followed a rather boring conversation discussing: (1) blood pressure, (2) serum lipid estimation, (3) smoking, (4) diabetic screening– I mentioned urine and blood and gave ranges[1] (mine were apparently a little on the generous side, i.e. I'd have missed approximately 25% of diabetics on screening!).

Although I didn't have much of a problem in keeping talking, I did feel that the information was being rather dragged out of me.

Fifteen minutes were spent discussing screening and then I changed examiner for the final five minutes. We discussed the **medical complications of splenectomy.** Again, I felt the information was dragged out of me.

Impressions: I really thought that I'd fared poorly in the viva. However, in retrospect, I suppose that despite my personal disappointment with my performance, at least I kept talking and didn't put my foot in it too much. I do wish, however, that the viva was geared a little more to the treatment of a particular medical problem or emergency. It was the end of the day and I thought the examiners were perhaps as happy as I was when the final bell went.

(*Passed*)

---

[1]   p. 212

71

Examiner: **'What investigations would you perform on a 40-year-old woman with diplopia?'**[1]

I was tempted to make a facetious remark about hazelnut yoghurt since it was the time of the botulism scare but I thought better of it. I said I would take a history and examine the patient before any investigations (his expression suggested that he was pleased I'd said that). I then said I'd be looking for symptoms and signs of **multiple sclerosis** since that was the most likely diagnosis. I then suggested **visual evoked responses**[2] (he asked how these were performed), CSF studies and then mentioned an MRI scan in passing. We then discussed prognosis and what the patient should be told. The emphasis was on the social aspects, disability and employment.

Examiner: **'What advice would you give to someone going to Egypt next week?'**

I started with vaccination, but said that one week was too short a time to fully **vaccinate**, and mentioned **malaria prophylaxis** in passing. Then I mentioned that I would advise him about not drinking **contaminated water**. He asked about the **prophylaxis of diarrhoea**. I didn't know what he was getting at and I said it would be easier to treat **giardiasis**. I then mentioned swimming in rivers because of **schistosomiasis** and was asked how to treat this. I admitted I didn't know and would ask an infectious diseases specialist. He replied with a grin, **'That's the trouble about the membership, isn't it, dear? You're supposed to know everything!'** He then commented that I was obviously not an ardent traveller to Egypt and passed the questioning to the other examiner.

The next question was about what I would do with an **unconscious** 40-year-old male patient in casualty. After mentioning various diagnoses and 'first aid' we got on to **subarachnoid haemorrhage**. I said I would like a CT scan before doing a lumbar puncture, especially if there was no history

---

1   A *Ghost* Story with a rather weak *ghost-link* (viz., a 40-year-old female), and the examiner's diagnosis was probably **myasthenia gravis.** The candidate should have started the discussion by presenting a differential diagnosis, e.g. myasthenia gravis, multiple sclerosis, mononeuritis of the 3rd, 4th or 6th nerve, Wernicke's encephalopathy, thromboembolism, etc. As the subsequent discussion reveals, the candidate treated it as a *Detective* Story, and suggested a single diagnosis of multiple sclerosis; the examiner took up the cue and asked further questions. Although multiple sclerosis is slightly commoner in females and the peak age is around 35, the question was not specific enough for a single diagnosis.

2   *Visual evoked response* (VER) measures the pattern and latency of the response from the occipital cortex evoked by photic stimulation. A prolonged latency indicates an abnormality in the visual system, most commonly in the optic nerve in multiple sclerosis which may be evident before any abnormalities can be seen in the optic fundi.

available regarding trauma,[3] etc. I was asked about **CT scans and strokes**[4] and who should have a CT scan and why? I mentioned previous head injury and the possibility of an intracranial haematoma. He asked why I should want to know about that (he'd got the wrong end of the stick and thought I was talking about CVAs) and raised an eyebrow when I said they were eminently treatable. We went round in circles for a few minutes and I was pressed again about the indications for a CT scan. He then said, **'So you think everyone with a CVA should have a CT scan?'** I stood my ground and he suddenly realised that we were talking at cross purposes and praised me for sticking to my guns. We talked briefly about **anticoagulation and strokes** (I got into hot water because I hadn't read the recent *Drug and Therapeutics Bulletin* on the subject!)[5] and then about the **complications of hemiplegia**. He made me finish the discussion on that even though time had been called. I don't think he was particularly satisfied by my handling of the CVA question and wanted to be sure I had at least some grasp of the problem!

Before moving on we discussed the management of a **cardiac arrest**. I started with the airway but he moved me on to the **treatment of ventricular fibrillation**, the use of lignocaine and at what stage I would use bicarbonate. I think he had expected me to say I'd use bicarbonate straight away, but I explained that the UK Resuscitation Council[6] now recommended that its use be delayed. He looked as if he didn't know a lot about the subject and shut up very quickly at the mention of the UK Council recommendations!

On the whole, the viva was a relaxed discussion (especially since it was 4.30 p.m. on a very hot day). I clearly got away with saying I didn't know how to treat schistosomiasis. The confusion over CT scans was disconcerting but, because I was so tired by then, I was more aggressive than I would otherwise have been and therefore stuck to what I'd said. The second examiner didn't look impressed by my answers and I think that had I changed my mind he would have been unhappier still. The first examiner was obviously very keen on the social impact of debilitating diseases and was very pleased to see that it was something I had considered. They were pleasant and their attitude put me at ease to start with.

(Passed)

---

[3]   We suspect that the candidate meant to say meningitis rather than trauma.

[4]   **Main indications for a CT scan in strokes** (Br Med J 1988; 297: 126; Hospital Update 1990; 16: 726)

1. Uncertainty about the diagnosis of a stroke – the onset may be gradual or there may be no clear history of sudden onset because of coma, confusion, speech disorder and the lack of a witness. There may be no definite lateralising neurological signs suggestive of a stroke

2. Current or contemplated anticoagulation, antiplatelet treatment or both – one would need to exclude intracranial haemorrhage before either of these therapeutic options can be adopted; a CT scan is the only means by which infarction and haemorrhage can be reliably differentiated as causes of a mild stroke

3. Suspected cerebellar haematoma

4. A possible candidate for carotid endarterectomy

5. Stroke in a young patient (age < 45 years).

[5]   Drug and Therapeutics Bulletin 1989; Vol 27: No 12

[6]   Advanced Life Support: Revised recommendations of the Resuscitation Council (UK) Brit Med J 1989; 299: 446. Also see p. 35.

72

It was a large hall with a series of tables for each pair of examiners. I had to wait for about 20 minutes after the time given for the viva so inevitably I was tense. I was directed to a table and was met with a cool reception. There was no effort to put me at ease and the first question started as I was sitting down.

Examiner 1: **'You are called to see a 26-year-old man from the poor part of the town—a block of flats in the low socioeconomic group.'** He seemed at pains to emphasise social background before telling me that the man had become **jaundiced** and was **complaining of pain in the left iliac fossa.** He commented that he had had a throat infection a few days earlier which may or may not be of relevance. **'What is going through your mind on your way to see this chap?'**

I started with **drugs, alcohol** and **hepatitis** in view of the poor social background. **'Yes, but what about the pain in the LIF?'** I couldn't relate social circumstances to pain in the LIF and the examiner kept emphasising that there was no hepatic tenderness or enlargement.

He then helped me by saying that the young chap was tender in the left upper quadrant, which made me wonder if I'd misheard him initially when he said LIF. Anyway, obviously the chap had **splenomegaly** but, instead of going through the differential diagnosis of splenomegaly, I was preoccupied with the relevance of the social circumstances.

I was not getting anywhere, and so the next clue was **'There are spherocytes on the blood film'** and having more or less given me the diagnosis, I was able to answer the remaining basic questions on **hereditary spherocytosis.** However, I felt annoyed that the social circumstances had been emphasised as these were irrelevant and had distracted me.[1]

Examiner 2: **'What are your thoughts on the *treatment of myocardial infarctions* nowadays?'**

I started to talk about the changes with the advent of thrombolysis but was cut short with, **'No, the fellow in front of you has had an MI—what are you going to do?'** I thought, 'Fine, but at least decide what question you want answered!' He quickly lost interest once I appeared to know the answers.

---

[1] *Anaemia, jaundice* and *splenomegaly* are the hallmarks of hereditary spherocytosis, and the structure of the scenario suggests that it was an effort at presenting a *Detective* Story. The examiner probably did mention the pain in the left upper quadrant which the candidate misheard as the left iliac fossa. It was probably a true story and the examiner narrated the entire account, including the social aspects, without pruning it to suit a good *Detective* Story!

Examiner 2: '**Tell me about the *JVP waveform*.**'[2]

This was an easy question, but I couldn't see what he wanted in asking about the cause of the *v* wave. In fact, he just wanted me to say 'opening of the AV valve'.[3]

Examiner 2: '**You see *a young man in outpatients with 1% sugar in urine – what do you do?*'**

I said, 'Ultimately I'd check the blood sugar.' '**Yes, but before that.**' They clearly wanted me to discuss all the other reasons for the urinary glucose before mentioning diabetes mellitus.

Examiner 2: '**Tell me something about *Clinistix* and compare it with *Clinitest*.**'[4]

I could give all the differences but he said that I was being too complicated. He wanted me to say that *Clinistix* gave a quantitative measure, whereas *Clinitest* did not. It seemed so obvious that I didn't mention it.

Overall, I felt that the questions were on very reasonable topics but that they could have been delivered more clearly when they seemed interested in specific points.

(*Failed*)

---

[2]   This examiner asked the same question to successive candidates which even his coexaminer found a little tedious! The candidate should have treated it as a *Bedtime* Story, and described the waveform freely without giving a reason to the examiner to interrupt.

[3]   The *v* wave results from the rise in right atrial pressure when blood flows into the right atrium at the time when the tricuspid valve is shut, i.e. during ventricular systole.

[4]   Basic questions like this one suggest that the candidate is on the pass/fail borderline.

73

The viva examination was conducted in a small, single, well-lit room beside the examination ward. I waited for about three minutes outside the room before being called in. The examiners introduced themselves but had mask-like faces; one of them had a hawkish attitude and he started the viva.

Examiner 1: 'You are the 'on call' registrar and a patient is admitted with a *blood urea of 30 mmol/l.*[1] **How will you proceed?'**

I answered, 'I will take a history' and was interrupted immediately by the examiner: **'He is 45 years old and previously a fit man'.** I said I would proceed with the examination and was told that nothing was abnormal on the clinical examination (I had the impression at this stage that the examiner was either pushing me or that he had something specific in his mind). 'I would proceed with the laboratory investigations.' He again interrupted immediately, *'What is the most important investigation?'* I said, 'Urinary and blood electrolytes, urea and creatinine.'

Examiner 1: 'It's the middle of the night. Will the lab technician entertain your request for urinary electrolytes?'

'He might do.'

Examiner 1: 'What are you looking for?'

Answer: 'To differentiate between dehydration and acute renal failure.'[2]

Examiner 1: 'Can you differentiate clinically?'
Answer: 'No.'

Examiner 1: 'What are the signs of dehydration?'

Answer: 'Dry tongue, decreased skin elasticity, tachycardia and low BP.'

Examiner 1: 'Anything else you would like to do between 11 pm and 9 am?'

I realised that he seemed to be looking for some other thing. I said 'I would go for a fluid challenge.'

Examiner 1: 'What do you mean?'

Answer: 'I would give three litres of fluid with a high dose of frusemide and see the results of the urine output.'[3]

---

[1]   From the reported details, it is clear that the examiner presented an incomplete scenario; the candidate would have been within his right to enquire about the serum creatinine level, and whether the serum electrolytes were within normal limits. Acute renal failure and dehydration are both unlikely if 'nothing abnormal' was found on clinical examination. We suspect that the examiner had intended to present a *Ghost* Story with polycystic kidneys, chronic glomerulonephritis, analgesic nephropathy and obstructive nephropathy (e.g. retroperitoneal fibrosis) as the initial possibilities for a discussion. This differential diagnosis represents a distillate of the views from six international nephrologists from Europe and North America, who commented that the examiner should have given a more detailed clinical scenario.

[2]   p. 51
[3]   p. 105

Examiner 1: 'Any other investigation or procedure?'

Answer: 'I would catheterise the patient and arrange an urgent abdominal ultrasound examination to exclude an obstructive cause.'
In summary, what he had wanted was catheterisation, fluid challenge with frusemide, and an abdominal ultrasound.

Examiner 1: 'What are the *side effects of the phenothiazines*?'

I took 15 seconds to think, as the question was very abrupt and my brain was still thinking about the raised urea.

I answered, 'Photosensitive rash, anticholinergic effects (dry tongue, urinary retention), postural hypotension,[4] involuntary movements, obstructive jaundice.'

Examiner 1: 'Obstructive!' (I corrected this to cholestatic jaundice).

Examiner 2
(looked pleasant): '*A middle-aged female presents with joint pains.* How would you manage?'

Answer: 'I would take a history.'[5]

Examiner 2: 'What will you look for in her history?'

Answer: 'I would like to know which joints are affected, I'd ask about morning stiffness, the duration of the pain and for any associated illnesses.'

Examiner 2: 'Then what would you do?'

Answer: 'Examination.'[5]

Examiner 2: 'Nothing to find except some tenderness in the joints of hands.'

Answer: 'Then I'd do investigations such as FBC, ESR, rheumatoid factor, and X-ray of the hands.'

Examiner 2: 'What are the earliest changes of RA on X-ray?'

Answer: 'Soft tissue swelling and periarticular osteoporosis of the distal and proximal interphalangeal joints.'

Examiner 2: 'What is rheumatoid factor?'[6]

Answer: 'It is IgG against IgM!' (I didn't realise what I had said until the end of the viva.)

Examiner 2: 'How would you treat?'

Answer: 'I would explain to the patient about the illness. Then I'd start with NSAIDs and if they don't work then I would try second line drugs.'

---

[4] Hypotension may be marked and not only postural, particularly with parenteral chlorpromazine.

[5] This experience is a good illustration of how short, snappy and nonspecific answers lead to disaster.

[6] Rheumatoid factors (produced by the B cells) are autoantibodies of IgG and IgM classes directed against immunoglobulin G (located in the F_c portion of the IgG molecules) as the autoantigen. Only IgM rheumatoid factors can be measured routinely by agglutination reactions such as the latex test.

Examiner 2:   'What are they?'

I told him, and I then went into their side effects.

I was also asked about **DNA and the recent advances in its research**. In spite of having read recent *BMJ*s and *Lancet*s I had to say 'I don't know.'

Before leaving he asked me again, **'What is rheumatoid factor?'** I said the latex agglutination test.

(*Failed*)

74

The viva followed the long and short cases and was held in a decent sized room with a view over Harrow (which I spent a fair time studying!).

The first question was about the **advice** I would give to a colleague who was **planning to travel to Central Africa in** *six months time*.[1] My heart sank, as I had never been fond of such topics. I had not revised it after the written section, assuming that it would be confined to that. Anyway, I muttered about **malaria prophylaxis** with difficulty and did manage to convey that travellers should be warned about **social and sexual behaviour**. It was obvious that the examiner wanted to talk about something else – he kept stressing the six months part of the question. It wasn't until he said, **'It's something that** *you* **should have had'** that I realised he meant **hepatitis B**. I couldn't remember much about the antibody/antigen so he changed the subject.

The same examiner asked me then about the **side affects of the oral contraceptive pill**. I talked about the sort of things that one reads in women's magazines until he started hinting again. It became clear that he wanted to talk about cholestatic jaundice, and ended up by telling me that the pill is **contraindicated in women** who have had **cholestatic jaundice in pregnancy**. By then he appeared a little exasperated!

The other examiner took over and, much to my relief, asked me about **carcinoma of the bronchus** and how one assesses whether someone with it is suitable for surgery. He particularly pressed me about the question of age and appeared to approve of my answer that age was immaterial, provided that the patient was suitable by other criteria. The second examiner appeared more benign than the first, though that may simply have been because I could answer his questions!

(*Failed*)

---

[1]   Our italics; six months is rather a long time ahead of a planned trip to seek advice! In the modern jet age, travellers to Africa would not need six months to prepare themselves, unless they were considering a vaccination which would need that duration to be completed.

75

The viva was the last part of my clinical – long case, short cases, then viva. I was feeling very positive and confident as the short cases had gone extremely well. The viva was held in a small office with the examiners behind a desk which almost filled the room. We said hello and shook hands; they were polite and slightly distant, neither friendly nor antagonistic.

The first examiner laid **two cards** on my side of the desk, **one with a set of U&Es, the other with a blood gas analysis**. He asked me to comment: *'Your houseman phones you with these results from an ill patient.'*

I noted, and said, that the K^+ was very high with a normal urea and creatinine, and suggested repeating the test as the sample may have been haemolysed. I was asked how else the K^+ may be artificially high; I suggested a sample from a drip arm, and was prompted by the examiner to come up with the alternative of a sample left lying around for hours. To regain the initiative (and avoid having to give the causes of a true high K^+ with normal urea![1]), I moved on to the other card and commented on the low PO_2 and normal PCO_2. I ran through a short list of possible causes including a **severe asthma attack**, which was what I was meant to say.

I was then asked for a standard, *'How would you manage acute severe asthma?'* including all the complications. This was followed up by, *'What problems might you come up against in the management of a young chronic asthmatic?'* Having done a respiratory medicine job, I was able to talk about the social and psychological problems which again seemed to be what was expected. Then, lulled into a false sense of security, I was asked a series of questions on the **ventilation of asthmatics**, **indications**, **complications**, how it differed from routine ventilation, perioperative, etc. This culminated with the examiner producing (with a flourish) a graph of **BP** *vs*

---

[1] **Causes of hyperkalaemia with normouraemia**

1. *Pseudohyperkalaemia* – stored blood sample due to cell lysis and release of intracellular potassium; confirmed by finding normal *plasma* K^+ in the next sample. It is usually associated with haemolysis, thrombocytosis or leucocytosis
2. *True hyperkalaemia*
a. Reduced tubular secretion
   i   Potassium-sparing diuretics, e.g. triamterene, spironolactone and amiloride
   ii Addison's disease
   iii Hyporeninaemic hypoaldosteronism
b. Transcellular shifts
   i   Tumour lysis
   ii Haemolysis
   iii Hyperkalaemic periodic paralysis
   iv Anaesthetic agents (succinylcholine) causing depolarising muscle paralysis
c. High potassium intake
   i   Oral potassium supplementation
   ii Intravenous potassium administration
   iii Rapid transfusion of aged blood
   iv Increased extracellular osmolality, e.g. sudden hyperglycaemia in a diabetic patient.

time in a patient with severe asthma prior to ventilation and for 2 hours after. I was asked to explain the large fall in BP on ventilation and I muttered vaguely about it revealing dehydration, but essentially I floundered.[2]

I was then passed over to the next examiner: '**As you know, the NHS is having to become increasingly accountable. You, as a consultant physician, are the unit general manager of a large hospital. Your haematology colleagues would like the hospital to purchase a *plasmapheresis* machine. You have to decide whether this would be money well spent and so you go on a tour of the hospital, asking each department how much use they would make of this machine which costs several hundred thousand pounds. Where would you start?**'

My recollection of the rest of the viva is slightly hazy due to a state of mild shock. I remember we covered renal diseases (especially immune complexes), neurology (Guillain-Barré and myasthenia) and cardiology (rheumatic fever and familial hyperlipidaemia) before time ran out. I was asked about the **genetics of familial hyperlipidaemia**. Two other candidates that I know of were asked the same question – one in Glasgow and the other at Northwick Park, London. We had all read recent journals without coming across anything about the developments in the genetics of hyperlipidaemia. It was probably a coincidence.

Specific memories of the second half of the viva include, firstly, that I was constantly trying to reassure myself that this was not a 'pass or fail' type of question in terms of specific items of knowledge. It seemed much more a test of 'thinking on one's feet'. Secondly, the examiner did a lot of prompting and encouraging to extend the line of questioning. For example, I talked about **Guillain-Barré and the value of plasmapheresis** but then dried up so he asked, '**And what else might the neurologists use plasmapheresis for?**' Pause, '**More a muscular problem.**' At each stage I had to come up with the alternative treatment and comment on their relative merits. Thirdly, I remember the point where I felt I had passed: the examiner was effectively teaching me, saying that plasmapheresis had been shown to be particularly effective in controlling symptoms of myasthenia before thymectomy (I had talked about conventional treatment of myasthenia but confessed to not knowing the value of plasmapheresis). I commented that prednisolone treatment (which I did know about) was also very effective and considerably cheaper than a plasmapheresis machine. The examiner seemed slightly taken aback then smiled and said, '**You'd obviously make a good general manager**'. He thanked me and said that he had no further questions.

(*Passed*)

---

[2] Positive pressure ventilation will increase the intrathoracic pressure thereby decreasing the venous return and causing a fall in blood pressure. Normally, the fall in the blood pressure is compensated by a reflex increase in peripheral venous pressure, which re-establishes the venous return and the blood pressure returns to normal. However, in patients with a low blood volume (haemorrhage, dehydration) or with impaired reflex vasoconstriction (elderly patients), the compensatory mechanism may be inadequate and the blood pressure may remain low.

76

The venue was the main hall in the Royal College of Physicians of Edinburgh. There were many examiners at desks around the outside of this hall, probably about 20 candidates. The examiners were friendly, smiling and polite (I thought I must already have failed and they were just being nice to me).

The viva began with a question from the first examiner (the younger of the two) about the **effects of alcohol on the nervous system**. I discussed the obvious depressant effects of alcohol on the central nervous system. The examiner then asked about the **peripheral effects of alcohol**. I discussed **alcoholic polyneuropathy**, mentioning in passing that vitamin deficiency was an important factor which led me to **Wernicke's encephalopathy** and **Korsakoff's psychosis**. The examiner seemed satisfied with these two and changed the subject.

'**What if a patient presents saying that he has *difficulty walking up stairs*?**' I said I would think of a **proximal myopathy** and he said '**Good**'. He asked for the causes and I mentioned iatrogenic, such as steroid therapy, and endocrine causes, such as Cushing's syndrome or thyrotoxicosis. He stopped me and asked whether I knew how long the myopathy took to reverse in young people with thyrotoxicosis.[1] I guessed several months and he said, '**Yes, it does, doesn't it?**' I continued with the causes, mentioning alcohol again, a nonmetastatic effect of carcinoma and then began to struggle.

He changed the subject. He asked me about a patient presenting with **nocturia**[2] and about my approach to this problem. I said, 'Of course, I would take a full history and perform a full examination but I would proceed primarily according to whether they were male or female.' I discussed the possibilities from prostatism in men, urinary tract infections in men and women, urethritis, chronic renal failure, hyperglycaemia and hypercalcaemia. He seemed pleased because I had mentioned hypercalcaemia and asked about its treatment. I mentioned i.v. saline, diuretics and steroids, and said that rehydration was most important and that the use of **diphosphonates**[3] was increasingly popular and effective.

---

[1] Metabolic myopathy, particularly the one associated with hypokalaemia, is reversible with restoration of the plasma K^+. In **thyrotoxic myopathy** with *muscle wasting* (mostly occurs in male thyrotoxic patients), some muscle strength returns when the metabolic state has been restored, but the muscle wasting takes much longer to improve. In this variety, light microscopy shows atrophy and infiltration of the muscle fibres by fat cells and lymphocytes; abnormal mitochondria and a dilated tubular system are seen on electron microscopy; electromyography shows decreased duration of the action potentials and an increased percentage of polyphasic potentials.

[2] **Nocturia** may be a manifestation of known **polyuria** (diabetes mellitus, central and nephrogenic diabetes insipidus, compulsive water-drinking and diuretic therapy) or may point to an *unsuspected polyuria* (chronic renal failure, hypercalcaemia, hypokalaemic nephropathy, sickle-cell anaemia and chronic pyelonephritis). In normal subjects, nocturia may occur after excessive beer or tea ingestion in the evening, during cold nights and after or during an episode of supraventricular tachycardia. Nocturia may also occur after some stressful situations such as an attack of angina, asthma or migraine.

[3] See p. 157

The second examiner took over, and asked about the **management of a small pneumothorax** in a young patient, **'Would you admit them?'** I said I would and he said I was being prudent.

His major question was, **'A 75-year-old man with *angina on a flight to Australia*, 32 000 feet over Bahrain, develops severe chest pain. What would you do?'** [4] I waffled about history and examination which irritated the examiner. **'I have told you it is angina, what are you going to do? Do you ruin his last chance of seeing his family in Australia? What does he need?'** It struck me then and I said, 'Oxygen, descend[5] and give him oxygen'. Big smile. **'That actually happened to me.'**

(*Passed*)

---

[4] Modern jet aircraft are pressurised to have a cabin pressure of 565 mmHg (equivalent to a height of about 8000 feet). Under these circumstances the arterial oxygen tension may be around 65–70 mmHg in normal subjects, but this may fall much lower if the patient has some degree of ventilation/perfusion mismatch due to, say, chronic obstructive airways disease. In this patient, the arterial oxygen tension may have fallen critically to have precipitated the angina.

[5] Descent would not be beneficial since it would not change the cabin pressure.

77

The examiners were friendly and reasonable. I was initially asked about the **management of a 45-year-old woman who is breathless with a Hb level of 4.1 g/dl and an MCV of 106.**[1] I said that the most likely diagnosis would be **pernicious anaemia** and I would investigate and take blood samples for serum B_{12} and folate levels, examine a bone marrow aspirate and do a Schilling test,[2] if appropriate. They told me that the B_{12} and folate levels were both low and the marrow was megaloblastic. I said I would treat with B_{12} injections and give folate and iron as indicated. The examiner said that the next day her Hb was 3.8 g and the following day 3.1 g.[3] What would I do? I said that in a symptomatic lady with a falling Hb, despite B_{12} injections, I would have to consider cautious transfusion. They pressed me on any particular risks of this but I could only give the general risks of transfusion. I felt they were after specific risks for B_{12} deficient patients.

I was then asked about **a 22-year-old lady with three generalised convulsions in three months**. I said I'd treat with carbamazepine (least toxic alternative) and that I would not investigate unless there were focal signs or if the epilepsy was resistant to treatment. They asked, **'What if she wanted to have a baby and wished to defer the drug treatment?'** I answered that the risks to the fetus from carbamazepine would be less than from further fits and they agreed.

They then asked me about **a 63-year-old-man with low back pain and a high ESR**. They were after **myeloma**.

Finally they asked about the **management of an elderly lady who was 'off her legs'**. If I wanted to start her on an ACE inhibitor, how would I do it and which one would I use? They accepted that if the indication was congestive cardiac failure she should be in hospital, the dose of the diuretic should be reduced beforehand, and her BP should be monitored for postdose hypotension.

Impressions: My viva was merely a commonsense discussion of regularly encountered clinical scenarios.

(*Passed*)

---

[1] A friendly *Detective* Story!

[2] This test is not necessary unless other causes of poor vitamin B_{12} absorption are suspected, e.g. pancreatic disease (lack of proteases in the duodenum may interfere with the formation of intrinsic factor–vitamin B_{12} complex), blind-loop syndrome, organic disease of the ileum (site of vitamin B_{12} absorption), infestation with *Diphyllobothrium latum* (rare nowadays), etc.

[3] Since the response to the administration of vitamin B_{12} occurs within two to three days, it is seldom necessary to subject the patient to the risks, discomfort and expense (in the current financial climate!) of blood transfusion. However, a falling haemoglobin state should be investigated (e.g. blood loss from the gut or heavy menstruation). Blood transfusion may become necessary if the anaemia becomes symptomatic (i.e. cardiovascular or neurological manifestations).

78

The viva followed a mediocre performance in both the long and the short cases.[1] The examiners started off very politely, then became increasingly hostile.

The opening question was, **'What would you understand by the term $p < 0.001$[2] if you read an article in the *Lancet?*'** I explained this, which they seemed to accept; I was then asked to explain the **null hypothesis**[2] which I was also able to do. The examiner then asked me about the **chi square** test and the **Students *t*-test** and the advantages/disadvantages of each.[2]

He then changed the subject and asked, **'How would you go about establishing the diagnosis of Cushing's syndrome?'**[3] I started with the conventional history, examination and investigations, but he became impatient and asked about what routine and specific biochemical tests I would do. I said that there may be a hypokalaemic alkalosis – again he got impatient and asked me about more specific tests. I said that the random serum cortisol may be elevated. I was told that this wasn't very helpful. I then suggested the loss of the diurnal cortisol variation – again he seemed agitated. The bell sounded and the examiners changed around.

The second examiner asked, **'What are the different types of shock you know of?'** I said cardiogenic, traumatic, septic, obstetric, etc. I was asked how I would **manage septic shock**. Once again, I said history, examination and investigations, all of which irritated him. I think he wanted me to talk straight away about the appropriate fluid replenishment and the use of a broad-spectrum antibiotic cover. When asked how I would *accurately* assess the circulating volume I said, 'By insertion of a CVP line'. At this he retorted, *'Well, you would look at the veins first, wouldn't you?'*

The bell sounded.

Impressions: I think it is important to attempt to establish a rapport with the examiners even though it is supposed to be a neutral atmosphere. I felt I made no great mistakes, and yet I couldn't say a thing right!

(*Failed. The candidate was given 4/10 in the viva*)

---

[1]   The long case was a postgastrectomy patient (30 years after the operation) who had received no vitamin B_{12} replacement for the last five years. The candidate demonstrated the signs of peripheral neuropathy and the examiners agreed, but they disputed his demonstration of the ankle clonus, particularly as there were no other pyramidal signs (they made an issue of this). He was shown six short cases (a palpable gall bladder, spastic paraparesis, type III hyperlipidaemia, diabetic retinopathy, necrobiosis lipoidica diabeticorum, and fibrosing alveolitis). He missed palmar xanthomata in his third short case and was less than confident in his last case. In retrospect, he had obtained a bare fail (4/10) in each of these two sections, and badly needed a good viva.

[2]   See Appendix I

[3]   p. 63

79

The viva was the last part of my examination, and as I waited to go in I was saying to myself, 'Don't blow it', because I was sure that I had passed up until then. While I was thinking all this I was called in. The examiners were pleasant but not overfriendly and they did not smile.

Examiner 1: **'Tell me about the symptoms of nocturia.'**

I gave a list of the causes – chronic renal failure (CRF), diabetes mellitus, prostatism, and urinary tract infections. The discussion centred on CRF.

Examiner 1: **'Why does nocturia occur in CRF?'**

She was not impressed with my answer that there was a loss of the concentrating ability, and she eventually answered her own question –'**Loss of reactivity at the nephron to ADH.**'

Examiner 1: **'Tell me about how drugs can produce kidney disease.'**

I talked about interstitial nephritis, e.g. due to nonsteroidal anti-inflammatory drugs (NSAID), glomerulonephritis due to penicillamine and urate nephropathy secondary to cytotoxics.

Examiner 1: **'What is the difference between the disease caused by NSAIDs now and in the past?'**

There followed a discussion of the differences in the pathology of interstitial nephritis and papillary necrosis!
  (I might add that all these questions come from a renal physician!)

Examiner 1: **'Tell me something about pellagra.'**

My mind went blank! I said I was sorry but I couldn't remember the vitamin that is deficient,[1] but I could describe the clinical signs. She asked if I knew any **conditions associated with pellagra**. I said Hartnup's disease and the carcinoid syndrome.[2]
  The examiners then swopped over and the second part of the viva was much more straightforward.

Examiner 2: **'Tell me how alcohol affects the body?'**

I was able to talk for a long time on the different systemic manifestations of

---

[1] The candidate had forgotten niacin, which is often used to refer collectively to nicotinic acid and nicotinamide.

[2] Hartnup's disease is a rare inborn error in which pellagra may develop because of a defect in the intestinal and renal tubular transport of tryptophan and of several other amino acids. Malnourished patients with the malignant carcinoid syndrome occasionally exhibit clinical features of pellagra because of diversion of dietary tryptophan to serotonin.

alcohol – on the heart, liver, stomach, peripheral nerves, CNS, bone marrow and so on.

Examiner 2: '**Tell me which drug you would choose to treat a young girl with epilepsy?**'

I said carbamazepine and we talked about it and the alternative drugs, which basically entailed me listing the side effects of these drugs.

Impressions: I get the impression that they want to see how you react to questions, and you don't have to get all the questions 100% correct.

(*Passed*)

80

Examiner: 'An 8-year-old girl attends my clinic complaining of sore ankles and a sore knee. She and her family had returned from a holiday in Spain two weeks previously. What is the likely explanation?'[1]

I immediately recognised the 'reactive arthritis' problem and gave an excellent answer. I knew a great deal about this as I had written my only publication on this topic!

Examiner: 'Define a normal population.'[2]

I answered this well.

Examiner: 'How do you define a normal range of a skewed distribution?'[2]

I answered this badly and I was told the answer by the examiner.

Examiner: 'The portrait on your left is of Mr Argyll Robertson. What is he famous for?'

I said for describing the pupillary changes in syphilis, and he was satisfied.

Examiner: 'How do you diagnose tertiary syphilis?'

I answered comprehensively, including all the serology.

Examiner: 'How do you treat tertiary syphilis?'

I told him 1 mega unit of procaine penicillin intramuscularly daily for 10 days.

Examiner: 'You have a patient in the admissions room with a clinical diagnosis of acute pancreatitis. How would you manage him?'

My answer included intravenous fluids, intravenous antibiotics, assessment of blood gases, calcium and the importance of resuscitation.

Examiner: 'Would an antispasmodic such as atropine be helpful?'

I answered badly (I couldn't remember the physiology of the sphincter of Oddi with respect to atropine).

(Passed)

---

[1] An excellent example of a *Detective* Story with a single diagnosis (**reactive arthritis**) in the examiner's mind, and correctly picked by this 'expert' candidate. The only odd feature in this scenario was that the patient was a young *female*. Like Reiter's syndrome, reactive arthritis mostly occurs in a young male; the male:female ratio is 20:1. HLA-27 is present in up to 80% of cases. The examiner had managed to pack *three* other clues in this story: the arthritis began *two weeks* after a holiday in Spain, it occurred in *lower limbs* and it was *asymmetrical*. Reactive arthritis begins within two weeks after a venereal or enteric infection, which may have been mild or asymptomatic (as in this case). Although the wrist and other joints of the upper limbs are occasionally involved, the arthritis mostly occurs in the weight-bearing joints.

[2] See Appendix I

What did I mean by saying that there was no such thing as a tough question, only tough answers? I was putting into a nutshell a little-known 'law' of interviewing, that whether a question is regarded as 'tough' is often determined not by the content of the question, but by the tone and manner of the answer.[1]

[1]   *Grand Inquisitor*
Memoirs of Sir Robin Day
London 1989, p. 238

Section 4
Anecdotes and suggestions

It is important to put mistakes behind you and to take each question afresh.[1]

I really filled in the gaps while he did most of the talking.[2]

[1] p. 104
[2] p. 237

I know the idea is to see how one performs under stress, but it is a wholly different type of stress to that in a busy casualty or with a sick patient.[1]

Of the several hundred reports we have received from the MRCP candidates, we chose eighty interchanges for Section 3, but there are many others which contain interesting anecdotes and experiences. In this Section we have assembled a small collection of these to provide light relief to the busy reader. Some of these reveal the idiosyncrasies of both the candidates and the examiners, but there is a self-evident lesson, or a message, in each extract. These represent candidates' views, and their selection does not necessarily signify our agreement; our views and suggestions about how to cope with the viva have been presented clearly throughout the book. These short experiences illustrate (as do the longer ones in Section 3) the well-known fact that the viva is a dynamic interchange, and the candidates must adjust their response to the evolving situation.

---

[1]   p. 237

1. The discussion about a 68-year-old healthy man with swollen ankles led on to cyclical oedema in women, and to what other cyclical conditions I knew of. The second examiner took over and asked about secondary prevention of myocardial infarction. I really filled in the gaps while he did most of the talking! My overall impression was one of dissatisfaction; although I did not feel that I had clearly failed, the examiners (never aggressive) really offered little feedback. (*Failed*)

2. I really was not impressed with the first examiner, a clinical pharmacologist, who asked me about aspirin overdose. I knew that he had written textbooks on aspirin poisoning and I felt intimidated by this. However, in general the questions were fair and wide ranging. (*Passed*)

3. After an unsatisfactory discussion about what advice I would give to my psychiatric[1] colleague going to East Africa (malaria prophylaxis, yellow fever, typhoid, etc.), the other examiner asked me about the management of an acute asthmatic attack. This went well except when he went on about the follow-up management. I mentioned the use of bronchodilators but he persisted with an **'Anything else?'**[2] routine followed by pathetic silence from me. When the bell went, they excused me. I said, 'I'm sorry,' and left. (*Passed the exam*)

4. The examiners were very pleasant and friendly. They gave me a lot of nonverbal (the eyebrows went up when I said something silly) and verbal (**'Yes, that's correct'**) feedback. (*Passed*)

5. Both the examiners asked about things that were topical or had recently appeared in the journals (a scenario of relapsing fever leading to Lyme disease, and autosomal dominant diseases leading to genetic counselling). A commonsense approach was very useful when I didn't know all the answers. (*Passed*)

6. The first examiner (a real *hawk*) presented a clinical scenario of pulmonary oedema in a patient with a myocardial infarction, and then proceeded to ask me about the nerve supply to the pericardium. I gave the root supply but couldn't remember the name of the nerve. The examiner pointed this out and asked me to name the nerve. I still couldn't remember but he kept on and on. In the end I said I didn't know. He shouted, **'You don't know?'** My own consultant, seated at the next desk, glanced round and there was **'What the hell is she doing?'** written all over his face! The other examiner mouthed **'phrenic nerve'** and I felt dreadful! I was very shaken up but managed to answer the other examiner's questions (opportunistic infections, hyperlipidaemia and population screening) reasonably well, though I could have done better but for the unhappy experience with the first examiner. I was very angry. I know the idea is to see how one performs under stress, but it is a wholly different type of stress to that in a busy casualty or with a sick patient. (*Failed the viva, passed the examination*)

---

[1] This was a deliberate cue to encourage the candidate to give comprehensive details of the medical problems likely to be encountered in East Africa, to a colleague who would be less likely to know them.

[2] This candidate did not address the various social, psychological and environmental triggering factors.

7. The second examiner plucked out a small notebook from his inside jacket pocket with a flourish, wrote down some urea and electrolyte results, and pushed it across to me for my opinion. I was thinking aloud, which he didn't mind, and I soon said the words he wanted to hear, 'Adrenal insufficiency.' After we had spent a few minutes discussing the management of acute hypoadrenalism, he drew a graph and asked me to comment. I felt very uncomfortable but managed to tell him a little about the *P* value, I waffled a bit about the *r* and that there was a good correlation. At this point he jumped off his chair, **'That's right, that's right, there is a good correlation.'** I passed the viva but failed overall because of the short cases.

8. We discussed the management of raging thyrotoxicosis in a 30-year-old woman who was 20 weeks pregnant. I felt on a decidedly sticky wicket and mentioned beta blockers. He seemed reasonably happy and said, **'She's delivered the baby and a week later develops malignant thyrotoxicosis. What are the signs?'** Frankly, I knew very little about this and he had to drag answers out of me. He kept pressing me to mention pyrexia[3] but I couldn't see what he was getting at. He said, **'What happens if you're waiting at the traffic lights and your girlfriend puts her foot on the accelerator?'**
'The engine races,' I said.
'That's right. What happens next?'
'It blows up,' I said.
'No,' he continued, **'It overheats.'**
Boy, what a terrible end to a viva! (*Failed*)

9. My start was poor (I couldn't say anything about myalgic encephalopathy) but I was able to finish better on questions about postural hypotension, tuberculous meningitis and malaria prophylaxis. The bell went in the middle of a question but there was no 'I've started so I'll finish',[4] and I was asked to leave immediately with no hint of the adequacy or otherwise of my responses. (*Passed*)

10. Beware the jovial, relaxed examiner – play it by the book! (*Failed*)

11. The whole examination seemed to espouse the principle of knowing the basic stuff very well. I was asked nothing esoteric; I only introduced it myself whenever appropriate. I realised on one or two occasions that I had either misunderstood them or given the wrong information. I explained the misunderstanding and corrected myself without getting flustered, even when we had moved on to another topic. (*Passed*)

12. They appeared impressed by a confident plan of action in the investigation of patients, starting with the basics. I did not know the answers to very specialised questions and they seemed happy to tell me about them. (*Passed*)

---

[3] **Hyperpyrexia** is a cardinal feature of *thyroid crisis* (also known as *thyroid storm* or *malignant* thyrotoxicosis). Fortunately, the condition is rare but carries a high mortality. See also p. 114.

[4] The expression has been borrowed from the television question master of the prestigious programme, '*Mastermind*', who invariably finishes the question that starts before the bell.

13. Overall, the viva went appallingly. The first examiner was very aggressive and disbelieving (even about the things I subsequently looked up and found to be correct!). He did not agree that alcohol had an adverse effect on hypertension. The second examiner was pleasant but continually corrected my errors, which increased my anxiety. (*Failed*)

14. I was asked about a young man who had been referred to the outpatients with a letter from his GP who had found glycosuria on routine urine testing,[5] and about another gentleman found to have proteinuria. The whole interview was friendly and seemed straightforward but I failed it!

15. On the whole, the examiners appeared to be more interested in what I would do in a particular clinical situation than in my knowledge of the current literature. All the questions were related to problems commonly seen and they wanted to know about my approach, and how I would investigate and manage them. (*Passed*)

16. I said, 'I don't know', in reply to at least five questions. When I had said all that I felt was relevant on a subject, I looked the examiner in the eye and waited for the next question without embarrassment. When I did not know a subject I talked as much as possible and did not allow them to interject without seeming rude. I passed in spite of being asked about three subjects I had not prepared, or even thought about, since my finals. I kept inwardly cool in spite of a certain amount of harassment from the second examiner. Please, advise future candidates to read the current leaders in the *Lancet* and the *BMJ*. (*Passed*)

17. I did the viva last. I thought I had fluffed the short cases but deliberately forgot about that and went in there as if nothing had happened. As I passed, I can say that one should try and put other sections of the examination out of one's mind, and concentrate on the bit one is doing. I came away with grateful thanks to the postgraduate tutor who advised me to read the recent *BMJ* and *Lancet* leaders, and to the nephrologist for his reminiscences in ward rounds. (*Passed*)

18. My recommendation to others would be to study the examination itself rather than the subject of medicine. There is no substitute for seeing patients every day; working in a district general hospital gave me the opportunity to see more patients than I would have done in a teaching hospital.

19. The viva can be strenuous and it is sometimes difficult to get on 'their wavelength'. Having the viva first in the morning is worse than when it is later in the day, as in Edinburgh (my second and successful attempt).

20. The examiners were very pleasant and helpful. They seemed to ask questions based on the 'guess what I'm thinking about' idea, and tried to guide me towards their diagnosis, or at least along their lines of thinking! (*Passed*)

---

[5] A *Biblical* referral story.

21. Both examiners were friendly and polite throughout. However, I felt as if it took me ages to get on to their train of thought for each topic; as soon as I did it was plain sailing. (*Passed*)

22. Do not be put off by (apparently) ridiculous questions such as: **'Are 'CCUs worthwhile?' 'Should patients with transplanted hearts be allowed to smoke?' 'Which ten drugs would you take to a desert island?'** Be prepared to offer a philosophical answer! (*Passed*)

23. The examiners were looking very unimpressed, but just after the bell rang they showed me a graph with a load of statistical twaddle underneath it. Fortunately, I have a degree in statistics and I was able to interpret this in about thirty seconds. The examiners looked amazed and, after a very mediocre performance, I'm sure that this persuaded them to pass me!

24. The second examiner then painted a further scenario of a 40-year-old businessman returning from Nigeria, having been there a month, and who had *been back in this country a fortnight*. He presented with a high fever and I was asked to outline my differential diagnosis and management.[6] Having discussed that the temperature may not be related to his foreign travel, I talked about malaria, hepatitis and diarrhoeal diseases. He seemed happy to hear me through but made it obvious that I was missing something. At the end he commented, **'Have you never heard of the viral haemorrhagic fevers, doctor?'** However, he did not seem too concerned that I could not recite 'chapter and verse' about them. We then discussed the management of an acute thyrotoxic crisis, which luckily I had had the occasion to manage 36 hours before the exam! That saved the day. (*Passed*)

25. This was by far my worst viva out of my five attempts at the exam! I annoyed one of the examiners at the beginning by my response to a clinical scenario of a 60-year-old obese lady with upper abdominal pain.[7] I started talking about peptic ulcer disease, chronic pancreatitis, gastritis, and irritable bowel syndrome. I was interrupted and asked for commoner causes. It was several moments before the two main causes they were looking for came to mind; namely gall-bladder disease and ischaemic heart disease. After that it was an uphill struggle. (*Failed*)

26. Both my examiners were *hawks*. Whatever happened to the pairing of a *hawk* and a *dove*? (*Failed*)

27. I felt that I had not performed at all well, partly through ignorance and partly because of stress. However, the behaviour of Examiner A was *ungentlemanly* as he kept nodding or shaking his head during my answers to Examiner B. I followed his prompting with disastrous consequences. (*Failed*)

28. Both my examiners looked stern but polite. It is probably best to assume that both are *hawks*, as trying to spot which is which before the start of the viva can lead one astray. (*Passed*)

---

[6] An interesting *Ghost* Story with the incubation period of at least two weeks (our italics) as the *ghost-link*. The incubation period of Lassa fever (West Africa) is 3–16 days, for Marburg virus 3–9 days and for Ebola virus 3–18 days.

[7] A *Ghost* Story with obesity as the *ghost-link* for gall-bladder disease.

29. I found this part of the exam the most difficult, as it revealed large gaps in my knowledge of the fundamentals. I think some practice with 'severe' consultant colleagues is helpful and, having done that second time round, I found the viva easier to handle. (*Failed*)

30. Some examiners are awful (my Number 2) but try not to be put off. If they ask a vague question, try to get them to be more specific even if they seem to be getting annoyed. I'm sure the other examiner becomes (partially) sympathetic. (*Passed*)

31. He started off with a question regarding brain death[8] and how you would approach relatives regarding organ donation. I immediately started on the brain death criteria, as I knew them well. As far as the relatives were concerned, I just used my common sense and imagined myself in this situation, using my vague recollection of the effects of bereavement from my undergraduate psychiatry. The examiner appeared satisfied with this. (*Passed*)

32. Finally, he asked me how I could prove that a 'fit' was genuine or not. I went round and round in circles, and still did not get the nod of approval that tells you that you've got the right answer. I was given a clue, '**What blood test would you do?**' Suddenly, I remembered something I'd done myself (three years previously) as some sort of an experiment, but I had to be prompted – prolactin.[9]

---

[8] **Brain death**

Before proceeding to establish the diagnosis of *brain death* the following *four* criteria must be fulfilled:
1. There is structural irremediable brain damage which has been diagnosed with certainty
2. The patient is in apnoeic coma (unresponsive to noxious stimuli and on a ventilator) with no spontaneous respiratory effort
3. No chance of drug intoxication and no paralysing or anaesthetising drugs should have been administered recently for treatment. Hypothermia must be excluded as a cause of coma and the core temperature (measured rectally or in the external auditory meatus) should be more than 35°C
4. There must be no significant metabolic, endocrine or electrolyte disturbance either causing or contributing to coma.

Criteria for the diagnosis of brain death
a. Fixed and unresponsive (to bright light) pupils
b. Absent corneal, oculocephalic (p. 61), gag and cough reflexes
c. Absent vestibulo-ocular reflex. This is established by instilling 20 ml of ice-cold water on the tympanic membrane; there should be no nystagmus on the opposite side
d. There should be no motor responses within the cranial nerve territory to painful stimuli. Purely spinal reflexes may be retained
e. Systemic circulation may be intact
f. Apnoea during oxygenation for 10 minutes in the presence of an arterial PCO_2 of 50 mmHg.

The examination should be performed and repeated after a few hours by two doctors of senior status six hours after the onset of coma or, if due to cardiac arrest, 24 hours after restoration of an adequate circulation.

Cecil Textbook of Medicine. Eds Wyngarden and Smith. 18th edn Saunders 1988 p 2073

[9] Serum prolactin level rises within 10 minutes after a single generalised tonic-clonic seizure, and it has been used to differentiate between hysterical attacks and epileptic seizures.

33. If you don't know about a subject try and steer round to a related topic. In discussions about managing patients, keep your answers very clinical, i.e. what you would do in acute situations. If you are unsure about something don't waffle; I was challenged to justify a lot of my answers. (*Passed*)

34. He started, **'I'm in outpatients and a yellow woman comes in. She is not jaundiced, what could this be?'**[10]
'Hypothyroidism!"
'No, no, her TFT's are normal, but she is a little strange.'
'Carotinaemia!' This is what he was getting at, and for the rest of the viva he proceeded to tell me about this woman–an actual patient he had seen the day before! (*Passed*)

35. You must be aware of the recent important papers, editorials and reviews; they turn up in the viva, as they did in mine. (*Passed*)

36. The first examiner told me I had done very well and he was impressed. The second examiner asked me what I would do with a pregnant woman with a tachycardia of 200 beats per minute. I talked about different types of arrhythmias and drugs. At the end he said that *he* would call the cardiologist in! (*Passed*)

37. Know how to manage common medical emergencies; the viva is the only time they can examine you on these. Don't regurgitate the textbooks; say exactly what *you* would do as if *you* were describing an experience you had yesterday. If you don't understand the question, say so; it also gives you the time to think! (*Passed*)

38. Try to think clearly and structure your answers. Express safe and moderate views, and *do not* argue. (*Passed*)

39. You can never tell what you may get asked. One of the other chaps with me was asked about the histology of skin biopsies and he passed.

40. Don't express too radical or revolutionary ideas, especially if you cannot substantiate them. (*Passed*)

41. I was asked clinical questions which drew upon my experience of common situations in the outpatient clinic or in the ward management of patients. The answers they wanted were those that I would have suggested in practice to any of my colleagues. (*Passed*)

42. Keep up to date with the journals. (*Passed*)

43. Don't be put off by silent gaps and wild-eyed stares from the examiners. (*Passed*)

44. Don't panic if they ask an obtuse or esoteric question, but you must get every question on medical emergencies completely correct. (*Passed*)

45. They wanted to make sure that I was reasonably up to date on most things but I did not need to have an in-depth knowledge of the newer developments. (*Passed*)

---

[10] A *Wild* Story which allowed the candidate to become an appreciative listener!

46. Sound confident. The examiners don't necessarily know more than you do. Certainly mine didn't know much about head injuries and their relevant neurology. (*Passed*)

47. There is nothing wrong with apologising for nervousness. Try and be sensible about your answers. If you don't know, say so! (*Passed*)

48. I think there is very little you can do to prepare for the viva. You have to hope that they pick a subject about which you can talk a little. You can make mistakes and still pass.[11]

49. Try not to waffle and if you are not sure, say so. It is definitely not worth lying. My examiners asked questions on their own specialist subjects,[12] and one cannot afford to hoodwink them! (*Passed*)

50. Remember that the viva is easy if you don't panic. Answer the questions as if you are teaching a group of final year students; try to structure your answers, don't waffle, and *don't* try to fool them! If possible, practise for the viva on a one-to-one basis with a colleague who is also preparing for the viva. (*Passed*)

51. Revise statistics. If you don't know the answers, say so. By doing this you can save a lot of time and change to a subject that you know about. (*Passed*)

52. They seemed to be asking questions which sprang from my previous answers, thus creating situations where a proposed investigation or treatment may not be the wisest course. I believe the purpose was to see whether I had a flexible approach to the given clinical problem. (*Passed*)

53. If you are stuck try to make sensible *basic* statements, and show that you are trying logically to work out the problem. (*Passed*)

54. I said I had no idea when he asked me how I would measure TSH in the laboratory. He then said, **'What has been the biggest immunological breakthrough of recent years?'** With a tongue in cheek I said, 'monoclonal antibodies', as I knew nothing about these except the name! He said, **'A good guess. That's how one measures TSH.'** (*Passed*)

55. There were persistent offputting interruptions and I never really got my presentation flowing. A part of the way through my viva, one of the examiners threw up his hands in horror at one of my answers. (*Failed*)

56. My impression of the viva as a whole was that the discussion was geared to very practical aspects (e.g. how to educate a newly diagnosed insulin-dependent diabetic). It seemed that they were trying to ascertain whether I had really encountered some of the problems in everyday practice. (*Passed*)

---

[11] This candidate was asked about the causes and the emergency treatment of hypoglycaemia, the management of a 45-year-old man with chest pain, the complications of an acute myocardial infarction, and the biochemical control of the blood sugar.

[12] The candidate guessed this from the questions he was asked on renal failure.

57. The second examiner asked, **'Tell us about the recent papers you have read.'** This was a gift as I had read quite a few. I discussed fetal tissue transplantation[13] and the current thinking in thrombolytic therapy.'[14] They were not cardiologists (and I'd just finished a cardiology job) so it all went smoothly. (*Passed*)

58. The first examiner said, **'A general practitioner sends you a patient with a diagnosis of gout. What do you do?'** He seemed a little agitated when I said I'd take a history, including a family history, and measure the serum urate level. He said, **'I *told* you he has gout.'** I justified the need for obtaining a proper history. (*Passed*)

59. All the questions were clearly stated and phrased so as to allow me to influence (to some extent) the line of discussion. The examiners were polite and it was not hard to establish some rapport. (*Passed*)

60. I think I gave the viva the least practice before the exam. I had only three 'formal' five-minute vivas on courses in Manchester and in my own hospital. As far as the knowledge for the viva goes, I did prepare a lot by reading *Medicine International*, sections of the *Oxford Textbook of Medicine* and the last three years issues of the *BMJ, Lancet, New England Journal of Medicine, Hospital Update* and the *British Journal of Hospital Medicine*. My presentation was not very fluent, and I would advise people to have a lot of viva sessions with *senior* doctors, preferably consultants. (*Passed*)

61. Several of my friends spent many hours reading journals in the belief that viva questions demand a comprehensive knowledge of the literature. I am sure this is not necessary except perhaps for the 'newer' topics (e.g. coronary thrombolysis) which are not yet properly covered in textbooks. (*Passed*)

62. I felt that this viva was biased towards chemical pathology and physiology (e.g. the body's handling of salt, water, magnesium and H^+), and the examiners were trying to find the depth of my knowledge. They were in no mood to allow me to display my knowledge of other topics. I was a wreck at the end and was certain that I had failed in the viva. (*Passed the exam*)

63. Stop and think about the questions carefully before answering; remember you *are* allowed to make mistakes though I think I was fortunate to have 'nice' examiners! It is important to avoid looking blank and saying nothing; better to admit you don't know and go on to something else (if they let you!). (*Passed*)

64. I was initially asked about the causes of erythema nodosum and we then launched into a friendly discussion on the diagnosis and management of inflammatory bowel disease. The examiner then said, **'Of all the causes of erythema nodosum you mentioned, what do they all have in common?'** I explained that they were all multisystem disorders. Both examiners looked at each other and laughed. I later looked up the speciality of the examiner

---

[13] p. 91
[14] p. 31

who asked this question and found that he was a rheumatologist. I suppose he had hoped that I would have said that they are all associated with an arthropathy! (*Passed*)

65. The second examiner, who was rather aggressive, opened by asking me what my reaction would be if I was called to see a patient with a painful ankle. I suggested a DVT. The examiner retorted, '**DVTs do not give painful ankles!**' I then suggested an arterial embolism, which was clearly the answer he wanted. (*Passed*)

66. Express yourself clearly and emphatically.

67. Speak confidently! When I was wittering on about the lessons learnt from the trials on mild hypertension, the examiner remarked at one stage, '**Well, you said that quite confidently!**' I interpreted this more as a compliment than an insult.

68. Use a dictaphone and speak for two minutes on any topic or clinical problem (e.g. history, examination, investigation and management) without ums, errs, hesitation or deviation. Play it back, correct your mistakes, reorganise your spiel and repeat the exercise. Practise for half an hour every evening for a few weeks before the examination. (*Passed*)

69. Keep up to date for about six months with the *BMJ*, *Lancet* and the *New England Journal of Medicine* because you can always recruit in extra information and score a high mark. Revise basic statistics, as I was asked questions about it in two of my three vivas. (*Passed*)

70. My friend and I went through common topics in the main specialities to prepare a brief spiel to come out with. It didn't do me any good but it helped my confidence! (*Passed*)

71. Stay calm and keep things simple. Don't give the examiners tempting leads, e.g. cat scratch fever as a cause of lymphadenopathy, unless you are comfortable with that topic. (*Passed*)

72. I passed the viva on three occasions but passed the short cases only once. I remember noting after each viva that my cover-to-cover knowledge of *Lecture Notes in Clinical Medicine* by Rubinstein and Wayne provided *all* the answers to *all* the questions I was asked. (*Passed*)

73. There was no response from the examiners, neither negative nor positive. I just had to keep ploughing on. Revise recent important trials, especially on cardiovascular topics – aspirin/streptokinase/hypertension, etc. Say 'I don't know' when you don't. Don't get bogged down with medical politics. I was advised by an examiner in a 'mock' examination, that as there are about 60% of non-British graduates this will not be emphasised. (*Passed*)

74. On the whole, I felt in control and knew enough to be confident about what I was saying. This was different from my first attempt, when I felt uncertain and 'medical studentish'. You need to practise talking about medical emergencies with a colleague. *BMJ* editorials give a very good overview of topics and seem to be used by the examiners (happened in both my vivas). You need to make sure that you know enough to stand up to constant

questioning and interruptions. Smile when you go in, sit up straight, and look them in the eye! (*Passed*)

75. Honesty is the best policy—if you are unsure about something, say so. Never come down too strongly on one side of a controversial issue, as the examiner may favour the other side! Better to give both sides and be noncommittal unless pressed by the examiner. (*Passed*)

76. Remember that the more elderly examiners may require occasional, but polite, reminders about modern trends. In my viva I was discussing the management of prolonged hypoglycaemia, I said that after confirming it with a laboratory glucose measurement I would give dextrose and continue the BM monitoring. My examiner remarked, **'You seem to be placing a lot of store by BMs.'** I said gently, *'That's what we tend to do these days!'* (*Passed*)

77. I had one nice examiner whose questions about alcohol were easily identifiable. My other examiner was awful and it was difficult to make any sense of what he wanted, e.g. **'Tell me about pharmacogenetics and its relevance to practice.'**
     Vivas are really hit-and-miss affairs and the onus is on the examiner to enable you to show him or her what you know. If they fail to allow you to do this, then they are bad interviewers and you are unlucky! (*Passed*)

78. I was sitting cross-legged throughout my viva. At the end of 30 minutes my right leg felt 'dead' with numbness and tingling which led to obvious difficulty in leaving the room! Both examiners looked bemused, wondering whether I was performing some sort of ritual! (*Passed*)

79. If your examiners don't know each other then they may use you as a means of impressing each other. Just sit tight and let them talk to each other! (*Passed*)

80. The viva is like playing football for Liverpool – possession play; if you have the ball (keep talking) they can't score! (*Passed*)

Appendices

There is so much to learn, so little time to do it in, and no time to practise it!

Silence weighs heavily on the examiners' ears![1]

---

[1]   A candidate

Appendix 1
Statistical Terms

In presenting the definitions and explanations of various commonly quoted statistical terms, we have taken note of the examiners' questions and an estimate of the understanding they expect from the candidates. This is not an attempt at giving a comprehensive guide to statistical methods, for which the candidate should consult one of the several standard textbooks available, as suggested by us at the end of this section. Our purpose is simply to make you familiar with the commonly used statistical terms and to give you some understanding of these. We hope that this section will whet your appetite for learning more about statistics. Methods of calculation and detailed explanations of the statistics mentioned in this appendix are outside the scope of this book.

In the final preparation of this section, we have been influenced by the comments from Dr Robert Newcombe, a medical statistician, and Dr David Phillips, a physician with expertise in epidemiological methods, both of the University of Wales College of Medicine, and from several MRCP candidates. We are grateful to all of them.

Frequency curves and distribution

A frequency curve can be drawn by plotting the numbers for each *set* or *interval* of a continuous variable, e.g. a number of adults on the y axis against height in centimetres on the x axis (Fig. 1). Such a curve gives a

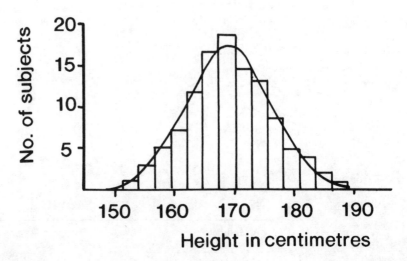

Fig. 1 Frequency distribution for height in one final year group of medical students

picture of the shape of a distribution of that variable. If we examine a population of 1000 adult males, we may find that the majority of them fall in the middle (i.e. between 165 cm and 175 cm), there are a few who are below 165 cm and a few who are more than 175 cm tall. The peak of this curve covering the most frequently occurring value of the population is called the *mode* and such a continuous symmetrical distribution is the Gaussian[1] *normal* distribution.

If a curve shows two humps, as would happen in this case if a large number of the adults were either more than 175 cm or shorter than 165 cm, causing a hump in either of these areas, then the technical term for this is a *bimodal* distribution (Fig. 2a). If, however, there are enough numbers to cause a distinct hump but the curve is asymmetrical, because there are a few more subjects either shorter or taller than those under the main hump, then the distribution is *skewed*. Such asymmetrical distributions are said to be positively or negatively skewed depending on the direction of the 'tail' of the curve. In a *positively skewed* distribution the 'tail' is at the upper end and the 'bulge' in the lower end, whereas in the *negatively skewed* distribution the long 'tail' is at the lower end (Fig. 2b).

Summarising data

Often we need to summarise in a single figure a spread of data across a unit of time or space. Most people are familiar with the idea of an *average*, which can be used to describe the 'general' level for a variable, e.g. the 'average'

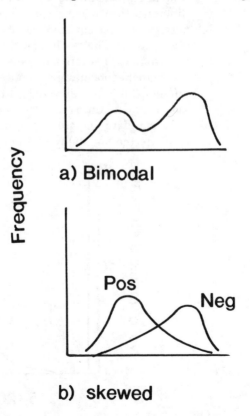

Fig. 2 Bimodal and skewed distributions

[1]   Named after the German mathematician, C F Gauss (1777–1855)

sunshine hours for a particular month. The average may be defined as a measure of the *central value,* which locates the middle or centre of a collection of values. The most common measure of the central value is the arithmetic *mean,* which is calculated by adding up the values of all the observations and dividing this total by the number of observations. The mean represents an average value for a collection of data. Another measure of the central value is the *median,* which is the value of that observation which, when the individual observations are arranged in ascending (or descending) order of magnitude, divides them into two equal sized groups. Thus, if 21 observations of age are arranged in ascending order, the middle observation or the median is the eleventh one. If the distribution of the data is normal then its mean, median and mode are interchangeable. In a skewed distribution the mean and median will not be the same but may approximate to each other (Fig. 3).

The mean of any set of values gives no idea about how widely dispersed the various observations are from the central value. In the same way that the mean actually represents the central value, it would be desirable to present the dispersion in a single summary figure. Giving simply the range of the values (i.e. the difference between the highest and lowest values) only gives the extreme values and ignores the others in the set; it also depends heavily on the sample size. A mathematical approach to defining a measure of dispersion, scatter or spread is to first find out how far each individual measurement is from the arithmetic mean, then square each difference (irrespective of its positive or negative sign) and then divide the average of these squared deviations by one less than the total number of observations. The resulting measure is called the *variance,* which is a most important expression of dispersion in statistics. The reason for using one less than the total number of observations is that in applying the statistical inference, it is useful to regard the collection of observations as being a *sample* drawn from a much *larger population.* The square root of the variance is the **standard deviation**, a commonly used term in statistics. In order to compare the variability of some measurements in two or more groups

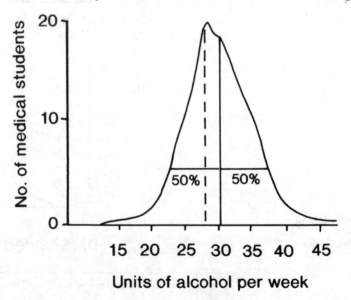

Fig. 3 Frequency distribution for alcohol intake among medical students.
Mean = – – – –
Median = ———

which may have different means (e.g. reproducibility of a laboratory method), the **coefficient of variation** is sometimes used; this is the standard deviation expressed as a percentage of the mean.

The standard deviation is a measure of the spread of a particular population but it does not indicate how precise a sample mean is as an estimate of a population mean. For this purpose the *standard error* of the mean is often used. This is obtained by dividing the standard deviation by the square root of the total number of observations. These two statistics–the standard deviation and the standard error–are frequently asked about in the viva. It will be clear from the above explanation that the standard deviation is a measure of the variability between individuals as regards the factor under investigation, such as the serum rhubarb level in a sample of rhubarb eaters. The standard error, on the other hand, reflects a measure of the uncertainty in a sample and depends on both the standard deviation and the sample size. Thus, the standard error of the mean indicates the uncertainty of the mean serum rhubarb concentration among the sample tested as an estimate of the mean value among the population of all rhubarb eaters. The level of certainty or *confidence* can be worked out from the sample mean ±2 (approximately) × standard error, and one can state that a sample mean lies within a certain range of the unknown population. In other words, there is a 95% chance that this interval will enclose the unknown population mean. This interval is known as a 95% *confidence interval*, and the values defining it are 95% *confidence limits*.

Tests of significance

Whenever we conduct an experiment or survey, whether in a test tube or on a group of subjects, we are attempting to explore Nature, with the hope that what we find to be true in the study group will be applicable to the larger unknown population. We are making a decision on the basis of a sample, and we face the danger that a potentially interesting result we have observed may have occurred merely by chance. In order to minimise this element of doubt, we formulate a hypothesis and test it. Since it is far easier to disprove a proposition than to prove it, we reformulate the medical hypothesis (e.g. that drug A is better than drug B in reducing blood pressure–which is what we set out to prove) to state that there is no difference between drug A and drug B, and then try to reject or disprove it! This reformulated hypothesis is referred to as a *null hypothesis*, and in most cases the investigators want to reject it.

Unfortunately, in real life a host of known and unknown factors operate and the rejection or acceptance of a proposition is never absolute. Rejection of a null hypothesis depends on the probability of getting the observed result. If the probability of getting an observed result by chance is small then the null hypothesis is rejected. In the scientific literature, the value of this probability is calculated and called the P value for the significance test. An arbitrary but universally used cut-off value for a rejection of the null hypothesis is 5% ($P < 0.05$) i.e. the chances of a spurious result are 5%. Many investigators use a significance level of 1% ($P < 0.01$) to reject the null hypothesis. In statistical language, a *significant* result is a result which is not well accounted for by chance.

The decisions about rejection and nonrejection of the null hypothesis may turn out to be incorrect. If the null hypothesis has been rejected in error (i.e. a significant difference was obtained when in reality there was no difference), this form of error is called an *alpha* or *type I error*. If a nonsignificant result is achieved and the null hypothesis is not rejected (i.e. a real difference is missed), this error is called the *beta* or *type II error*.[2] These considerations are very important in deciding about the validity of the results of a study. In particular, if the study gives a nonsignificant result at a specified level (e.g. 5%) the probabilities for a type II error, or the beta probabilities, should be considered for a range of possible values for the mean of the population from which the sample was taken. For example, the sample size may have been too small to show a significant result, which would have been obtained in a larger sample. The inadequacy of a study should be judged at the outset by examining the *power* $(1-\beta)$ of the study, to detect a specified clinically plausible and potentially important effect.

A variety of statistical methods are used to test a null hypothesis. A comparison of means between two samples is achieved with the use of the Student's *t*-test, and the significance is determined by reference to the *t* distribution. The *t*-test is strictly only valid if the distribution of the test sample is normal. However, the *t*-test is fairly 'robust' and gives a reasonable agreement with the result that would be obtained when a more appropriate test is applied. The *t*-test comparison may be made between *paired* (same population being tested for the drugs A and B) or *unpaired* (one population having drug A and the other drug B) samples.

A special test is required if the variable to be tested has more than two categories. For example, a survey of the smoking habits of 150 male doctors may reveal 23 (15%) current smokers, 60 (40%) exsmokers, and 67 (45%) nonsmokers. To compare these percentages with those obtained from males in the general population, we need to use the **chi-square** test which can accommodate the three categories of smoking in the two populations. The test is based on calculating expected numbers in the different categories of the variable if the null hypothesis were true, and comparing these with the numbers actually obtained (the observed frequencies). The chi-square test requires that the actual number, not merely the percentage, of the sample in the different categories of the variable be known.

Many expert statisticians criticise medical investigators for their use of inappropriate statistical procedures. Before deciding upon a procedure it is important to consider whether the various assumptions demanded by the procedure are fulfilled. For example, as stated earlier, the use of the *t*-test requires a normal distribution of the data, especially when the sample size is small. Such significance tests which make distributional assumptions about the data being analysed are called *parametric tests*. In contrast, *distribution-free* or *rank tests* are called *nonparametric tests*[3] p. 47. Their use is justifiable whenever there is clear non-normality of the variable to be tested, or the size of the sample is so small that one cannot establish whether or not the distribution is normal. These tests are also applicable for ordinal data when the measurements are graded categories, e.g. −, +, ++, for the degrees of clinical improvement.

---

[2]   p. 147
[3]   p. 47

Regression and correlation

The statistical methods of *correlation* and *regression* examine the association and comparison between two *quantitative* variables, e.g. systolic and diastolic blood pressures, weight and systolic/diastolic blood pressure, age and weight, etc. In all such comparisons, the underlying expectation which we want to test is that there *is* a relationship between the two variables. Often, the purpose of the experiment that generates the data is to find the degree of the relationship. For example, we expect that systolic blood pressure and age should be related and we wish to examine this relationship. To do this, we conduct a longitudinal experiment and measure systolic blood pressure in three subjects at regular intervals up to the age of 75 years and plot our recordings on the *y*-axis against each interval on the *x*-axis. This is a *scattergram* and gives us a visual impression that the systolic blood pressure increases with advancing age, but we need to know a more precise and definable relationship between the two variables. As the points fall close to a straight line, we can express this relationship numerically by means of an equation, Y=a+bx, where 'a' is the intercept of the line on the *y*-axis and 'b' is the slope of the line (Fig. 4). In this experiment we see that an increase of one year in age is associated with an increase of 1.33 mmHg in the systolic blood pressure. Such a relationship, where the change in one variable causes a predictable and specific (e.g. increase or decrease but continues in one direction) change in another variable is called a *linear relationship*.

The line showing this relationship is called a *regression line*, and the corresponding equation a *regression equation*. The coefficient 1.33 in the equation is called the *regression coefficient*. It means a change in *y* per unit change in *x* and is represented by 'b', or the slope of the line.

A measure of the degree of linear association between the two variables is provided by the **coefficient of correlation**, denoted by *r*. Values of *r* vary between +1 to −1, the sign of *r* depends on whether there is a positive or an inverse relationship between the two variables. The greater the

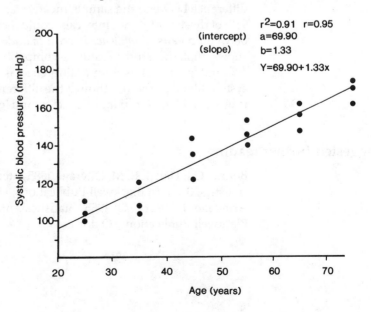

Fig.4 A longitudinal relationship between age and systolic blood pressure. In this regression there are multiple values for *y* for each value of *x*.

numerical value of r, the stronger the relationship between the two variables. In this example there is a strong relationship (denoted by r=0.95) between the age and blood pressure. Often, the square of r (the correlation coefficient) is used to express the relationship between the two variables; this is termed the *coefficient of determination*. For example, r^2 of 0.91 between x and y would suggest that 91% of the variation in y can be explained by the change in x. This provides a readily understandable interpretation when one is considering the influence of one variable on the other, e.g. height on weight, or weight on blood pressure.

Confidence intervals

The commonly used significance statement '$p < 0.05$' means that the observed result would occur by chance only 5 times out of a 100 experiments, and as such gives little information about the sizes of the differences between study groups. Nowadays, there is an increasing emphasis on calculating *confidence intervals*, which depend on the standard error and give the size of the difference of a measured outcome between groups. This statistic gives us a measured degree of 'confidence' that we would want to associate with the result. The confidence interval provides a formal expression of uncertainty which must be attached to the mean and standard error of a sample on account of the sampling errors.

Suppose that we are comparing systolic blood pressure in samples of 100 alcohol drinkers and 100 nondrinkers, and we observe that the mean difference is 8 mmHg in their systolic blood pressures and that the standard error of this difference between the sample means is 3 mmHg. Our calculated 95% confidence interval between the means is 1.5 to 12.5 mmHg. This means that there is a 95% chance that the difference would be obtained if the total populations of drinkers and nondrinkers were studied. In other words, if a series of identical studies were carried out on different samples from the same population, and a 95% confidence interval for the difference between the sample means was calculated in each study, then 95% of these confidence intervals would include the population difference between means. *Confidence interval indicates the width of the difference* and shows that the study result is compatible with a small difference of 1.5 mmHg as well as with a difference as great as 12.5 mmHg in mean systolic blood pressures, though the difference between population means is likely to be near the middle, i.e. 8 mmHg in the above example.

Suggested further reading

Bourke G J, Daly L E, McGilvray J 1985 Interpretation and uses of medical statistics, 3rd edn Blackwell Publications, Oxford
Armitage P, Berry G 1985 Statistical methods in medical research, Blackwell Publications, Oxford.

Appendix II
Eponyms

As in every other field of human achievement, great personalities in medicine are remembered and revered by having syndromes and signs named after those who first described them. While some have been lucky enough to have had greatness wrongly thrust upon them, there are others who have been deprived of the honour that they deserve. However, our purpose here is not to put the record straight but, rather, to present a selection of some of the famous dignitaries whose names commonly recur in the medical literature. In addition to the usual information that may be asked for by the examiners, in some cases we have also given some of their idiosyncrasies for light relief.

Robert ADAMS (1791–1875)
Professor of surgery, Dublin, and surgeon to Queen Victoria.
Stokes-Adams attacks (see Stokes).

William ADIE (1886–1935)
An Australian-born neurologist during the first world war. He worked at Queen's Square (London) until his death at the early age of 48.
Holmes-Adie syndrome (see Holmes).

Thomas ADDISON (1793–1860)
A physician at Guy's who became known as the founder of endocrinology. He was the first to realise that the adrenal glands are essential to life. However, in 1855 his monograph on 'The constitutional and local effects of disease of the supra-renal capsule' was much debated in England and Scotland and was largely dismissed. It was Trousseau who later named the condition of adrenal insufficiency after Addison. Addison suffered from depression in later life and it is thought that he committed suicide in Brighton in 1860.
Addison's anaemia – pernicious anaemia due to B_{12} deficiency.
Addison's disease – adrenal insufficiency, classically due to tuberculosis but autoimmune disease of the adrenals is the commonest cause nowadays.

Alois ALZHEIMER (1864–1915)
Born in Bavaria, initially a neurologist but later became a professor of psychiatry. He described the histological features in the atrophied brains of patients dying with dementia.
Alzheimer's disease – the term is applied to both presenile and senile dementia.

Julius ARNOLD (1835–1915)
Professor of anatomy at Heidelberg.
Arnold-Chiari malformation – a tongue of the cerebellum protrudes into the foramen magnum causing CSF outflow obstruction. There may be associated spina bifida, and syringomyelia may develop. Arnold's contribution was to describe one case; most of the work was done by Hans von Chiari who described the condition in 1891.

Joseph BABINSKI (1857–1932)
Born in Paris of Polish descent, he worked with Charcot and became a founder member of the Neurological Society of Paris. He devised the rapid alternating movements test for cerebellar disease (sometimes also called Babinski's sign). He wrote several hundred papers, mainly in neurology, but he also described acromegaly associated with a pituitary tumour. Later in life he developed Parkinson's disease.
Babinski's sign – extensor plantar response in upper motor neurone lesions.

William BAKER (1838–1896)
A surgeon at St. Bartholomew's Hospital, London.
Baker's cyst – popliteal cyst (clinically important in its rupture) commonly associated with rheumatoid arthritis.

Jean BARRÉ (1880–1967)
French neurologist who had worked with Guillain in the Sixth Army. He was also houseman to Babinski and wrote hundreds of papers on neurological topics.
Guillain-Barré syndrome (see Guillain).

Halushi BEHÇET (1889–1948)
Turkish dermatologist.
Behçet's syndrome – recurrent ulceration of the mouth and genitalia associated with arthralgia, inflammatory ocular disease and neurological disorders (e.g. aseptic meningitis, cerebral venous thrombosis, encephalitis, etc.).

Sir Charles BELL (1774–1842)
Professor of anatomy in London and later professor of surgery in Edinburgh. He was also a founder member of the medical school at the Middlesex Hospital and he was almost penniless when he died.
Bell's palsy – idiopathic lower motor neurone facial palsy.
Bell's law – motor and sensory functions are carried by the spinal nerves; the anterior root carries the motor and the posterior root the sensory fibres.
Bell's phenomenon – in Bell's palsy, the eyeball on the affected side rolls upwards when the patient attempts to shut his eyes.

Henry BENCE JONES (1818–1873)
Physician at St. George's Hospital, London. He was an excellent physician and a chemist, and insisted on the microscopic and chemical examination of the urine in diagnosing clinical disorders.
Bence Jones protein – low molecular weight protein found in the urine of patients with myeloma.

Arthur BIEDL (1869–1933)
German physiologist
Laurence-Moon-Biedl syndrome (see Laurence).

Theodor BILHARZ (1825–1862)
A German physician who later in life became a zoologist in Egypt.
Bilharzia–schistosomiasis.

BORNHOLM
The first documented cases of pleurodynia occurred on the Danish island
of Bornholm in the Baltic Sea between Denmark and Sweden.
Bornholm disease – epidemic pleurodynia (Devil's Grip).

Richard BRIGHT (1789–1858)
A physician at Guy's Hospital. Together with Addison and Hodgkin he was
one of the 'Great Men of Guy's'. He was also an artist and a naturalist.
Bright's disease – acute poststreptococcal haemorrhagic glomerulonephritis.
Bright's apparatus – a spoon to detect protein in the urine.

BROMPTON
Brompton cocktail – an analgesic mixture (cocaine, morphine/heroin,
alcohol) usually reserved for patients with terminal disease. It was first
introduced in Brompton Hospital (London) by H. Snow in 1896.

Charles BROWN-SÉQUARD (1818–1894)
Born in Mauritius, he worked in neurology and endocrinology at Queen's
Square, then at Harvard and finally in Paris. He was also an experimental
physiologist and contributed greatly to Claude Bernard's discovery of the
vasomotor system.
Brown-Séquard syndrome – hemisection of the spinal cord causing
ipsilateral motor weakness, loss of vibration sense and proprioception and
contralateral loss of pain and temperature sense.

Major General Sir David BRUCE (1855–1931)
A British army soldier who described brucellosis in 1887 while serving in
Malta. He also identified the trypanosome causing cattle plague, and
showed that the tsetse fly was the vector in sleeping sickness in man.
Brucellosis – undulant fever.

George BUDD (1808–1882)
Professor of medicine, King's College, London.
Budd-Chiari syndrome – hepatomegaly and cirrhosis due to occlusion of the
hepatic veins.

Denis BURKITT (b. 1911)
Formerly a surgeon in Uganda, he now works at the Medical Research
Council in London. He is well-known for his work in high-fibre diets in the
prevention and treatment of colonic disease.
Burkitt's lymphoma – malignant lymphoma of sub-Saharan Africa.

Louis Roger CELESTIN (b. 1900)
Consultant surgeon at Bristol.
Celestin tube – tube inserted for dysphagia caused by inoperable
oesophageal carcinoma.

Jean-Martin CHARCOT (1825–1893)

Born and worked in Paris where he became the first ever professor of neurology. He was the first to describe many neurological diseases and he gave world-famous lectures.

Charcot's joints – neuropathic joints, classically seen in syphilis but also in syringomyelia, diabetes mellitus and leprosy.

Charcot-Marie-Tooth disease – progressive peroneal muscular atrophy.

Maladie de Charcot – motor neurone disease (amyotrophic lateral sclerosis).

Charcot's biliary fever – intermittent fever with suppurative cholangitis.

Charcot's triad – intention tremor, nystagmus, and scanning speech in multiple sclerosis with brain-stem involvement.

Charcot's laryngeal vertigo – cough syncope.

Charcot-Leyden crystals – colourless, needle-like crystals seen in bronchial asthma.

Charcot-Wilbrand syndrome – visual agnosia and inability to revisualise images once seen due to posterior cerebral artery occlusion in the dominant hemisphere.

Charcot also made the distinction between gout and rheumatoid arthritis.

John CHEYNE (1777–1836)

Scottish physician.

Cheyne-Stokes respiration (see Stokes).

Hans von CHIARI (1851–1916)

Professor of pathology at Strasbourg.

Arnold-Chiari malformation (see Arnold).

Budd-Chiari syndrome (see Budd).

Mr S. CHRISTMAS

Christmas disease – named after the patient in whom factor IX deficiency was first detected.

Frantisek CHVOSTEK (1835–1884)

A physician in Vienna. He described the bone lesions in parathyroid disease and wrote about myasthenia gravis and tetanus.

Chvostek's sign – hyperexcitability of the facial nerve on percussion in patients with hypocalcaemic tetany.

Jerome William CONN (b. 1907)

American physician.

Conn's syndrome – primary hyperaldosteronism.

Robin Royston Amos COOMBS (b. 1921)

Professor of biology at Cambridge. He is reported to have said that erythrocytes were made by God primarily as tools for the immunologist and only secondarily as carriers of haemoglobin.

Coombs' test – antiglobulin test to detect Rh antibody on the surface of red cells.

Sir Dominic John CORRIGAN (1802–1880)

One of Dublin's most popular physicians who also became physician to Queen Victoria.

Corrigan's pulse – collapsing carotid pulse in aortic incompetence.

Hans Gerhard CREUTZFELD (1885–1964)
A psychiatrist in Munich.
Jakob-Creutzfeld syndrome (see Jakob).

Burrill Bernard CROHN (1884–1983)
Chief of gastroenterology at Mount Sinai Hospital, New York.
Crohn's disease – regional ileitis. Morgagni had also described this condition as far back as the middle of the 18th century.

Harvey Williams CUSHING (1869–1939)
Founding father of neurosurgery and worked at Harvard and Yale. He travelled widely throughout Europe with his great friend William Osler. He also produced one of the original anaesthetic records. He was a meticulous writer and won the Pulitzer Prize for his biography of Osler. He described the pituitary gland as the 'conductor of the endocrine orchestra'.
Cushing's syndrome – hyperadrenocorticism in the adult.

Henri Alexander DANLOS (1844–1932)
A dermatologist in Paris.
Ehlers-Danlos syndrome (see Ehlers).

Glenn A. DRAGER (1917–1967)
Neurologist in Maryland, USA.
Shy-Drager syndrome (see Shy).

William DRESSLER (1890–1969)
New York cardiologist.
Dressler's syndrome – post-infarction pericarditis.

Guillaume DUPUYTREN (1777–1835)
French surgeon. He had the misfortune to be kidnapped twice as a child. He was described as rude, ambitious and arrogant. He was born poor and died a millionaire – famous but very unpopular. He is said to have seen 10 000 private patients annually in addition to his hospital work.
Dupuytren's contracture – palmar fibrosis with contracture.

Wilhelm EBSTEIN (1836–1912)
Professor of medicine in Gottingen.
Pel-Ebstein fever (see Pel).
Ebstein's anomaly – the deformity is characterised by a downward displacement of the tricuspid valve into the right ventricle due to the anomalous attachment of the tricuspid leaflets. The right ventricle is under-developed and has reduced pumping capacity.

Edvard EHLERS (1863–1937)
A Berlin dermatologist.
Ehlers-Danlos syndrome (cutis laxa) – congenital collagen disorder giving hyperelasticity of the skin and connective tissue.

Victor EISENMENGER (1864–1932)
German physician.
Eisenmenger complex – VSD with pulmonary vascular disease and a right-to-left shunt.
Eisenmenger syndrome – any communication between the systemic and pulmonary circulations that produces pulmonary hypertension and reversal of the left-to-right shunt.

Edwin Horner ELLISON (1918–1970)
Professor of surgery in Ohio, USA.
Zollinger-Ellison syndrome (see Zollinger).

W. EWART (1848–1929)
English physician.
Ewart's sign–dullness to percussion, increased fremitus and bronchial breathing below the angle of the left scapula in a pericardial effusion.

Andre FEIL (b. 1864)
French neurologist.
Klippel-Feil syndrome (see Klippel).

Augustus FELTY (1895–1963)
American physician.
Felty's syndrome – splenomegaly, lymphadenopathy and leucopaenia associated with rheumatoid arthritis.

Austin FLINT (1812–1886)
One of the leading American physicians of his time. He founded Buffalo Medical College and wrote one of the standard medical texts of the 19th century.
Austin Flint murmur – the apical mid-diastolic rumbling murmur in pure aortic incompetence. He attributed the murmur to functional mitral stenosis due to impingement of the anterior leaflet caused by the regurgitant stream. Modern echo- and phono-cardiography support this view.

Nikolaus FRIEDREICH (1825–1882)
Both a neurologist and a professor of pathological anatomy in Heidelberg.
Friedreich's ataxia – progressive spino-cerebellar ataxia.

Nicolas GILBERT (1858–1927)
A Parisian physician.
Gilbert's disease – benign familial non–haemolytic hyperbilirubinaemia.

Ernest GOODPASTURE (1886–1960)
A pathologist at the Johns Hopkins Hospital in America. He described his syndrome at the time of the big 'flu epidemic in 1919.
Goodpasture's syndrome – glomerulonephritis associated with intra-pulmonary haemorrhage.

W. R. GOWERS (1845–1915)
Educated at Christchurch School, Oxford and took his MB in London in 1869. He became a fellow of the RCP and the RCS. At University College Hospital, London he was a student of Sir William Jenner. He was an inspiring teacher, an excellent neurologist and an ardent naturalist.
Gowers' myopathy – distal muscular dystrophy.
Gowers' phenomenon – passive dorsiflexion of the foot produces pain along the sciatic nerve when the nerve is compressed.
Gowers' sign (1) – irregular contraction of the pupil in early tabes dorsalis.
Gowers' sign (2) – inability of a patient with a proximal myopathy to stand from a sitting position with the arms outstretched.

Robert GRAVES (1796–1853)
A physician in Dublin, he described primary thyrotoxicosis in 1835. He also described angioneurotic oedema, scleroderma, erythromelalgia and the pinpoint pupils of pontine haemorrhage. Spoke German fluently. He introduced clinical, ward-based teaching for undergraduate medical students.
Graves' disease – primary thyrotoxicosis characterised by diffuse enlargement of the thyroid gland and by the presence of TSH-receptor antibodies in the blood.

George GUILLAIN (1876–1961)
French neurologist who worked at one time in the Sixth Army with Jean Barré.
Guillain-Barré syndrome – acute infective polyneuritis.

Hakaru HASHIMOTO (1881–1934)
A Japanese surgeon. His thyroiditis was confirmed as an autoimmune condition 20 years after his death. Since his account on 'struma lymphomatosa' was published in a German surgical journal, his compatriots were unaware of his discovery. He died of typhoid.
Hashimoto's thyroiditis – autoimmune thyroiditis.

William HEBERDEN (1710–1801)
A London doctor who became physician to George III. He was the first to describe the differences between smallpox and chickenpox, angina pectoris and the features of night blindness.
Heberden's nodes – swellings at the terminal IP joints in osteoarthritis.

Eduard HENOCH (1820–1910)
Professor of paediatrics in Berlin.
Henoch-Schönlein purpura – a syndrome affecting children and characterised by the acute development of joint, gastrointestinal and renal abnormalities together with a nonthrombocytopenic purpura.

Thomas HODGKIN (1798–1866)

Born in Tottenham, trained in Edinburgh. He was one of the first doctors in Britain to use a stethoscope, which he brought back from Paris where he had studied with Laennec. He described the first few cases of Hodgkin's disease. Later in life he became a missionary. Whilst visiting Palestine he died of typhoid and is buried there. He annoyed a very wealthy patient of his by filling in £10 on a blank cheque; the patient never consulted him again. He also wrote an original account of aortic regurgitation in 1829.

Hodgkin's disease – malignant lymphoma with distinct histological features.

Johann HOFFMANN (1857–1919)

A neurologist in Heidelberg.

Hoffmann's reflex – a positive reflex indicates a pyramidal tract lesion. It is elicited by snapping the terminal phalanx of the middle finger which results in sudden flexion of the terminal phalanx of the thumb.

Hoffmann's syndrome – muscular hypertrophy with weakness and delayed relaxation in adult hypothyroidism.

Sir Gordon HOLMES (1874–1965)

An Irishman who became a consultant with the British Expeditionary Force and who had an interest in both neurology and endocrinology.

Holmes-Adie syndrome – myotonic pupils with absent tendon reflexes. The affected pupil is smaller than the other, often does not react to light, and reacts slowly but completely to accommodation.

Johann HORNER (1831–1886)

A professor of ophthalmology in Switzerland who established that red–green colour blindness was a sex-linked disorder.

Horner's syndrome – ptosis, miosis, anhydrosis and enophthalmos associated with damage to the cervical sympathetic nerve.

James Ramsay HUNT (1872–1937)

New York neurologist.

Ramsay Hunt syndrome – herpes zoster of the ganglion of the facial nerve with vesicles and pain in the ear. It is associated with a lower motor neurone facial palsy and loss of taste on the anterior two-thirds of the affected side of the tongue.

George HUNTINGTON (1850–1916)

Born, and spent his working life, in New York State. He wrote only one paper, at the early age of 22, describing families with the condition which now bears his name.

Huntington's chorea – autosomal dominant condition of chorea and progressive dementia starting in middle age.

Hughlings JACKSON (1835–1911)

A Yorkshireman who became the father of English neurology. He worked at Queen's Square and wrote many papers on focal fits. He enunciated a number of fundamental principles concerning the brain functions, and was one of the founder editors of 'Brain' in 1878. He was an eccentric lover of thrillers; he would buy a book, rip it into two halves, put one half in his pocket and throw the other half away! He was a contemporary of Bell and Brown-Séquard.

Jacksonian epilepsy – focal fits starting in one muscle group.

Alfons-Maria JAKOB (1884–1931)

German neurologist who served in the first world war and was a visiting professor in South America. He also described the neuropathological features of yellow fever.

Jakob-Creutzfeld syndrome – cerebral atrophy starting in mid-life and thought to be due to a slow virus. It is known to have been transmitted to children in growth hormone made from pituitary extracts.

Harold JEGHERS (b. 1904)

Professor of medicine, Boston.

Peutz-Jeghers' syndrome (see Peutz).

John KANTOR (1890–1947)

A New York gastroenterologist.

Kantor's string sign – constriction of the terminal ileum seen on barium studies in Crohn's disease (narrowing of the lumen is shown by a thin line of barium).

Moricz KAPOSI (1837–1902)

Born in Hungary, he was professor of dermatology in Vienna.

Kaposi's sarcoma – multiple skin neoplasms which occurred with greater frequency in Italian Jews and are now associated with AIDS.

Foster KENNEDY (1884–1952)

Born in Belfast, he qualified in 1906 from the Royal University of Ireland. He worked in the National Hospital, Queen's Square and was much influenced by Sir William Gowers. He was a kind man but was known for his cutting remarks and aphorisms.

Foster Kennedy syndrome – unilateral optic atrophy with contralateral papilloedema and anosmia usually due to a frontal lobe tumour.

Paul KIMMELSTIEL (1900–1970)

German-born pathologist who worked mainly at Harvard.

Kimmelstiel-Wilson disease of the kidney – diabetic glomerulosclerosis.

Theodor KLEBS (1834–1913)

Worked as a bacteriologist in many parts of Europe and then in America. He discovered both *Klebsiella* and the *diphtheria* bacilli. It is said that he was at the forefront of every advance in bacteriology but that he had the misfortune to miss out on every great discovery.

Klebsiella – a gram-negative bacteria.

Klebsiella pneumonia – also known as Friedlander's pneumonia.

Harry KLINEFELTER (b. 1912)

A physician in Baltimore.

Klinefelter's syndrome – hypogonadism with XXY chromosomes and associated with aberrant behaviour.

Maurice KLIPPEL (1858–1942)

French neurologist.

Klippel-Feil syndrome – congenital fusion of the cervical vertebrae.

Nicolai KOROTKOFF (1874–1920)

A Russian physician and naval surgeon.

Korotkoff sounds – heard when recording blood pressure.

Adolf KUSSMAUL (1822–1909)
A German physician who described hemiballismus and word-blindness. He wrote a book on aphasia and introduced pleural tapping and gastric lavage.
Kussmaul breathing – 'air hunger' in diabetic ketoacidosis.

Norten A. KVEIM (b. 1892)
Norwegian-born pathologist in Copenhagen.
Kveim test – intradermal test for sarcoidosis.

Rène LAENNEC (1781–1826)
Born in Brittany, France, he became professor of medicine at the College de France. In 1819 he invented the stethoscope. He died at the early age of 42 from tuberculosis.
Laennec's cirrhosis – fatty degeneration of the liver seen in malnutrition and alcoholism.

J. Z. LAURENCE (1830–1874)
A London ophthalmologist.
Laurence-Moon-Biedl syndrome – autosomal recessive condition of obesity, polydactyly, mental retardation and retinitis pigmentosa.

Ernst von LEYDEN (1832–1910)
German neurologist.
Charcot-Leyden crystals (see Charcot).

Emil LOOSER (1877–1936)
Swiss surgeon.
Looser's lines – lucent lines on the X-rays of long bones and pelvis in osteomalacia.

Bernard MARFAN (1858–1942)
He was the pioneer of clinical paediatrics in France and, whilst professor in Paris, he described the condition from which Abraham Lincoln is thought to have suffered. His doctoral thesis was on tuberculosis and he developed the so-called Marfan Law which stated that pulmonary tuberculosis was rare following the healed, local lesion because of immunity.
Marfan's syndrome – tall stature, arachnodactyly, high-arched palate, lenticular dislocation, hyperextensibility and cardiovascular involvement.

Joseph MEIGS (1892–1963)
Professor of gynaecology at Harvard.
Meigs' syndrome – ovarian fibroma with pleural effusions.

Prosper MÉNIÈRE (1799–1862)
He had hoped to become the professor of medicine and hygiene but instead was chief physician to the Imperial Institute for Deaf-Mutes. He was an expert on orchids and was the casualty officer on duty on the day in 1830 when 2000 casualties from the Paris riots were admitted to the local hospitals.
Ménière's disease – progressive deafness with episodic vertigo, tinnitus and vomiting.

Louis MILKMAN (1895–1951)
An American radiologist.
Milkman fractures – multiple stress fractures in osteomalacia.

Richard MOON (b. 1926)
An American pathophysiologist.
Laurence-Moon-Biedl syndrome (see Laurence).

Campbell de MORGAN (1811–1876)
English surgeon at the Middlesex Hospital, London.
Campbell de Morgan spots – cherry-red spots in the skin, especially in the elderly. He originally thought they were a marker of cancer.

Albert NIEMANN (1880–1921)
German paediatrician.
Niemann-Pick disease – autosomal recessive lipid storage disorder, commonest in Jewish children.

Sir William OSLER (1849–1919)
Born in Canada, he became professor of medicine at McGill at the early age of 25. He became professor at Oxford and was the first to see platelets. He is best known for his textbook '*The principles and practice of medicine*'.
Osler's nodes – cutaneous nodules in bacterial endocarditis.
Osler-Rendu-Weber syndrome – hereditary haemorrhagic telangiectasia.
Osler-Vaquez disease – polycythaemia rubra vera.
Some of the observations were undoubtedly made by his colleagues, but Osler is reputed to have said that 'in science the credit does not go to the one who makes the discovery but to the one who convinces the world'. He was an excellent teacher and his own epitaph was 'He taught medicine in the wards'.

Sir James PAGET (1814–1899)
Born in Yarmouth, one of 17 children. He was surgeon to Queen Victoria as well as being surgeon at Bart's. He became President of the Royal College of Surgeons and had the largest private practice in London.
Paget's disease of bone – osteitis deformans.
Paget's disease of the nipple – a slow-growing duct carcinoma.
Paget's disease of the penis – carcinoma following longstanding balanitis.

Henry PANCOAST (1875–1939)
An American professor of radiology.
Pancoast tumour – apical carcinoma of the bronchus associated with a T1 sympathetic lesion.

James PARKINSON (1755–1824)
Born in the East End of London, he became a general practitioner. He had an interest in palaeontology and was the founder of the Geological Society In London. He was also known as 'Old Hubert' when campaigning with politicians – another of his interests. He wrote his classic essay on paralysis agitans ('the shaking palsy') in 1817. It was 40 years later that Charcot actually named the condition after him. He also described the first case of appendicitis in 1812.
Parkinson's disease – a condition affecting the basal ganglia; it classically produces the triad of tremor, rigidity and bradykinesia.

Sir John PARKINSON (1885–1976)
London cardiologist.
Wolff-Parkinson-White syndrome (see Wolff).

John PEUTZ (1886–1957)
Physician in The Hague, Holland.
Peutz-Jeghers' syndrome – familial, autosomal dominant, intestinal polyposis with circumoral pigmentation.

Friedel PICK (1867–1926)
A laryngologist in Prague.
Pick's disease – chronic constrictive pericarditis.

Ludvig PICK (1868–1935)
A German physician who described the arrhenoblastoma.
Niemann-Pick disease (see Niemann).

PICKWICK
Pickwickian syndrome – obesity, day-time somnolence, alveolar hypoventilation with hypoxia and hypercapnoea. The term is derived from the character in Charles Dickens' 'Pickwick Papers' and was first applied by Osler.

J E von PURKINJE (1787–1869)
A famous Czech doctor who became a popular hero in his country. He had many other interests, working, for example, on the development of the animated cartoon, as co-editor of a Czech paper and as translator of Shakespeare into his native language. His studies on vision were influenced by Goethe (Farben-Lehre), who wrote regarding his series on vision 'and should you fail to understand, let Purkyne (the correct Czech spelling) give you a hand'.
Purkinje fibres – subendocardial muscle fibres.
Purkinje cells – cerebellar cortical cells with lots of dendrites.
He discovered sweat glands in the skin, the uniqueness of fingerprints, and wrote papers on colour vision.

Q (for query)
Q-fever – a systemic rickettsial infection caused by *Coxiella burnetti* and characterised by headache, malaise and interstitial pneumonitis. In the chronic form there may be hepatitis and endocarditis.

Maurice RAYNAUD (1834–1881)
Paris physician.
Raynaud's disease – abnormal sensitivity of the upper limbs to cold resulting in vasospasm.
Raynaud's phenomenon – vasospasm in the peripheral parts of the limbs due to an organic disorder of the main artery, or secondary to vibration or a connective tissue disorder.

Friedrich von RECKLINGHAUSEN (1833–1910)

Assistant to Virchow for six years and a professor of pathology in Germany. He described haemochromatosis and opposed Koch's concept that the tubercle bacillus was the cause of tuberculosis. He is best remembered for:

von Recklinghausen's disease – neurofibromatosis.

von Recklinghausen's disease of bone – osteitis fibrosa cystica (associated with parathyroid adenoma).

Hans REITER (1881–1969)

Born in Leipzig he became an enthusiastic Nazi. He was professor of hygiene and discovered the causative organism of Weil's disease.

Reiter's Disease – urethritis, arthritis, conjunctivitis (nongonococcal). This condition was first reported by Sir Benjamin Brodie (1783–1862), a London surgeon, in a textbook (*Joint diseases*) in 1818. Reiter's contribution was a case history of a single patient with bloody diarrhoea, conjunctivitis and arthritis (1916).

Henry RENDU (1844–1902)

Paris physician.

Osler-Rendu-Weber syndrome (see Osler).

Ralph D. K. REYE (1912–1977)

Australian histopathologist.

Reye's syndrome – encephalohepatitis secondary to aspirin ingestion during a viral infection and usually seen in children and young adults.

Argyll ROBERTSON (1837–1909)

Ophthalmologist in Edinburgh and also became surgeon-oculist to Queen Victoria. He described an operation for ectropion.

Argyll Robertson pupil – tabetic (small and irregular) pupil that reacts to accommodation more than to light.

Moritz von ROMBERG (1795–1873)

A German neurologist who was the uncle of Eduard Henoch. He looked after the Berlin cholera hospitals during the epidemic.

Romberg's sign – loss of balance with the eyes closed and feet together, classically in tabes dorsalis due to lack of joint position sense (posterior column).

David SALMON (1850–1914)

A veterinary pathologist in New Jersey, USA.

Salmonella – Gram-negative rods, including the organisms that cause typhoid and paratyphoid.

Robert SCHILLING (b. 1919)

American professor of medicine.

Schilling test – used for testing vitamin B_{12} absorption.

Johann SCHÖNLEIN (1793–1864)

Physician in Berlin.

Henoch-Schönlein purpura (see Henoch).

Robert SENGSTAKEN (b. 1923)
Surgeon in New Jersey, USA.
Sengstaken tube – tube with inflatable balloons used to stop the bleeding from oesophageal varices. The tube was actually developed under the direction of A. H. Blakemore (1897–1970), a US surgeon, in 1954, and is sometimes referred to as the Sengstaken-Blakemore tube.

Harold Leeming SHEEHAN (b. 1900)
A Manchester graduate who became professor of pathology at Liverpool.
Sheehan's syndrome – postpartum pituitary necrosis.

G. Milton SHY (1919–1967)
Neurologist in Maryland, USA.
Shy-Drager syndrome – primary autonomic failure with features of Parkinson's disease and postural hypotension.

Morris SIMMONDS (1855-1925)
A general practitioner in Hamburg who became an honorary professor of pathology.
Simmond's disease – panhypopituitarism.

Henrik Samuel Conrad SJÖGREN (b. 1899)
Professor of ophthalmology in Sweden. In 1935 he developed the technique for corneal transplantation.
Sjøgren's syndrome – rheumatoid arthritis with keratoconjunctivitis sicca and a dry mouth (xerostomia).

H. SNELLEN (1834–1908)
Dutch ophthalmologist.
Snellen's chart – used for measuring visual acuity.

Reginald SOUTHEY (1835–1899)
Born in Harley Street and educated at Oxford, he became a physician at St. Bartholomew's. Apart from being a diligent clinician he had a keen interest in clocks, which he collected and repaired.
Southey's tubes – fine tubes used in the past for draining subcutaneous fluid from the lower limbs in cardiac failure.

Ernest STARLING (1866–1927)
He was born in Bombay (India) and studied medicine at Guy's Hospital, London. He was professor of physiology at University College, London. Among his multiple contributions are the demonstration that serum proteins exert osmotic pressure, the discovery of secretin and his heart–lung preparation.
Starling's law – within certain limits, the force of cardiac contraction is a function of fibre length.
Starling's curve – the cardiac output is plotted against the venous filling pressure (right atrial pressure minus the negative intrathoracic pressure); the ascent represents a compensated state (increased stroke output due to an increased filling pressure causing ventricular dilatation at the end of diastole), and the descent represents a decompensated state (a critical point in ventricular dilatation beyond which further dilatation results in a fall of output).

Graham STEELL (1851–1942)
Manchester physician.
Graham Steell murmur – diastolic murmur in pulmonary regurgitation.

Sir George STILL (1868–1941)
Having studied at Guy's, he went on to work at Great Ormond Street and King's College and became the greatest paediatrician of his day. He was physician to the Royal Household and also to Dr Bernardo's Homes.
Still's disease – juvenile polyarthritis associated with splenomegaly and lymphadenopathy.

William STOKES (1804–1878)
A physician in Dublin and one of the leaders of the Dublin school of medicine.
Stokes-Adams attacks – syncope in complete heart block.
Cheyne-Stokes respiration – cyclical periods of apnoea followed by hyper-pnoea and seen in cerebrovascular disease, respiratory and cardiac failure.

William Allen STURGE (1850–1919)
London physician.
Sturge-Weber syndrome – port-wine stain on the face associated with angiomatous malformations intracranially as well as in other parts of the body.

Mikito TAKAYASU (1860–1938)
Japanese surgeon who later became a professor of ophthalmology.
Takayasu's 'pulseless' disease – obliterative arteritis affecting the aortic arch, carotid and subclavian arteries of young women.

Jules TINEL (1879–1952)
A Paris neurologist. He wrote a text on the autonomic nervous system and described the paroxysmal hypertension in phaeochromocytoma. He was also a resistance fighter in the second world war.
Tinel test – distal tingling on percussion of the median nerve at the wrist in cases of compression of the nerve (e.g. carpal tunnel syndrome).

Howard Henry TOOTH (1856–1926)
London physician and neurologist.
Charcot-Marie-Tooth disease (see Charcot).

Armand TROUSSEAU (1801–1867)
French physician. He gave one of the early descriptions of haemochromatosis, adopted the term 'aphasia' and introduced thoracocentesis in 1843. He was an outstanding clinician and one of the greatest French teachers.
Trousseau's sign (1) – thrombophlebitis migrans associated with visceral carcinoma, especially gastric and pancreatic. He noted this sign on himself.
Trousseau's sign (2) – carpopedal spasm (main d'accoucheur) induced using a tourniquet in hypocalcaemic tetany.

Henry TURNER (1892–1970)
Physician in Oklahoma, USA.
Turner's syndrome – XO chromosome pattern, short stature, webbed neck, cubitus valgus and gonadal agenesis.

Antonio VALSALVA (1666–1723)
Italian anatomist.
Valsalva antrum – mastoid antrum.
Valsalva manoeuvre – forced expiration against a closed glottis which raises the intrathoracic pressure.
Valsalva sinus – aortic sinus.
Valsalva test – during the Valsalva manoeuvre, air passes into the tympanic cavity if the auditory tubes are patent.

Jan WALDENSTRÖM (b. 1906)
Swedish physician.
Waldenström's hepatitis – chronic active hepatitis.
Waldenström's macroglobulinaemia – a dysproteinaemia with a monoclonal increase of IgM. The patients often present with bleeding disorders, visual disturbances and hepatosplenomegaly.
Waldenström's hyperglobulinaemia – a polyclonal increase in gamma globulin which characteristically occurs in women and runs a benign, protracted course.

Frederick WEBER (1863–1962)
London physician.
Osler-Rendu-Weber syndrome (see Osler).
Sturge-Weber syndrome (see Sturge).

F. WEGENER (b. 1907)
German pathologist.
Wegener's granulomatosis – acute midline necrotising granulomas associated with periarteritis nodosa.

H. Adolph WEIL (1848–1916)
German physician.
Weil's disease – leptospirosis caused by *L. icterohaemorrhagiae*. It is characterised by jaundice, fever, oliguria, haematuria, epistaxis, headaches and muscular pains.

William WELCH (1850–1934)
A pathologist at Johns Hopkins, USA and later professor of the history of medicine. He travelled widely collecting old medical textbooks.
Clostridium welchii – causes gas gangrene.

Marel WENCKEBACH (1864–1940)
Dutch-born physician who practised mainly in Vienna.
Wenckebach phenomenon – progressive increase in the PR interval on the ECG in second degree heart block.

Karl WERNICKE (1843–1904)
Professor of neurology and psychiatry in Breslau. At the age of 26 he published a book on aphasia in which he described sensory aphasia as well as agraphia. Although aware that a toxic factor may be involved in the aetiology of Wernicke's encephalopathy, he did not realise that this was nutritional.
Wernicke's encephalopathy – deterioration of mental function with confusion, ophthalmoplegia, nystagmus, ataxia and peripheral neuropathy in thiamine deficiency, especially in chronic alcoholics.

Paul WHITE (1886–1973)
Boston cardiologist.
Wolff-Parkinson-White syndrome (see Wolff).

Louis-Frederic WICKHAM (1861–1913)
Paris dermatologist.
Wickham's striae – network of lines over the papules of lichen planus.

H. WILBRAND (1851–1935)
German neuro-ophthalmologist.
Charcot-Wilbrand syndrome (see Charcot).

E. A. von WILLEBRAND (1870–1949)
Finnish physician.
von Willebrand's disease – factor VIII deficiency, prolonged bleeding time and autosomal dominant inheritance.

Robert Miltan ZOLLINGER (b. 1903)
American surgeon.
Zollinger–Ellison syndrome – gastric-secreting adenoma of the G cells of the pancreas associated with peptic ulceration. These peptic ulcers occur in unusual places in the stomach, duodenum and sometimes jejunum.

Appendix III
Questions from the surveys

It is often said that the examiners have a vast field of medicine to draw from and that they can, and do, ask anything. However, our surveys during the last four years have shown that this is a misconception: the examiners mostly ask about common and important clinical problems and we have endeavoured to show this in Sections 2–4. The range of the topics covered, however, is still wide. The phraseology also tends to vary from time to time and from examiner to examiner, depending on the particular aspect of the topic the examiner wishes to probe into. We felt that the candidates would find it interesting to have a glimpse of this wide range of questions but we could not accommodate *all* the questions asked in this Appendix. In order to cover most of the topics, and to include the maximum number of questions, we have had to make three alterations. First, we have excluded repetitious questions but have indicated the frequency of the topic either in bold (occurred in one or two surveys frequently), or in italic bold (when the topic occurred in most surveys at various centres). Second, we have summarised each question by removing extra sentences and words, but have preserved the objective of the examiner. Third, the Appendix is in smaller print in order to accommodate as many questions as possible.

For easy reference we have listed the questions under their relevant systems. Although the main stems of the questions have been condensed, it is still possible, in most cases, to fit them into our classification (see Section 2). The focus of the discussion, which is not necessarily the correct answer, has in certain cases been put in brackets after the question. Many of the questions have already been dealt with in detail in Sections 2–4; here, as the questions may be out of context with the discussion between the examiner and the candidate, we have limited our comments to an occasional footnote. We hope that this Appendix will provide a 'loose' syllabus for you to work on, and to give you some idea of the viva encounters.

General medical topics

Discuss the *value of screening*.

We hear a lot about screening in the general public – what are your opinions on screening? If you were a GP what sort of a 'screen' would you wish to perform?

Community screening – what conditions are appropriate to screen for? What could we screen for in respiratory medicine? What general and specific population groups are suitable for screening?

A small company asks you to screen and offer health promotion for their employees. You are allowed ten minutes per patient, what would you do?

Tell me what you think about a screening service for diabetes in pregnancy.

Do you think that health screening by BUPA is a cost-effective exercise for a company?

You see a 35-year-old man with a raised gamma GT on a BUPA screen. He takes no alcohol. What do you think? (Hepatitis B)[1]

Is routine cholesterol measurement indicated in general practice?
Are there any dangers in having a low cholesterol level?

What proportion of the population die before the age of 65?
What conditions are the major causes?
If I were Secretary of State for Health, what measures might I be looking at to reduce these deaths?

Tell me about screening in the middle-aged population. How do we test the usefulness of a screening test?

What do you know about **osteoporosis**? (Recent *BMJ* article)

Discuss the recent developments in *hormone replacement therapy* in post-menopausal women. (Recent review articles in the *BMJ*, *Lancet* and in the *Journal* of the RCP)

What is the differential diagnosis of **low back pain** in a 50-year-old woman? (Osteoporosis)

What are the biochemical findings at the menopause? (This led to a discussion on osteoporosis)

A GP does a fasting lipid profile on a patient and finds raised chylomicrons, cholesterol and triglycerides. How would you manage the patient?

Discussion on *lipids*.

Cholesterol production and metabolism. What is the mechanism of action of the lipid-lowering agents and name their drug interactions?

Who should be screened for hypercholesterolaemia?

What are the causes of secondary hyperlipidaemia?
What is the genetic defect in type IIa hyperlipidaemias?

What is the relationship between lipids and hypothyroidism?

How would you divide up the different lipoprotein fractions? A 30-year-old man with raised cholesterol level. Tell me about the dietary management and the modern drugs that are now available.

What are the drawbacks of a lipid clinic on 1st January?

What drugs can raise lipid levels?

What are your views about the facility to get a cholesterol level done at a chemist's shop?

Ascertain from this man's history whether or not he is an alcoholic. (Broad question on alcohol)

What are the nonhepatic manifestations of *alcohol abuse*?

Tell me how alcohol affects the body.

---

[1] A raised level of gamma GT may be found in the presence of a variety of inducers of hepatic microsomal enzymes (e.g. barbiturates, phenylbutazone, phenytoin, chronic ethanol ingestion, etc.), and sometimes in normal healthy subjects.

What is the management of a 40-year-old unkempt man with pyrexia and signs of right upper lobe consolidation? (Lobar pneumonia, alcoholic, *Klebsiella*, Wernicke's, etc.)

How would you advise a man drinking one bottle of whisky per day?

You are invited to a Women's Institute meeting to talk about alcohol. How do you structure the talk?

What is the treatment of acute alcohol withdrawal?

You are on ITU with an adult patient who has had a major head injury. What would you do to confirm and certify **brain death**?[2]

What are the prognostic factors for a patient on the intensive care unit?

The ethics of **organ transplantation** and the role of the medical registrar in this. Immunosuppression and its complications.

Management of **septicaemic shock** on the ITU.

What different types of shock do you know of?
How do you manage septic shock?
How would you accurately assess the circulating volume?

There is a diabetic on ITU, ventilated and ketoacidotic. He starts to pass blood – what would you think of? (Rhabdomyolysis)[3]

The physiology of shock: changes in the microcirculation; causes of septic shock; what happens to the oxygen tension?; what is the best treatment?

Disseminated intravascular coagulation.

Acute respiratory distress syndrome and theories of its causation.

What do you think about **epidemic myalgic encephalitis**. Is it a real entity?[4]

Do you believe in the 'Royal Free disease'?[4]

A young woman with two children comes to you complaining of lethargy, lassitude, sleepiness and just not feeling well. What do you think?[4]

What is the best way of investigating tiredness?[4]

Tell me about the paraneoplastic syndromes.
Have you ever seen a cerebellar syndrome?

What is the use of **tumour markers**?[5]

Tell me about oncogenes.[6]

What do you tell a woman in her forties who has disseminated cancer about her disease in various different situations, i.e. if she is single, married, with a son of 15 years, etc.?

A medical student has a node in her neck. Investigations show that it's an anaplastic carcinoma. How do you tell her?[7]

---

[2]   p. 241
[3]   p. 210
[4]   pp. 18, 24, 87
[5]   p. 197
[6]   p. 197
[7]   p. 136

What is the differential diagnosis of a young man with cervical lymphadenopathy, night sweats and weight loss? How would you investigate the cause?

Pathological fractures. (Led to a discussion on **multiple myeloma** and its treatment)

A 63-year-old man with low back pain and a raised ESR. (Myeloma)

Treatment of hypercalcaemia.

How would you investigate a milkman who starts putting bets on horses after the races have been run? (Hypercalcaemia)

How would you manage someone with **malignant hypercalcaemia**?

Management of disseminated breast cancer.

What advice would you give to an asthmatic about driving?

Tell me about patients and driving.

How would you test for porphyria?

What is the differential diagnosis of a red eye?

Causes of bilateral red eyes. (The examiner just wanted a list of the causes)

What problems can be encountered in anaesthetising patients?

What are the causes and management of postoperative confusion?

How would you recognise a **DVT**?
What are the complications? (Pulmonary embolism)
What would be the indications for thoracotomy and embolectomy?

Investigation of a patient with multiple DVTs.

What are you interested in? (Discussion was on ulcer treatment and the role of prostaglandins in medicine and, in particular, in renal disease)

You are the registrar and you see a 14-year-old boy who is blind in both eyes with general malaise of 72 hours duration – what is the differential diagnosis? (The candidate had no idea what the examiner was getting at)

What are the causes of visual failure in a middle-aged man?[8]

Tell me about the management of sudden unilateral loss of vision in a middle-aged woman.

What are the features and causes of Lyme disease?[9]
What sort of arthritis occurs?
What's the commonest neurological complication?

Let's talk about the complement cascade.

What is Kussmaul's respiration?

---

[8] Visual failure needs to be specified, e.g. a visual acuity of 6/60 or less in the better eye or a visual field reduced to a small area around the fixation point. Myopia, neurological disorders, cataract, glaucoma, diabetes mellitus and trauma are the principal causes in the age group between 40–60 years.

[9] p. 25

You see a woman aged 52 years with weight loss, mild anaemia and a raised ESR – what would you think of? (Polymyalgia rheumatica)[10]
If the alkaline phosphatase is also raised what do you think of? (Discussed the possibility of polyarteritis)
Does polymyalgia rheumatica affect the liver? (Yes!)

Weight loss in a person with a good appetite. (Thyrotoxicosis, diabetes mellitus, malabsorption)

Weight loss in a young girl. (Anorexia nervosa)

What are the causes of gynaecomastia?

What do you know about 'multi-resistant *Staph. aureus*'?

Paget's disease – how common?, symptoms, etc.

Homocystinuria – specific features and treatment.

You see a lady with atrial fibrillation and a swollen tummy. (Mesenteric ischaemia)

I saw a young biochemistry student in the OPD last week. He was doing a practical and noted that his plasma was yellow. What thoughts do you have? (Gilbert's syndrome)

You see a young West Indian male in his twenties with severe pleuritic chest pain and cyanosis. The next day he is jaundiced. What is the diagnosis? (Sickle-cell disease)

Clinical scenario – a woman with sickle-cell anaemia and meningitis.

Tell me about *meningococcal outbreaks*. What are the complications of meningococcal septicaemia? (Examiner wanted to include meningopericarditis)

What is the care needed for the terminally ill patient?

Lactic acidosis. (This led to a discussion about the differences in the mode of action of metformin and the sulphonylureas)

Investigations of a 30-year-old woman with loin pain. (Urolithiasis – hypercalcaemia, sarcoid, use of steroids)

Tell me about the use of activated charcoal.

Give some causes of why a woman cellist was having to climb up her cello. (Proximal myopathy)

What do you know about *Streptococcus bovis* septicaemia?

How do you manage a 30-year-old woman with **nocturia**?

Tell me about nocturnal incontinence.

Tell me about mountain sickness.

What is the management of a 10-year-old boy who has been rescued from the swimming pool in an unconscious state?

Tell me about the Riley-Day syndrome.

---

[10] The subsequent questions suggest that the examiner was expecting the candidate to say 'giant cell arteritis' in which alkaline phosphatase and other liver function tests may be moderately abnormal. The liver is less often affected in straightforward polymyalgia rheumatica.

A GP rings you on a Friday evening. He saw a lady on Tuesday who had difficulty in swallowing. She's worse now. She's a previously fit, 58-year-old spinster who lives in a country cottage and is fond of her roses. (Tetanus)

A patient becomes unwell soon after catheterisation. He then develops a petechial rash. What would you do?

What is the differential diagnosis of a petechial rash in a young girl? (Idiopathic thrombocytopaenic purpura)

Which malignancies that present on a CXR are of value diagnosing?

What is the differential diagnosis of delirium and fever in a previously fit, young construction worker? (Heat stroke, meningitis, encephalitis)

You are called to a patient's house. His wife has been unable to wake him. What do you think of? (Carbon monoxide poisoning)[11]

What is the short- and long-term management of a patient with postthyroidectomy tetany?

What is Ortner's syndrome?

Tell me about the haemolytic-uraemic syndrome.

Name a dominantly inherited condition, then a recessive one and then any sex-linked dominant conditions. (Vitamin D resistant Rickets)

Causes of periostitis.

Tell me about stimulating antibodies in autoimmune disease. (Graves' disease)

Tell me about curative and palliative chemotherapy.

What is the differential diagnosis of a young woman with a lumpy purplish rash on her legs? (Differential diagnosis of erythema nodosum)

What are the genetics of polycystic disease (infantile and adult) and cystic fibrosis? What's the importance of the gene loci?

A 70-year-old retired, diabetic, paediatric surgeon goes fishing and comes to see you two weeks later with a painful shoulder. What do you think of? (Septic arthritis)[12]

What are the complications of intravenous drug abuse?

What do you understand by immune complexes?

There has been a lot written recently on bovine spongiform encephalopathy. What do you know about it?

A 35-year-old woman who had lived in a remote Highland cottage for several years becomes unwell and tired with a Hb level of 8g/dl. Several other inhabitants in this area had also been unwell of late. (Lead poisoning from the ancient water supply!)

What diseases might be found in immigrants? (TB, haemoglobinopathies, vitamin D deficiency)

What is your approach to an Asian man with a PUO?

---

[11] An overdose of sleeping tablets would be a more likely possibility.
[12] The story would logically have suited a diagnosis of a tenosynovitis of the shoulder joint or, more commonly, of the extensor tendons of the wrist joint. However, the two-week incubation period should direct the suspicion to a septic arthritis.

What are the medical problems of West Indians? (Including bush tea and veno-occlusive disease)

Tell me about the bends.[13]

Tell me about the NHS review.

Emergency medicine

How would you deal with a cardiac arrest?[1]

Doctors have been accused of not knowing enough about cardiopulmonary resuscitation – can you prove that wrong?

Here are the ECG findings from a 40-year-old man presenting in casualty with chest pain and dyspnoea. How would you manage this patient? (Myocardial infarction)

The examiner produced an ECG which had anterior ST elevation but with no q waves. It was of a 45-year-old man with a 3½ hour history of chest pain who presented in casualty. What would you do? (Discussion about thrombolysis and the recent trials) What would you look for when examining a man with an acute myocardial infarction?

What would you do with a 42-year-old in casualty with a **definite anterior myocardial infarction**? (Streptokinase)

How would you differentiate, in an emergency situation, between acute left ventricular failure and acute respiratory failure?[2]

What is the management and investigation of a patient seen in casualty who is acutely short of breath with a pleural effusion?

A patient aged 40 comes into casualty with severe breathlessness of two hours' duration. What would you do? What do you think the cause was?[3] (Toxic fumes)

Which clinical situations would you regard as absolute emergencies requiring immediate action? (Cardiorespiratory emergencies, Addisonian crisis)

You are called to casualty where a hysterical mother has brought a child of 10 years who is very breathless. What would you do? (Acute asthma)

What is the management of an *acute asthmatic attack*?

What is the clinical assessment of acute, severe asthma in the casualty department?

How would you deal with a 22-year-old man presenting in casualty with a **sudden onset of left-sided chest pain?** (Spontaneous pneumothorax)

A 14-year-old boy with acute onset SOB and cyanosis arrives at casualty with a distraught mum. What is your management? (Tension pneumothorax)

You see a healthy young man with acute SOB. What goes through your mind? Suppose he has a history of asthma–what are the indices of severity, what is the treatment and how does each drug work?

---

[13] p. 127
[1] p. 35
[2] p. 38
[3] p. 76

How would you manage an acutely breathless middle-aged man who has no past history of any respiratory problems?

You are asked to see a young lady who is hyperventilating. What do you do? (Lactic acidosis)[4]

A 55-year-old man is admitted with **severe back pain of sudden onset**. What would you do? (Dissecting aneurysm)

Discuss the management of a 53-year-old man who is known to have hypertension and who presents acutely with hypotension and back pain. (Aortic dissection)

What would you do for a 60-year-old man with a lobar pneumonia in casualty? (This led to a discussion of the merits of different combinations of antibiotics)

Management of a young woman in casualty with a tachycardia and breathlessness.

You see a patient in casualty with a murmur that has changed. (SBE and its causes)

You are called to casualty to see a middle-aged man in atrial flutter and cardiogenic shock.

A woman who is over 70 years presents in casualty. She is confused and 'off her legs'. What are your first thoughts and impressions?

What is your management of an *unconscious* patient in casualty?[5]

Consider the problem of a 60-year-old woman who is a respectable, retired lawyer but known to be fond of drink. She is found unconscious at home – how would you manage her?

What is your management of a comatose drunk?

A previously well, 46-year-old man wakes in the night and feels unwell. In the morning he is rousable but tired. At 5 p.m. he is unconscious. You see him in casualty. What do you think? (Epileptic fit, CVA, hypoglycaemia, SAH, SOL. Examiner kept saying, 'Yes, but what else?')[6]

What is your management of an unconscious 20-year-old girl in casualty? (Subarachnoid haemorrhage)

Management in casualty of an unconscious patient who may have had a fit. (Hypoglycaemia)

Management of an *aspirin overdose*.[7]

How would you manage a *paracetamol overdose*?[8]

What is the commonest self-poisoning? Tell me about it. (Paracetamol)

We discussed the management of an unconscious, hypotensive tricyclic overdose.

A girl in her twenties comes into casualty with a swollen calf/leg. What would you do?

I was given a case history of someone with a **pulmonary embolus** and asked to discuss.

---

[4]   This is somewhat of an unusual diagnosis for the given story. More commonly, a young lady may have psychogenic hyperventilation.

[5]   p. 60

[6]   Encephalitis should be a serious possibility

You rush down to casualty to see a 40-year-old man with chest pain. What's going through your mind? (Pulmonary embolus)

A man arrives in casualty in shock with chest pain. What would you do? (Streptokinase)

A young woman suddenly collapses in the supermarket. What is the differential diagnosis?

A known COAD patient is brought into casualty comatose. How would you manage?

Management of a breathless, nondiabetic girl. (Hyperventilation)

What is the likely cause of a patient under anaesthesia who goes rigid with a high temperature? (Malignant hyperpyrexia and rhabdomyolysis)

You are asked to see a patient on a surgical ward. It's a 70-year-old woman who is deaf with a high alkaline phosphatase. What do you think?

A 70-year-old man admitted to a surgical ward is found to have a low sodium. What's the management? (Addison's)

You are called to see a patient with a suddenly painful red foot the night after a cholecystectomy. What is the cause? (Gout)

How do you manage a collapsed, postoperative patient on the urology ward?

You are called to see a postoperative patient on a surgical ward whose symptoms and signs suggest shock. What is your differential diagnosis? (Sepsis, bleeding, myocardial infarct, pulmonary embolus, inadequate fluid replacement)
How would you manage and monitor the patient?

Investigation of a patient with a sodium of 115 mmol/l after an operation.

A postsurgical patient presents with a urea of 30 mmol/l and a creatinine of 400μmol/l. How do you proceed? (Acute renal failure)

You are called to see a patient on a surgical ward five days after an operation. He has a painful ankle. What do you think of? (Arterial embolus)

Management of a collapsed patient on a surgical ward. (Pulmonary embolus)

You are called to see a surgical patient who is anuric after surgery. What would you do as the medical registrar on call?

What are the postoperative complications of a partial thyroidectomy?

You are called to the surgical ward to see a lady who had a partial thyroidectomy that day and now complains of paraesthesiae. How would you manage?[9]

The orthopaedic team asks you to see a young man who has suddenly deteriorated after a motorcycle crash and a fractured femur. What would you do? (Fat embolus)

As a medical registrar in renal medicine you have been called to see a 38-year-old man who has been in a road traffic accident. He has multiple injuries and his urine output has gone off. How will you approach the problem and manage the case?

---

[7] p. 44

[8] p. 42

[9] Hypocalcaemia – hypoparathyroidism as a complication of neck surgery.

You are asked to see a patient urgently on the ENT ward who has had what sounded like an oculogyric crisis.[10]

As duty medical registrar you are called to the gynaecology ward to advise on whether a patient is fit for operation. Discuss what you would do and why.

You are the medical registrar called to see a 40-year-old man admitted 12 hours previously with severe abdominal pain and vomiting. He is now blue. What would you do?
How do you confirm a diagnosis of **pancreatitis**?
What is this syndrome called and its treatment? (adult respiratory distress syndrome)
What is the pathophysiology of ARDS?

What is the management of an acute GI haemorrhage?

A patient with ulcerative colitis presents unwell to casualty. Discuss the possible diagnoses and clinical signs.

Tell me about the management of a patient arriving in casualty with total amnesia.

A 50-year-old is admitted with a left hemiparesis. There is nothing else to find. However, you are called two hours later as he has suddenly become dyspnoeic and cyanosed. (Aspiration pneumonia)[11]

What is the management of a patient in casualty with a sodium of 110 mmol/l? I was asked what 'beer drinker's potomania' was.[12]

What is the investigation and treatment of a 35-year-old man presenting in casualty fitting?

You are in casualty and a child is brought in who had fallen into a frozen pond, been dragged out from under the ice, and who is now not breathing. He has had 15 minutes of CPR by the time of arrival. What would you do? (Epileptic fit by the lakeside)

Management of a confused, aggressive 45-year-old in casualty. (Cerebral abscess)

A 50-year-old man presents with sudden headache to casualty. What would you do? (Subarachnoid haemorrhage)

You are asked to see a patient in casualty who has collapsed and is not breathing and who has had what sounds like a myasthenic crisis.

What will you do for a man who collapsed in the toilet in the early hours of the morning? (Autonomic diabetic neuropathy)

You see a college student who is unwell and who notices blue areas on his hands. He doesn't go to lectures and the next day is found by a friend confused, drowsy with purple areas on his hands. You are the casualty officer. What are your thoughts? (Meningococcal septicaemia)

How would you manage an alcoholic with nystagmus? (Wernicke's)
What are the side effects of *parentrovite*?
Tell me about the various vitamin deficiencies in alcoholics.

---

[10] The ENT ward is a *ghost-link* for the use of prochlorperazine in a patient with Ménière's disease. This drug can cause extrapyramidal side effects even in small doses.
[11] p. 186
[12] p. 126

Outline the management of a patient who presents to the casualty department with shock and pyrexia together with purpura and a peripheral neuropathy late on a Friday night.

You are called to see a patient in casualty who has shaking of the left leg and right arm which is worsened by knocking the bed. What do you think of? (Tetanus)

How would you manage a young woman with angiooedema of the larynx and who is just about to obstruct?

What is the management of a patient arriving in casualty with a snake bite?[13]

You see a woman in her forties with a Hb of 5g who is asymptomatic apart from a pulse of 110 and tiredness. There is no evidence of bleeding seen in casualty. What do you do?

What is the management of a 45-year-old woman who is short of breath with a Hb of 4.1g and an MCV of 106?

You are called to see a young man in casualty who is drowsy and jaundiced. He is an intravenous drug addict. He is hypotensive and warm. (Management of gram-negative shock)

A ward sister asks you, as the registrar, to see a nurse who has had a needlestick injury in casualty. What do you do? The patient had tattoos and was a drug addict.

Cardiology

How would you deal with a BP of 160/100 in a man of 60 years?

Management of a patient with headaches and a BP of 200/140.

Investigation and management of *moderate hypertension.*
(Discussion about proteinuria and phaeochromocytoma)

What initial treatment would you use for *mild hypertension* in an asymptomatic 70-year-old man?
Do beta-blockers work in a different way in the elderly?

Management of a high blood pressure in the early stages of a stroke.

Management of a patient in the GP surgery with a high BP.

What do you understand by borderline hypertension? What have the recent trials taught us?

Case history of a patient with postoperative hypertension. (Porphyria)

You see a case of a young hypertensive woman. What would be your differential diagnosis? What would you do next in clinic?

What do you understand by the term 'accelerated hypertension'?

What are the side effects of some of the antihypertensive drugs and which ones would you use in different situations, e.g. asthmatics?

Discussion on the EWPHE study.[1] Has it made a difference to your prescribing habits?

What is the definition of malignant hypertension.

---

[13]   p. 86

[1]   p. 203

Tell me about some of the **major hypertension studies**.

You see a patient who is hypertensive and hypokalaemic. What do you think?[2] (Further discussion on renins and cortisols)

Treatment of mild hypertension, side effects of drugs, effect of drugs on risk factors, e.g. lipids, and why are ACE inhibitors possibly the best treatment?

How would you treat a patient recently admitted to CCU? (Thrombolytic agents and streptokinase in particular)

What is the initial management of a patient with a myocardial infarction?

Mortality from a myocardial infarction. Causes of initial mortality.

Management of a 50-year-old man with **cardiogenic shock** following a myocardial infarction.

The **reduction of mortality in myocardial infarction**.

What interventions do you know of that can reduce the mortality from a myocardial infarction?

What is the disadvantage of using r-tpa (recombinant tissue plasminogen activator)? (Cost)

Would you give thrombolytic therapy to someone with a history of indigestion?

What are the effects of immediate postthrombolysis angioplasty?

Thrombolytic therapy **and the contraindications to its use.**

Tell me about the trials of beta-blockers in acute myocardial infarction.

You see a 40-year-old man ten days **after a myocardial infarction**. What **investigations** will you do?[3] (Lipids)

What is the **value of a coronary care unit**?[4]

What is the management of a patient who has persistent pain after a myocardial infarction?

Poor prognostic indicators in myocardial infarction.

What would you tell the wife of a 50-year-old man who was going home after a myocardial infarction when she asks about his prognosis?

You are a registrar in the cardiology department. You have a 57-year-old man 10 days after an uncomplicated anterior myocardial infarction. You need his bed, so you decide to discharge him.[5] What do you do?

Management of heart failure in a patient in the coronary care unit with a recent myocardial infarction.
Some detailed basic questions, e.g. 'What is the cellular mechanism of nitrates?' Also discussion of aortic balloon counterpulsation.

How would you manage a patient who two days after a myocardial infarction becomes oliguric on the coronary care unit? (Management of cardiogenic shock)

---

[2]   Primary aldosteronism (Conn's syndrome) should be at the top of the list.
[3]   p. 32
[4]   p. 89
[5]   Most physicians would not need a special reason to discharge a patient with an uncomplicated myocardial infarction after 10 days in hospital.

How would you assess the **size of a myocardial infarction** and which parameter is the most accurate?

You have a 45-year-old man in **congestive cardiac failure after an anterior myocardial infarction**. He's on no drugs. What do you do?

What is the **follow-up assessment of ventricular function after a myocardial infarction**?

Role of oxygen free radicals and their relation to coronary artery thrombosis.

What do you think is the **value of exercise ECG testing**?

What protocol do you use for exercise ECGs? If abnormal, what do you do next?

In my home town of Dublin we have the highest rate of coronary artery disease in the world. Tell me what I should do about setting up a screening service.

How would you organise a campaign to reduce the mortality of coronary heart disease?

What are the risk factors for ischaemic heart disease?

You see a patient with *crescendo angina* who is taking beta-blockers and calcium antagonists but who is unkeen on surgery. What might be suggested?

Given that the headaches of nitrates wear off, do the beneficial effects not do so as well? When were the transcutaneous nitrates first used?

Current use of nitrates in ischaemic heart disease.

Definition of crescendo angina and what is its modern treatment? (Angioplasty and intracoronary streptokinase)

Management of a 45-year-old man with chest pain. (CCU and the purpose of it, complications and arrhythmias)

Chest pain in a young man. (Ruptured oesophagus)

Investigation of chest pain.

Airline pilot with chest pain – what will you do?

Management of unstable angina.

I'm 45 years old, overweight but a nonsmoker. I drink 10 pints a week and I come to see you to ask for aspirins to prevent a heart attack. What would you advise me?

How do you investigate patients with angina?

The use of ACE inhibitors in congestive cardiac failure.

Treatment of acute LVF.

Treatment of resistant cardiac failure.[6]

You see a man with acute CCF and atrial fibrillation who has a heart rate of 112. What is the acute management of CCF? Discuss the use of digoxin in heart failure.

Tell me about diuretic resistant oedema.

A 40-year-old man comes to see me with cardiac failure. What is the likely aetiology? What are you thinking of? (Treatment of heart failure)

---

[6]   p. 64

Changes in prevalence of infective endocarditis over the past 20 years.

Talk about the **antibiotic prophylaxis for infective endocarditis**.

Imagine I am a dentist and I have a patient with a heart murmur. What advice are you going to give me?

How do you approach a febrile patient with known valvular heart disease?

Management of a patient attending the outpatient department complaining of palpitations.

Investigation of a tachycardia in a young female.

A 55-year-old man comes to the outpatient department in established atrial flutter resistant to antiarrhythmics. How do you manage him? (Discussion included the side effects of quinidine)

What are the likely causes of a woman aged 50 years being aware of her heartbeat at night?

How would you establish the **cause of palpitations**?

Cardiopulmonary resuscitation and the drugs used in ventricular fibrillation.

Management of ventricular tachycardia.

What is the management of broad complex tachycardia?

What would you do for a fit 40-year-old man who has atrial fibrillation and no obvious cause clinically?

Management of atrial fibrillation.

Functions of the atria.[7] (Presentation of atrial fibrillation. Who should be anticoagulated?)

Anticoagulation in AF. What are the indications and dangers?

Investigation of postural hypotension. (Recent *BMJ* leader)

Management of a patient presenting with hypotension. (Drugs as the aetiology)

What do you know about **mitral valve prolapse**?

What is the biggest cause for the recent improvement in prognosis in cardiomyopathy? (Heart transplants and antiarrhythmics. The examiner really wanted the side effects of amiodarone)

Tell me what you understand by the term *cardiomyopathy*.
What are the causes of cardiomyopathy?

You see a young man in clinic with cardiomyopathy. His GP has been increasing his *frumil* but he is still in failure. What do you do?[8]

Discuss the management of a 35-year-old man unwell presenting with his second pulmonary embolus.

Pericardial effusion and tamponade.

---

[7]   p. 49

[8]   p. 64

An ECG which showed atrial flutter, RAD and RVH. (Cor pulmonale)
(We discussed the causes and treatment of cor pulmonale with a little about the physiology of heart failure)

Physiological basis for and ECG findings in SVT.[9]

ECG criteria for left ventricular hypertrophy.[10]

What do you understand by the term 'venous pressure'? What are the normal values?

Explain the mechanisms of the Valsalva manoeuvre and its clinical importance.[11] Postulate on the mechanism of cough syncope.

A clinical setting was given of a case of **aortic dissection** ripping off one of the spinal arteries.

Name the complications of ventricular aneurysms.

What is syndrome X?

What are the uses of elective DC cardioversion?

What is your opinion regarding **cardiac transplantation**?

Which patients should be selected for heart transplants?

What are the neurological complications of a coronary artery bypass graft?

What is the role of an ECG machine in casualty?

What is the clinical use of the stethoscope?

What cardiac problems do **drug addicts** have?

Gastroenterology

What are the mechanisms of *peptic ulcer disease*?

Treatment of a resistant peptic ulcer not responding to six weeks of H_2 antagonists. (Zollinger-Ellison syndrome, malignancy)

Management of a 55-year-old man with a large *gastric ulcer* on barium meal.

Campylobacter duodenale and *pylori*.

What drugs are used to treat peptic ulceration?

Discuss benign peptic ulcer disease and oesophagitis. What is the new 'scientific' evidence for the mechanism of action of bismuth?

Treatment of a duodenal ulcer with reference to *Campylobacter pylori*. (Discussion included the side effects of bismuth)

How would you investigate and manage a case of suspected Zollinger-Ellison syndrome?[1]

Discuss the role of proton pump inhibitors in Zollinger-Ellison syndrome. What is the aetiology of gastric cancer?

---

[9] p. 49
[10] p. 51
[11] p. 48
[1] p. 67

How would you investigate a man of 40 years who presents with indigestion?

What is the emergency management of a haematemesis?

How would you manage a 22-year-old boy with a haematemesis due to varices? What are the likely causes?

How is a Sengstaken tube used?

What are some rare causes of gastrointestinal haemorrhages?

You see a middle-aged woman with a gastrointestinal haemorrhage who is on warfarin because of mitral stenosis (or mitral valve replacement). What are the likely causes of bleeding and what is the role of endoscopy? What are the drug interactions with warfarin?

Tell me, doctor, about **oesophageal reflux**. Do you think it is overrated as a clinical condition? (*BMJ* leader that week)

Tell me about the recent *BMJ* article on Barrett's oesophagus.

What is the usefulness of the term 'nonulcer dyspepsia' and how would you manage such a patient?

What are the effects of alcohol on the GI tract? (The examiner wanted a detailed discussion from the mouth to the anus)

Effects of alcohol on the liver.

Describe the histology of alcoholic liver cirrhosis.

How might a patient present with cirrhosis? How would you manage ascites? Tell me about viral hepatitis.

What are the causes of chronic hepatitis?

In hepatitis B infection what is the only situation where immunisation is absolutely vital? (Babies born to mothers who are HbsAg or HbeAg positive must be given immunisation and antihepatitis B globulin)

How would you pick up the small proportion of patients with acute hepatitis B infection who were going to do badly?[2]

How do you diagnose viral hepatitis and what is the most likely mode of acquisition?

You see a young man with needle marks, jaundice and septicaemia. What are the likely causes and management?

Acute liver failure – drugs involved and treatment.

Investigation of a patient with obstructive jaundice.

Chronic active hepatitis, the histology, presenting complaints and the Mayo study.

Questions about **primary biliary cirrhosis** and its treatment.

---

[2] Patients who are either too young or too old, those on dialysis or on immunosuppressive drugs, those with Down's syndrome, those with HBeAg during the acute stage, and those with persistent HBsAg beyond six months may fare badly and go on to develop chronic persistent or chronic active hepatitis.

What are the causes of a very elevated bilirubin level on a biochemical profile with no other abnormal results?[3]

Classification of pancreatitis.

The management of a patient with the *irritable bowel syndrome* and discussion about other causes of diarrhoea.

What is the likely cause of a patient presenting with a five-year history of intermittent abdominal pain, constipation and diarrhoea? (Irritable bowel syndrome)

You see a male aged 20–30 years who has had diarrhoea for several months. What do you think of? What is the immunology of AIDS?

Discussion about the **differential diagnosis of diarrhoeal illnesses** and the irritable bowel syndrome. Also discussed were the management of ulcerative colitis, and pseudomembranous enterocolitis.

Investigation and management of rectal bleeding.

Examiner produced a barium enema which showed diverticular disease and a fistula. Discussion about the complications of diverticular disease.

Management of constipation in (a) a patient aged 25 and (b) on a geriatric ward.

What is subtotal villous atrophy? What conditions cause it?

What is the aetiology of **coeliac disease**?

Tell me how coeliac disease presents in an adult.
This coeliac patient has absent reflexes. What might be the cause? (Hypokalaemia secondary to diarrhoea, myopathy)

Management of acute ulcerative colitis.

What are the radiological and histological differences between Crohn's disease and ulcerative colitis?

The use of cholestyramine in diarrhoea associated with Crohn's disease.

Investigation of Crohn's disease.

What are the extra-articular features of Crohn's disease?

You see a young boy with vomiting and weight loss. What is the differential diagnosis?

I was given a case history. How would you investigate chronic abdominal pain in this patient who has had normal radiological investigations?

Discuss malabsorption and lactose intolerance.

You see a patient with '*main de coucheur*' and abdominal pain. What are your thoughts? (Pancreatitis)

Discuss angiodysplasia of the colon.

---

[3]   The phrase 'very elevated' suggests a level of bilirubin in excess of 100 μmol/l and thus excludes Gilbert's disease and a compensated haemolytic anaemia (see p. 66). Hereditary hyperbilirubinaemia (Crigler-Najjar type II, Rotor's syndrome, Dubin-Johnson syndrome) and liver storage disease are consistent with high bilirubin levels and normal liver function test results.

In which conditions is regular screening for colonic neoplasia clearly warranted? (Ulcerative colitis, Crohn's, familial polyposis)

How does carcinoma of the bowel present?

Discuss the two types of hiatus hernia.

What are the causes of oral ulceration?

Discuss the sensible and rational use of an endoscopy service.

Examiner produced a sequence of ERCP films which demonstrated a dilated common bile duct with stones in it and then subsequent postsphincterotomy X-rays. What is this examination, what does it show, what has happened in the latter films and what are the complications of sphincterotomy and ERCP?

Here is the barium enema of a 35-year-old, previously fit man. It was taken two days after a routine hernia operation. He has had profuse watery diarrhoea with no blood. What do you think? (Pseudomembranous colitis)

Describe the blood supply of the gut.
Discussion of small vessel diseases of the bowel. (Polyarteritis nodosa)

Tell me about *Shigella* and *Salmonella* dysentery.

Discuss atypical bowel infections and the relevant organisms producing opportunistic infections.

Endocrinology

What is the *treatment of diabetic ketoacidosis*?

I am the parent of a newly diagnosed diabetic child and I am worried about hypoglycaemic attacks. What advice will you give me?

What is the management of a 19-year-old newly diagnosed diabetic?

Complications of diabetes mellitus, particularly retinopathy.

Are there any regulations regarding diabetes mellitus and driving?

Management of a patient with hyperosmolar nonketotic diabetic precoma.

Tell me about diabetic emergencies.

What is the most beneficial therapeutic measure in treating diabetes mellitus overall? (Diet) I was then asked questions on the oral hypoglycaemic drugs.

You are looking after a diabetic woman in her seventies who develops a pyrexia. What possible causes must you think of? (DVT, infected pressure sores)

We are going to talk about diabetic ketoacidosis – start by giving me some 'numbers' that we are dealing with.[1]

What are the steps required to diagnose diabetes mellitus in a young man with glycosuria?[2]

Detailed questions concerning diabetic retinopathy.

What are the eye complications in diabetics? Discuss diabetic microvascular disease.

How might diabetes mellitus affect the gut?

Why do people die from diabetes mellitus?[3]

What would you tell a newly diagnosed diabetic (insulin-dependent) about his treatment, complications and the likely prognosis for life?

Question on diabetic **microalbuminuria.**

You see a young diabetic man with a lump on his chest which 'looked like an abscess but is not an abscess'. What do you think of? (Atypical infections, osteomyelitis of a rib, infected injection site)

A well-controlled diabetic starts having hypoglycaemic attacks. What do you think of? (Associated hyperthyroidism)

What is the emergency treatment of hypoglycaemia and the possible causes of hypoglycaemic coma?

Mechanisms of hypoglycaemia and liver enzymes.

How is the blood sugar controlled biochemically?

How do you perform a clinitest?

---

[1]   p. 161
[2]   p. 212
[3]   Macrovascular disease (CVA, ischaemic heart disease), microvascular (renal failure), sepsis and diabetic coma.

What is the value of measuring early morning urinary cortisol in diabetics?[4]

You see a 23-year-old Swedish *au pair* with polydipsia. What do you think of? (Eosinophilic granuloma, diabetes mellitus, compulsive water drinking)

How would you investigate a child of 14 years of age who is brought by his parents with a complaint of short stature?[5]

Investigation of a male of normal height but with no secondary sexual characteristics at the age of 17 years. (Pituitary causes or testicular causes)

Investigation of **Cushing's syndrome.**[6]

Investigations of obesity in the OPD.

Investigation of thyrotoxicosis.

Discuss thyrotoxicosis as a cause of congestive cardiac failure. What is the appropriate treatment? How do you prepare a patient who is to be treated with radioactive iodine?

A patient comes to you complaining of pain during swallowing. What do you think of? (Subacute thyroiditis)

Acromegaly and pituitary tumours.

What are the two commonest causes of amenorrhoea? (Hyperprolactinaemia, anorexia nervosa)

Causes of galactorrhoea in a 32-year-old woman.

You see a man in the OPD with impotence and headaches – does this mean anything to you? (Prolactinoma)

What is the difference between prolactin and the other pituitary hormones? (Prolactin is the only hormone regulated by the *inhibitory* action of dopamine) What is the differential diagnosis of a 20-year-old man with gynaecomastia?

What is the BMI formula?[7] (Discussion about the health problems of obesity)

---

[4]   The examiner's bees were probably stress hyperglycaemia, coincident hypopituitarism and hypoadrenalism.

[5]   p. 17

[6]   p. 63

[7]   Body Mass Index=weight in kg divided by the square of height in metres; kg/m^2

Neurology

Management of a 24-year-old man who suddenly becomes unconscious during a football match.

Management of a first epileptic fit.

A 50-year-old man has one witnessed epileptic fit. What would you do? What about driving restrictions? What about **therapy**?

What is the management of an epileptic, normally well-controlled on phenytoin, who has an increased fit frequency?

Epilepsy and driving.

Discuss temporal lobe epilepsy.

Management of resistant status epilepticus in a known epileptic who was usually well-controlled.

Management of a 22-year-old woman with three generalised convulsions in three months.

A man in his fifties presents with a fit. **How useful is an EEG?**[1] What advice would you give about his driving licence?

What is the management of a young footballer who is fitting on the football pitch?

I saw a patient in the long cases this morning who was on phenobarbitone for epilepsy. What are your views on this?

What is the choice of anticonvulsants in various situations?

What are the rules pertaining to driving, work, etc. in epilepsy?

How could you prove that a fit was genuine or not? (Serum prolactin)[2]

Management of subarachnoid haemorrhage.

How would a patient with a subarachnoid haemorrhage present?
What investigations would you do if the patient is unconscious?
What would be the typical appearances on a CT scan? (Long discussion on sub-arachnoid haemorrhages)

A clinical setting was given of a young student with a headache. (SAH)

You see a boy of 12 years of age who has photophobia and neck stiffness. What is the likely diagnosis? What is the geography of the West Country? Why has there been an outbreak of meningitis in that area? Are the people different?

A child presents very ill with purpura. (**Meningococcal meningitis**)

What is the long-term management of stroke patients?

Stroke rehabilitation – what factors may cause problems?

It is not unusual to find an element of depression in patients who have had a stroke. Discuss.

A case history of a patient with a recent stroke. How does one localise the lesion in a CVA?

---

[1]   p. 73
[2]   p. 241

You see a 22-year-old female with a stroke. What are your thoughts? (Contraceptive pill, hypertension, infective endocarditis, atrial myxoma, a-v malformation, space-occupying lesion, brain abscess)

Transient ischaemic attacks – investigations and prognosis.

Discuss the pathogenesis, diagnosis and *management of TIAs.*

A 55-year-old man presents with neurological symptoms suggestive of a TIA. (This led to a discussion about the risk factors and the general assessment of the patient and about hypertension in particular)

What action do you take on discovering a carotid bruit in a patient?

I'm a 20-year-old woman and I've had bad headaches for two weeks. Ask me some questions. (Contraceptive pill)

What is the management of a unilateral headache? (Temporal arteritis, migraine)

Classification of *headaches.*

You see a patient in clinic with a headache. What features would lead you to suspect raised intracranial pressure?

There is a patient with a six weeks' history of headache. Discuss the differential diagnosis.

Have you read about 'thunder headache' in the correspondence columns? What is your understanding of it?

The examiners gave a classical history of migrainous neuralgia and this was discussed.

What are the visual defects that can occur during migraine attacks?

Treatment of migraine.

You are looking after a young woman with newly diagnosed disseminated sclerosis. What are you going to tell her?

What is the management of a patient with *multiple sclerosis*? (Treatment options and prognosis)
Discuss the value of hyperbaric oxygen and diet.

What is the aetiology and pathology of multiple sclerosis?

A young woman presents with unilateral optic neuritis. What do you think of? (This led to a discussion about multiple sclerosis)

What is the management of a patient with **Parkinson's disease** in an OP consultation?

What is the natural history of Parkinson's disease and what is the treatment? What drugs can be used and what are their side effects?

A patient found he kept bumping into things while out walking. What do you think of? (Visual field defect)
What are the origins of the basilar and vertebral arteries?

How do you manage a patient with a headache and double vision? (Discussed the range of differentials and the positive signs that might be present)
The patient has a third cranial nerve palsy. What do you think? (Aneurysm of the posterior communicating artery)
What investigations would you do? (Angiography, CT scan)

You get a call from a colleague who had a severe headache on getting up. On your way to see him, what are your thoughts?

Tell me something about **myalgic encephalitis**.[3]

What do you know about myalgic encephalitis? Do you think it really exists?

How do you explain to someone that they have **motor neurone disease**?

What is the management of a patient who presents in OPD with difficulty swallowing liquids?

What are the **neurological complications of excessive alcohol intake**?

How do you differentiate between a confusional state and dementia?
Can a young man become demented?
How would you diagnose a frontal lobe tumour?

What is the differential diagnosis of dementia in a man of 40 years of age?

What are the causes of a painful neuropathy?

Chorea in a 24-year-old woman.

A young man of 25 years of age presents with foot drop and is also found to have an absent ankle jerk. What do you think? (S1 lesion)

A 50-year-old man presents with paraesthesiae in his arm. What investigations would you do?

What is the lateral medullary syndrome?

Tell me about the methods available for imaging of the brain.

What are the methods of clinical and electrocardiographic detection of autonomic neuropathy?

What are the causes of, and how would you manage, someone with an acute cord compression?

What do you know about benign intracranial hypertension?

What do you know about tropical spastic paraparesis?

Diagnosis of brain death.[4]

What do you know about hydrocephalus?

Tell me about neurosarcoidosis.

What do you know about the neuroleptic syndrome?
What is the most important laboratory test? (CPK)

What is the course of the seventh cranial nerve? What is the differential diagnosis of bilateral palsy?

---

[3] p. 18, 24, 87
[4] p. 241

Nephrology

What are the causes of *proteinuria* and how does it come about?

You see an adult male patient with heavy proteinuria. What investigations would you perform?

What is orthostatic proteinuria? What is its significance?

Renal failure – clinical diagnosis, management of acute and chronic renal failure.

Renal transplantation and its indications, followed by a discussion about diabetics and transplants.

How would you investigate a man with a blood urea of 15 mmol/l?

Management of **haematuria**.

Discuss the investigation of a patient with haematuria and its association with a sore throat.
What might be wrong with a young man who develops haematuria every time he has an URTI? (Berger's disease)[1]

How would you investigate a patient who presents with microscopic haematuria which was found at an insurance medical?

You see a patient in the rheumatology clinic with a urea of 25 mmol/l. What do you think?

What is interstitial nephritis?

Discuss amyloidosis and its causes.

Tell me about familial mediterranean fever.

Discuss **urinary tract infections in women**.

Management of recurrent urinary tract infections in a woman with sterile urine and normal investigations. (The size of the problem; general measures, including good fluid intake and long-term cyclical antibiotics)

What are your views on the treatment of asymptomatic bacteriuria in nonpregnant subjects?[2]

What are the recent advances in the treatment of renal stones?

What are the causes of urinary stones?

What is the treatment of CAPD peritonitis?

Discuss the various aspects of renal bone disease.

Discuss the management of a previously well 30-year-old man who is admitted with diarrhoea and vomiting, has a raised urea, and has passed little urine overnight. (Prerenal *vs.* established renal failure)

A man in his forties presents with pain at the end of micturition. How would you treat him? (Prostatitis)

Tell me about the symptom of **nocturia**. Why does nocturia occur in CRF?

What is an IVP used for in modern medical practice?

What are the renal manifestations of hypokalaemia?

---

[1]   p. 152
[2]   p. 29

AIDS and infections

I was asked to define a rotavirus and to give an example. (HIV)[1]

You are a consultant in charge of an infectious diseases unit and a patient with **AIDS** and who has diarrhoea is admitted. How would you manage him?

HIV tests – what do you think about having the patient's consent?

I was asked a question regarding practising dentists who have HIV infection.

What do you know about counselling? (Questions about HIV)

What would you do as a doctor if you were found to be HIV positive?[2] Would you still work? Would you tell your patients?

A man comes to your clinic who is HIV positive. Do you tell him and discuss his prognosis, etc.? What do you tell his wife and GP?[3]

How could you identify a case of AIDS at the OP clinic?

You see a 32-year-old man with a cervical lymph node. What are the causes, management and investigation of AIDS?

How do you counsel a colleague who is homosexual and who has had a recent unprotected contact?
What tests are available? Are they helpful in this situation?

What is the natural history of HIV-positive patients?

What drugs are useful in the treatment of atypical mycobacterium infections in AIDS patients?

What are the neurological complications of AIDS? (*Cryptococcal* meningitis)

Have you heard of the new drug for the treatment of AIDS?
Tell me about the recent developments for the AIDS vaccine.

Have you ever looked after AIDS patients?
Tell me about any available prophylactic therapies.

Do you think that there is going to be an AIDS epidemic? Is there any precedent against which your suspicions can be justified?

Botulism – diagnosis and management. (Hazelnut yoghurt)

What are the symptoms of botulism? How would you differentiate it from the Guillain-Barré syndrome?

What is the treatment of *Salmonella* septicaemia?

What are the current risks of *Salmonella*? (Edwina Currie)[4]

What is the presentation of typhoid fever?

Give some examples of diseases caused in man by *Chlamydia*.

What can you tell me about nosocomial infections?

---

[1] The candidate has confused rotavirus (causing gastroenteritis) with retrovirus (causing HIV).
[2] p. 36
[3] p. 34
[4] A Junior Health Minister at the time who said all eggs carried *Salmonella*.

Tell me about leprosy.

The rubella syndrome.

Tell me two signs that may be found in rubella.

Listeria *infections.*

Rabies and rabies vaccine.

Tell me about cholera.

Which diseases are caused by *Campylobacter* bacteria?

Discuss the merits of vaccinations for immunocompromised patients.

Let's talk about malaria – how does it kill you, how do you diagnose it and what's the treatment?

You see a giraffe-keeper with diarrhoea. What do you think of? (Cryptosporidiosis)

What would you do with a young nurse who has just has a needle-stick injury? (from a drug addict)

The portrait on your right is of Mr Argyll Robertson.[5] What is he famous for? How would you diagnose and treat tertiary syphilis?

You see an adolescent with conjunctivitis and swollen cervical lymph nodes. What are the possibilities? (*Chlamydia*)

Tell me about diseases which birds transmit to humans. (*Chlamydia*, pigeon fancier's lung, etc.)

What is the rash of measles?

What are the manifestations and treatment of giardiasis?

---

[5]   p. 267

Statistics

Tell us about the different ways of analysing experimental data.

How would you evaluate statistically a trial of a new antihypertensive drug?

How would you design a phase III clinical trial of a new NSAID?

Design of clinical trials. What is a double-bind cross-over trial?

What are **type 2 errors** in clinical trials?[1]

Have you taken part in any clinical trials? How would you set up a clinical trial, e.g. testing drug A *vs* drug B?

How would you compare 'unmatched' data? (Student's *t*-test)

The examiner drew a graph and asked about various statistical factors – *P* value, *r* value, **coefficient of variation**.

Define '*p* value' and '**regression coefficient**'.[2]

What is the **specificity and sensitivity of a test** with relation to an exercise ECG?

Discussion of a graph with lots of statistics underneath it.

Interpretation of some basic statistics and explanation of some statistical symbols.

The examiner drew two graphs and asked about the available tests to compare the data.

Calculation of the correlation between two groups that were not normally distributed. Also the definition of **mean, median** and **mode**.[3]

What is the meaning of mean/mode/median?[3]

What is the definition of **standard deviation**?[4]
Is there any other way of describing the same sort of idea? (Confidence intervals)

What do you understand by the terms 'standard error of a mean' and 'standard deviation of a mean'?[4]

What is the difference between a **parametric** and a **nonparametric statistical test**?[5]

How would you define correlation?

Discuss *t*-tests and probabilities.

The chi square test/Student's *t*-test and the advantages/disadvantages of each.

Define a normal population. How would you define a normal range of a skewed distribution?[6]

What would you understand by the term $P < 0.001$ if you read a research article in the *Lancet*?

Explain the null hypothesis.[7]

---

[1]   pp. 147, 252
[2]   p. 253
[3]   p. 250
[4]   p. 251
[5]   p. 47
[6]   p. 250
[7]   p. 251

Foreign travel

Tell me about *malaria prophylaxis* in chloroquine resistant areas.

What is the *treatment of malaria*?

What investigations would you do for a man returning from the Sudan complaining of headaches?

A 45-year-old man returns from West Africa with fever. Discuss the management in the GP surgery.

What do you know about lassa fever?

You see a male patient who has recently returned from Spain. He presents with a swollen and painful knee and diarrhoea. What would you do?[1]

Would you let a relative of yours go to Nigeria and, if so, what specific advice would you give?

What is the likely cause of drowsiness in an Asian man who has just arrived from Pakistan?

What is the **investigation of dysentery** in a 30-year-old man who has just returned from Egypt?

A man returns from abroad with a fever. What would you do and what is the differential diagnosis?

A man is brought to casualty unconscious. You are told that he has recently been to Africa. What do you think? (Cerebral malaria)

A 40-year-old man returns home from a holiday abroad and later that day comes to your clinic complaining of a change of bowel habit and weight loss. What do you do?

Discuss the **medical problems of Asian migrants coming to this country**.[2]

You see an Indian boy with difficulty in walking. What might be the cause? (Osteomalacia)

What advice would you give to a colleague travelling to South East Asia and Bangkok?

What vaccinations are needed prior to going to Central Africa?

If I went to Nepal what drugs would I take with me?

What do you think about an 8-year-old girl returning from holiday with her family, all of whom have diarrhoea? She herself presents with a large joint arthralgia.[3]

A 34-year-old man returns from the USA with a toxic confusional state. What is the likely cause? (Legionnaires' disease)

---

[1]   Reactive arthritis. See p. 233

[2]   p. 81

[3]   p. 233

Clinic investigations

Investigation of a man with hypercalcaemia and an elevated alkaline phosphatase. What are the features of hypercalcaemia?

What would you do if faced with a 35-year-old woman who was referred by her GP because her serum calcium was 2.8 mmol/l?

A patient comes to the OPD with a severe *headache* – what do you think?

You see a 60-year-old man complaining of headaches. What is your approach? (Temporal arteritis)

In the OPD I have seen a 52-year-old smoker who has got a massive right pleural effusion. How would you manage him?

Investigation and management of an outpatient with a pleural effusion, including the technique of a pleural biopsy in detail.

A 19-year-old girl comes to the OPD with *weight loss.* How would you approach the problem?

You have an Indian lady in the OPD who speaks no English and her only complaint is of weight loss. What investigations would you do?

A 30-year-old patient in OPD complains of diarrhoea of one year's duration. What is the likely diagnosis? (Crohn's, ulcerative colitis, irritable bowel syndrome)

How would you investigate a healthy Nigerian with diarrhoea?

Management of a 30-year-old man with retrosternal *chest pain.*

You see a patient in clinic with chest pain. How do you differentiate between cardiac and oesophageal causes?

What is the management of 'funny turns' in the OPD?[1]

You see a patient with an incidental rise in AST and gamma GT. How would you proceed in the OPD? (Repeat LFTs, autoantibody screen, HBsAg, ultrasound scan, liver biopsy)

The management of a patient in OPD with an **elevated alkaline phosphatase.**[2] (Discussion about the distinction between bone and liver isoenzymes and then about the management of Paget's disease)

A middle-aged woman has just had an insurance examination. She is found to have three round **opacities** in the apex of her lung on **CXR**. History and examination are unhelpful. How would you investigate in the most cost-effective way? (Fine needle biopsy)

You are in the OPD and a GP refers a 45-year-old man with a BP of 160/110 mmHg found at an insurance medical and 150/105 mmHg in the surgery. What would you do?

A woman has a late systolic murmur. She is well but attends you for a medical. Would you reassure her?

A man in OPD complains of polyuria. What would you ask about?

---

[1]   pp. 18, 65
[2]   p. 14

You are given a case history of a 19-year-old man who is found at an insurance examination to have haematuria and mild hypertension. What is the diagnosis? (IgA nephropathy)

What is the differential diagnosis and management of a painful inflamed joint in an elderly patient found on a ward round?[3]

How would you manage a 60-year-old man in the OPD with a six-month history of low back pain? (Osteoporosis, myeloma)

What is the management of a 30-year-old woman with anaemia?

You see a 40-year-old woman in the OPD with anxiety and palpitations. How would you manage her? (Thyrotoxicosis, smoking, caffeine)[4]

Management of a patient in a GP surgery with swelling of the ankles. (Discussed causes, use of TED stockings)

A woman comes to you with a fever (for a week) and no specific localising complaints. What would you do? (Lyme arthritis)

Investigation and management of a man with **intermittent claudication** in the OPD.

What would you be thinking of if a patient came to clinic with tremor, memory loss and morning sickness? (Alcohol excess)

You see a patient in clinic with chronic obstructive airways disease who is complaining of increasing breathlessness. What would you do? (Look for chest infection, check inhaler technique)

What is the management of a woman presenting with hirsutism? (Polycystic ovary syndrome)

A girl comes to the OPD following a series of **blackouts**. What would you do? (Hyperventilation syndrome)

A 34-year-old North Sea diver comes to your clinic with a heart rate of 40. What would you do? (Stop him working)
What other conditions do you know which could prevent a man from being a professional diver? (Previous pneumothorax)

How would you manage an elderly man with a limp who walks into your clinic?

A 23-year-old boy, who feels well, attends your OPD referred by his GP with a Hb of 13.5 g and MCV 105. What are your initial thoughts? (Coeliac disease)[5]

What is the investigation of a jaundiced patient who walks into the outpatient clinic?

What goes through your mind if you see a patient in the OPD with cerebellar signs? (Alcohol, drugs, hypothyroidism, SOL, demyelinating disease, brain stem CVA, Friedreich's ataxia, manifestation of malignancy)

A 65-year-old woman is referred by her GP with a diagnosis of myxoedema and diarrhoea. The GP has already started her on thyroxine before she attends the OPD. Routine tests show a low folate. What are your thoughts? (Coeliac disease)

---

3   p. 69
4   p. 62
5   p. 185

Elderly Patients

Management of a confused 70-year-old woman.

Investigations of dementia.

What are the treatable and untreatable *causes of dementia*? What clinical features distinguish Alzheimer's from other dementias?

How do you assess the difference between dementia and an acute confusional state?

What do you know of the recent work on **Alzheimer's disease**?

A 70-year-old man has been admitted with a confusional illness of 5–6 months' duration. How would you manage him?
Do you know of any new treatment being proposed for Alzheimer's disease?

Alzheimer's disease – histology and the theories of its aetiology. (This led to a discussion about dialysis dementia and the other complications of dialysis)

An old lady presents with a low temperature. What is the management?

Define *hypothermia*.

Discuss thermoregulation in the elderly.

How do you investigate a 70-year-old lady who presents with dizzy spells?[1]

Discuss **blackouts in the elderly**. (Transient ischaemic attacks, Stokes-Adams attacks, postural hypotension, drugs)

What is the treatment of **temporal arteritis**?

You see an elderly man with a unilateral headache. What are you concerned about? (Temporal arteritis)
What would be the histology of a biopsy?[2]
How could a diagnosis of polyarteritis be made?

What are the causes of *back pain* in the elderly?

A 60-year-old man has back pain of sudden onset. What do you think of?

A 66-year-old woman has severe mid-thoracic back pain. What is the likely cause? **(Osteoporosis)**

An old lady has sudden onset of pain between the shoulder blades while cleaning windows. What do you think of?

Should an 80-year-old patient with iron deficiency anaemia have investigations to determine the cause?

An elderly man presents with a Hb of 9.0 g and an iron deficiency picture. What are the investigations for this?

What are the causes of a **macrocytic anaemia in the elderly** when the levels of B_{12} and folate are normal?

---

[1]   p. 65
[2]   p. 164

What is the diagnosis of a pale, elderly woman (Hb 4.2 g) who was previously getting 'liver injections' until ten years ago?

When did hydroxycobalamin injections first come on to the market?

What is the daily requirement of vitamin B_{12}?

How much is stored in the liver?

What is the terminal care of a man in his nineties who has had a dense cerebrovascular accident?

What is the differential diagnosis of a 'collapse' in an old lady?

You have a clinical situation of an elderly man presenting with a chest infection and a serum Na of 110 mmol/l. What is the likely cause?

(There was a discussion on the underlying mechanism of SIADH)

What are the causes of a low serum sodium in an old person?

Causes of **incontinence in the elderly**.

Management of a 70-year-old man with **Parkinson's disease**.

A 75-year-old patient has difficulty walking, speaking and is constipated. What goes through your mind? (Parkinson's disease)

A 75-year-old woman is referred to you with weight loss. What would you do? (Hyperthyroidism)

You are asked to do a domiciliary visit on a 70-year-old woman who has been treated by her GP for congestive cardiac failure with diuretics but has not improved. What would you suggest?

As a medical registrar you have to see a patient on the geriatric ward who is confused and has a serum calcium level of 3.3 mmol/l. What is the management?

Management of an elderly patient with a low serum folate.

Tell me about night sedation in the elderly.

Why is polypharmacy in the elderly a bad thing?

What is the differential diagnosis and management of an acutely breathless 70-year-old man?

Investigation and diagnosis of an 80-year-old lady who has an ejection systolic murmur in the aortic area. (Differences between stenosis and sclerosis)

What is the role of the ESR in the elderly?

Discuss the elderly in hospital and getting them home.

Treatment of hypothyroidism in an elderly patient with ischaemic heart disease.

An elderly patient is found unconscious at home, brought to casualty and has to be ventilated. No specific abnormality is found on tests or examination. The next day the pupils are dilated, the plantars are extensor and there are no reflexes, etc. What would you do? (Overdose, subdural haematoma, CVA)

Diabetic emergencies in the elderly.

Do you think an 80-year-old man with angina should be referred for a coronary artery bypass graft? (Age itself is not a contraindication)

What do you think are the major problems involved in the care of elderly patients?

Tell me about osteomalacia in the elderly.

What is the epidemiology of Paget's disease of the bone? Is there case clustering?

Which vitamin deficiency is most common in the elderly? (Vitamin D)

Basic sciences

Discuss the **physiology of cardiac failure**.

Tell me about preload.

What is the physiological basis of the treatment of heart failure? Do prophylactic antiarrhythmics work?

What are the haemodynamics of atrial fibrillation?

What is the anatomy of the third cranial nerve, including its origins in the brain stem?

Discuss the innervation of the urinary bladder.

What are **liver function tests**? What do they mean?

Tell me about the physiology of the formation of ascites.

Why is sodium bicarbonate made for use as an 8.4% solution? What is its molecular weight?

How is the glomerular filtration rate measured? What is meant by clearance?

What are the different fluid compartments of the body?

You have a patient with dehydration. What are the mechanisms of fluid and electrolyte balance?

How would you explain serum levels of Na 139, K 2.2, HCO_3 29? (Laxative abuse)

I was shown the following results – Na 129, K 3.3, urea 3.0. What do you think? (Induced labour with syntocinon)

I was shown some biochemical results which indicated a **dilutional hypo-natraemia**. I was then asked about the possible causes and treatment.

A set of U&Es and a FBC together with a short history were produced for discussion. (Chronic renal failure with a salt-losing picture)

Some laboratory data were presented which indicated that the patient had the **syndrome of inappropriate ADH secretion**. What investigations would you do?

Define cyanosis. Discuss the HbO_2 saturation curve.

The differences between central and peripheral cyanosis.

Examiner produced some arterial blood gas results of a patient with type I respiratory failure and these were discussed.

What sugars are we interested in measuring in the blood?

What substrate would you use to assay for antinuclear factor in the blood? (Mouse liver)

Nutrition and vitamins

What are the skin manifestations of nutritional deficiencies?[1]

Tell me about **nicotinic acid**.

Tell me about pellagra.
Do you know any conditions associated with pellagra?

If you were the Queen of England and could order the ideal diet, what would it be?

Tell me about **vitamin D** absorption and metabolism.

Where is most dietary iodine obtained from? (Dairy products)
Where do cows get iodine from?[2]

What is the role of the different diets in medicine (in particular for hyper-lipidaemia)?

Tell me about scurvy and its accompanying physical signs.

Discuss aluminium toxicity. (Chronic renal failure and dementia)

Discuss **zinc deficiency**. (Acrodermatitis enteropathica)

What do you know about **magnesium**?

---

[1]   p. 55
[2]   From seaweed in the feed and absorbed from cleansing iodoform on the udder

Rheumatology

Rheumatoid arthritis–discuss drug treatment and its side effects.

What is the secondary treatment of rheumatoid arthritis?

Rheumatoid is often described as rheumatoid disease and not rheumatoid arthritis – why?

Talk about **gout**.

What is the management of a patient with a raised uric acid level?

Management and diagnosis of gout/pseudogout.

Treatment of acute gout.

How would you investigate a 40-year-old woman with a short history of Raynaud's?

What is the treatment of Raynaud's disease?
How long does a cigarette act on the peripheral vasculature? (The examiner had done this piece of research himself!)
Can you name a vasodilator?

Discussion regarding systemic lupus erythematosus.

Give me a differential diagnosis for a 30-year-old man with a flitting arthralgia.

Paget's disease – indications for treatment, the drugs used and their side effects.

Tell me what you know about **polymyalgia rheumatica**.
What would a muscle biopsy show?

A middle-aged lady who has been on NSAIDs for six months for painful shoulders comes to see you with lethargy. She is found to be uraemic. What do you think?

What is the clinical use of the antinuclear factor in practice?

How would a young man with ankylosing spondylitis present?

What are the indications for steroids in rheumatoid arthritis?

Medical aspects of pregnancy

You have a management problem of an 18-year-old pregnant woman with a normal BP and proteinuria of 5 g/24 hours.

Management of a DVT in pregnancy.

Management of epilepsy in pregnancy.

What is the diagnosis of a 24-year-old woman three weeks postpartum who is taking metronidazole and furodantin for a urinary tract infection? She presents with dysarthria, weak legs and abdominal pain. (Acute intermittent porphyria).[1]

What are the main problems that you, as a medical registrar, could be called upon to deal with on an obstetric ward?

You are asked by the obstetric registrar to see a 38-week-pregnant woman who is vomiting and very unwell. What thoughts are going through your mind?

The treatment of a 26-week-pregnant woman with a BP of 140/90 and proteinuria of 2+.

Which drugs would you use to treat **hypertension in pregnancy?**

Discuss anticoagulation during pregnancy.

Discuss the medical consequences of pregnancy.[2]

You are referred a woman of 16 weeks' gestation who is having **palpitations**. How will you manage her?

What are the dermatological problems of pregnancy?

What is the management of a pregnant woman with a tachycardia of 200 beats per minute?

What would you do with a four months' pregnant woman who has a history suggestive of a pulmonary embolus?

How would you investigate a pregnant woman with a swollen hot calf who has a history of recurrent abortions? (Antithrombin III deficiency)

Management of thyrotoxicosis in pregnancy.

What infections can be passed from mother to baby? What are the effects of rubella, toxoplasmosis and cytomegalovirus?

What new techniques are available for prenatal diagnosis and treatment?

Discuss the management of **mitral stenosis in pregnancy**.

How would you approach the treatment of an Asian lady who presents at 20 weeks' gestation with mitral stenosis?

What is the management of a lady in the first trimester of pregnancy who has cyanotic congenital heart disease?

What is the use and safety of verapamil in pregnancy? What is the pharmacological action of calcium channel blockers on skeletal, smooth and cardiac muscles?

What are the problems of sickle cell disease in pregnancy?

---

[1]   p. 70
[2]   p. 154

Psychiatry

What do you know about *depression*?

The **biological markers of depression**.[1]

What are the recent research developments in **Alzheimer's disease**?

Investigation of presenile dementia.

What is the current aetiological connection between Down's syndrome and Alzheimer's disease?

How would you manage and investigate a case of **anorexia nervosa** in a 12-year-old girl?

What do you think about feigned illnesses?

A psychiatric patient gets polyuria. How would you investigate?[2]

What are the likely causes of a 50-year-old man presenting with **polyuria and polydipsia**? (Psychogenic and diabetes insipidus)

Tell me about your assessment of a **problem drinker**.

Tell me about alcoholism and the dexamethasone suppression test.

You are called to a psychiatric ward and asked to assess a patient for ECT. (Cardiovascular and respiratory assessment, any tendency to fractures)

Discuss chronic panic attacks and their management with benzodiazepines.

Discuss the manifestations of anxiety – somatic and psychiatric. Discuss the management of a phobic disorder.

---

[1]   p. 56
[2]   pp. 74, 139

Dermatology

Tell me about **retinoids** and what they are used for.

Tell me what you know about Behçets syndrome.

You see a patient with a bullous skin disorder. How do you differentiate between **pemphigus and pemphigoid**?

Tell me about the recent advances in the treatment of *psoriasis*.

How do you recognise psoriatic arthropathy clinically?

What do you know about **PUVA**?

Tell me about the causes and management of alopecia.

How would you tackle the problem of a 25-year-old woman who comes to see you with diffuse hair loss?

Tell me about **drugs and the skin**.

What are the causes of pruritus?

A young Irish woman has painful, red lumps on her legs. What do you do? (Erythema nodosum)

Respiratory medicine

What is your management of a 16-year-old girl who is a known asthmatic and who is admitted with breathlessness?

Management of a severe asthmatic attack. (Clinical features and when to ventilate)

What features in an acute asthmatic attack would suggest a severe episode?

Asthma and the causes of sudden deterioration.

What do you know of the recent reports on **asthma deaths** and what do you think are the **factors contributing to the increase**?

What would you do for a 50-year-old lady who complains of nocturnal and early morning wheeze and who hasn't improved with simple antiasthmatic medication from her GP? She refuses any investigations except for a CXR.

Definition and management of status asthmaticus.
What is the immunopathology of asthma?

The examiner pretended to be a 40-year-old man with disseminated lung cancer. The candidate was asked to **'break the news' in a role-playing situation**.

A 60-year-old man with lung carcinoma develops polyuria and polydipsia. What's the diagnosis? (Hypercalcaemia)
How do the diphosphonates work?[1]

What are the nonmetastatic neurological manifestations of **carcinoma of the bronchus**?
What is the treatment of a fit man with lung cancer?

Give me a list of complications that could be anticipated from a patient with carcinoma of the bronchus and mediastinal involvement.

How would you tell me that I had a pleural mesothelioma? What would be the management of my terminal illness?

I was asked about a patient with a slowly resolving pneumonia which was not really responding to antibiotics.

Atypical pneumonias.

What do you understand by the term 'atypical pneumonia syndrome'?

What is the use of antibiotics in **community acquired pneumonia**?

Treatment and investigation of a man admitted with a lobar pneumonia.

What is the presentation of tuberculosis in the present day, and the diagnosis of an atypical case especially in the elderly?

Management of a young girl diagnosed as having **pulmonary tuberculosis**.

Discuss **extrinsic allergic alveolitis**.

You see a 40-year-old woman with a shadow on the chest x-ray. How would you establish the cause?

Treatment and management of pneumothorax.

Management of a middle-aged man with pleuritic chest pain.

---

[1]   p. 157

What is the mechanism of tension pneumothorax?

What are the physical signs of hyperinflation of the chest?

Various questions on COAD and sleep apnoea including investigations and treatment.

What is your understanding of **cor pulmonale** and the use of domiciliary oxygen?

Define forced vital capacity. Discuss the value of lung function tests in discerning the nature of an underlying lung disease.

You see a patient with a pleural effusion that has been found by accident. He is otherwise fit. How would you manage?[2]

A 40-year-old man comes to see you complaining of increasing breathlessness and on examination you find bilateral basal crepitations. What are the likely causes?

Diagnosis of a pulmonary embolus.

What are the biochemical abnormalities in type I and type II respiratory failure? What are the main causes of CO_2 retention?

Basic questions on sarcoidosis.

Candidate was shown a CXR showing *Pneumocystis* pneumonia. What would you do in the casualty department?

Discuss asbestos exposure.

What diseases do farmers get?
What is the pathology of Farmer's lung?

Occupational asthma – what is it, what causes it, how would one diagnose it and treat it?

What investigations would you do to find the cause of breathlessness in a London roadsweeper?

What are the complications of bronchiectasis?

What are the criteria for home oxygen treatment?[3]

---

[2] p. 183
[3] p. 215

Haematology

Tell me about erythropoietin.

A 20-year-old woman presents to her GP with an *iron deficiency anaemia* which has not responded to oral iron treatment. How would you investigate?[1]

You see a patient with iron deficiency anaemia who has had a normal barium meal and barium enema. How would you proceed? (Crohn's disease)

Tell me how iron gets from the gut to the bone marrow; about iron overload; about management of chronic iron overload; about acute hepatic necrosis in such patients.

What is the commonest cause of a raised mean corpuscular volume in a blood film in the outpatient clinic? (Alcohol)
What are the other haematological abnormalities seen in alcohol abuse?[2]

What would be the most likely cause of a *macrocytic anaemia* if you excluded dietary causes? (Pernicious anaemia)

Why does alcohol cause a *macrocytosis*?[3]

Tell me about **vitamin B_{12}**.

Tell me how vitamin B_{12} deficiency presents.

How do we know that pernicious anaemia has an immunological basis?

Tell me about sideroblastic anaemia.

What is the ESR? What does it depend on? What factors affect it?

Imagine you are my registrar and I bring in a patient who is generally unwell with a very **high ESR**. How would you proceed with the investigations? (Discussion on myeloma and temporal arteritis)[4]

How would you manage a patient with an ESR of 100? How does myeloma present? Name four radiological features of myeloma. What do plasma cells look like?[5]

What is Bence Jones protein? Who described it and when?[6]

What are the presentations of **myeloma**?

Tell me about primary and secondary *polycythaemia* and its investigations.

What is the use of venesection?

What is a megakaryocyte?
What is a platelet and how does it work?
Do you know of things that make platelets less sticky?

How would you manage a patient with bruising?

---

[1] The diagnosis may have been wrong; the dose of iron may have been inadequate or not regularly taken by the patient; there may be an associated disease (e.g. chronic infection) causing marrow suppression; there may be continual and excessive blood loss; or, rarely, there may be malabsorption of iron.

[2] p. 106

[3] Through a direct toxic effect on the red cell precursors.

[4] p. 151

[5] p. 125

[6] See Appendix II

What is **haemophilia**? You are asked to counsel the sister of a patient with regard to having children.

How might the sex of a fetus be determined early enough for a therapeutic abortion?

Draw me the genetics of haemophilia.
Can women be affected?

What would you tell the father of a young boy with acute lymphocytic leukaemia about his prognosis?

Discuss chronic lymphatic leukaemia and its associated immunoglobulin (monoclonal) production and haemolytic anaemia.

Tell me about **bone marrow transplants**.

Tell me about the **staging of lymphomas**. Why do we do it?
How would you treat these cases?

What are the causes of a lymphocytosis?[7]

What are the features of infectious mononucleosis and how do you diagnose the condition?

Discuss **haemolytic anaemias**.

What do you know about acholuric jaundice?

Tell me about sickle cell disease.

What are the causes of a dimorphic picture on a blood film?

What are the causes of a pancytopaenia?

---

[7]   p. 154

Pharmacology

Tell me about all the *drug interactions* you can think of.[1]

Tell me about pharmacogenetics and its relevance to practice.

What is pharmacokinetics and what is pharmacodynamics?[2]
Tell me about first pass metabolism.[3]
What is the pharmacodynamics of digoxin?
What is the correct time after a dosage to take an aminophylline level?

Drug metabolism, in particular 'acetylator' and 'hydroxylator' states.

What happens to drug metabolism in chronic liver disease?

Tell me about drugs that affect the liver.

What is 'liver enzyme induction'? Give me an example of a drug.[1]

There has been a lot of publicity about the *dangers of NSAIDs*. Can you comment please?

What is the mode of action of the NSAIDs?

What are the side effects of NSAIDs? (Long discussion ending up with the role of prostaglandin in the kidney)

Tell me the different ways that antirheumatic drugs con produce kidney disease. What is the difference between the renal disease produced by NSAIDs now and in the past?

What are the principal side effects of benoxaprofen and why was it banned? (Examiner was related to the Irish physician who first exposed the deaths related to the drug!)

What are the side effects and problems of NSAIDs in the elderly population?

What kind of drug is penicillamine? What are its uses? (Wilson's, rheumatoid arthritis, cystinosis)
What are its side effects?

Tell me about the use of nonanalgesic drugs in the management of pain.[4]

Speaking of aspirin (previous question) tell me about Reye's syndrome.

What are the uses and cautions of ACE inhibitors in the management of heart failure?

Tell me about the ACE inhibitors and their mechanism of action.

What are the **side effects of amiodarone therapy**?

I am a patient who you wish to put on amiodarone. What advice would you give me?

What is the mechanism of action of diuretics?

Discuss the problems of diuretic therapy.

---

[1]   p. 55
[2]   p. 54
[3]   p. 57
[4]   p. 166

What are the indications for the use of digoxin nowadays?

I have a friend who thinks that digoxin should be withdrawn from the market. Could you support this assertion?

Tell me about warfarin and its important drug interactions and the mechanisms thereof.

Tell me about the use of inotropic drugs in the treatment of heart failure.

I don't believe in beta blockers. I think they're awful drugs. Can you persuade me that they have a use in clinical medicine?

What are the side effects of quinidine?

Can you name some vasodilators?

Have you heard of simvastatin? What do you know about it? Do you know how it works?[5]

Tell me about the different types of prophylactic antibiotics.

What do you know about the very early antibiotics, i.e. the prepenicillin era?

What type of drug is vancomycin? What are its uses and side effects? (The red-man syndrome)

A 23-year-old girl comes to me with a urinary tract infection and I give her a course of septrin. A week later she comes back with red spots on her arms. What do you think? (Toxic epidermal necrolysis)

Discussion on **antituberculous therapy**.

Tell me about the antiviral drugs.

What antifungal agents do you know of? What group of drugs do they belong to? Do you know any new ones?

What are the known interactions between the antiepileptic and antibiotic drugs?

Tell me which drug you would choose to treat a young girl with **epilepsy**.

What is the cheese reaction? (MAOI and tyramine-containing foods)

Do you know of an MAO B inhibitor? (Selegiline)

Tell me about dystonic reactions to certain drugs.

What are the side effects of lithium?

Tell me about the benefits of human insulin.

We went through a detailed discussion on the **role of the hypoglycaemic drugs** including their complications, uses, half-life, the role of the biguanides and the specific problems in the elderly.

The differences between the modes of action of metformin and the sulphonylureas, including their duration of action.

What do you know about calcitonin?

What is the chemotherapeutic treatment of Hodgkin's disease?

What are the side effects of cyclophosphamide?

---

[5]   p. 116

Which H^2 antagonist would you use in the elderly?

Treatment of a peptic ulcer. (Ranitidine *vs* cimetidine)

Tell me who you would give hepatitis B vaccine to.

Which drugs would you put on a crash trolley?

Tell me about controlled oxygen therapy.

What do you know about the use of recombinant DNA technology in drug manufacturing?

How do you monitor drug compliance?

What are the main precautions when prescribing drugs in the elderly?

What are borderline substances?[6]

What is a yellow card?[7]

---

6   Substances that are not drugs but are useful in the management of certain disorders and can be prescribed on FP10, e.g. Aminex biscuits, clinifeed, hycal, etc.

7   p. 54

Miscellaneous

What are the **medical consequences of a nuclear disaster** such as Chernobyl?

I am the mother of two young children and we live next to Dounray. I come to ask your opinion about **childhood cancer and nuclear power stations**. How would you reply?

Roy Plumley of Desert Island Discs has just died. Suppose you were on a desert island, which 10 drugs would you want to take with you and why?

Name three antibiotics to take on a **mountain expedition** to the Himalayas. **What other drugs would you take?**

You are asked by the editor of the *Lancet* to write an article on '**the heart as an endocrine organ**'.[1] What would you write about?

Which journals do you read? Discuss one article you have read recently.

What are the adverse effects of biomedical devices?

What is the **application of genetic engineering**?

How would you advise a patient with polycystic kidneys?[2]
(This led on to a discussion about Huntington's chorea and the implications of a genetic probe to indicate affected patients before the onset of the disease)
What is a genetic probe?[3]

What are the uses of **recombinant DNA techniques in medicine**? (Prenatal diagnosis, especially cystic fibrosis)

What is the commonest inherited disorder in the UK? (Cystic fibrosis)

Genetic counselling[2] and the genetics of diabetes mellitus.

Questions were asked about the different types of genetic diseases. Name an autosomal dominant condition.

Tell me about the use of **laser treatment in medicine** today.[4]

I was asked to name the single greatest advance in diabetes in the last 10 years.[5]

What major therapeutic advance has made a difference to patients in the last 5 years?[6]

What has been the most important single pharmacological advance in the last five years?[7]

What do you see as the major problems facing medicine in the 1990s? (Ageing population)

Do you know the mechanism of hypoalbuminaemia in inflammation?[8]
Tell me about the normal regulation of hormone-binding globulin levels and then what happens in inflammation.

---

[1] p. 29
[2] p. 169
[3] p. 170
[4] p. 79
[5] Continuous subcutaneous insulin infusion and the use of pens for self injection, insulin analogues and pancreatic transplantation are all possible answers.
[6] Cyclosporin
[7] Cyclosporin (major advance in the field of cardiac transplantation)
[8] p. 162

Name some diseases that are more severe (not merely more common) in women than men.[9]

What are the causes of a man falling asleep whilst watching the France v England rugby match on TV? (Narcolepsy)[10]

Tell me about diseases associated with fish.

What are the likely diseases to be found in a seaside port?[11]

What are the specific illnesses of Glasgow shipbuilders? (Asbestosis and the epidemiology of lung cancer)

I come from Glasgow. What would Dr X (Dumfries) see here that I would not see in Glasgow? (Dumfries is a rural area with specific rural industries – such as a shellfish processing factory and a polyvinyl chloride monomers factory)

Tell me about the **medical hazards facing farmers**.

What diurnal rhythms are there in the body?

Do you think malnutrition occurs in hospital?

How does the body respond to starvation? (Ketones, increased T3, gluconeogenesis in the liver)

What can you tell me about the **trace elements**?[12]

Tell me about the value of dieting.

What role does a dietician have in hospitals?

Tell me about total parenteral nutrition.

What is the treatment of obesity?

What are the biological effects of sunlight?
Tell me about vitamin D metabolism.

What do you know about acute phase reactants?

Tell me about monoclonal antibodies.

What do you think of a campaign called 'Sport for All'?

What are the medical complications of long distance running?

We know exercise is good for health, but are there any hazards associated with exercise?

A man presents complaining about bad breath. How would you manage him?

If you were an administrator how would you reorganise a Nuclear Medicine Department? What investigations would you keep and which would you get rid of?

If I were a hospital administrator on the finance committee and the consultants wanted a CT scanner, what would I say to them?
(This led to a discussion on the indications for CT scans)

What do we mean by institutionalisation?

---

[9] p. 87
[10] And the sleep apnoea syndromes
[11] p. 23
[12] p. 54

What are the harmful effects of smoking?

What are the medical complications of splenectomy?

What industrial, environmental and social causes of neoplasia do you know?[13]

Give some causes of enlarged lacrimal glands. (Connective tissue diseases, leukaemia, lymphoma)

I'm going to ask you a question out of interest which won't detract from your overall mark. Could you explain what you understand by 'linkage disequilibrium'?[14]

How would you teach 'immunity' to medical students?[15]

Why does the death rate go up in the winter?

What do you think of **medical audit**?

Tell me about 'opting out' of the NHS.

What do you know about the Community Care Act?

---

[13] p. 82

[14] Because of the process of crossing-over at meiosis, a particular combination of alleles on a chromosome changes in subsequent generations. The frequency of crossing-over depends on the distance apart of the alleles, such that those that are furthest apart are more likely to cross-over. In time, however, even closely linked alleles would cross-over so that every combination of different alleles should eventually occur. Thus the frequency of a particular allele would depend on its overall frequency in the population. This is *linkage equilibrium*. When alleles occur together more frequently or less frequently than expected from their individual frequencies, then they are said to be in a *linkage disequilibrium*. Linkage between two DNA markers which are close enough will result in disequilibrium during meiotic recombination.

[15] p. 85

Index